Harrison's

Principles of Internal Medicine

PreTest®
Self-Assessment
and Review

• NOTICE •

Harrison's

Principles of Internal Medicine

PreTest® Self-Assessment and Review

Twelfth Edition

For use with the 12th edition of
HARRISON'S PRINCIPLES OF INTERNAL MEDICINE

Edited by

Richard M. Stone, M.D.
Dana-Farber Cancer Institute
Brigham and Women's Hospital
Instructor, Harvard Medical School
Boston, Massachusetts

McGraw-Hill, Inc.
Health Professions Division
PreTest Series

New York   St. Louis   San Francisco   Colorado Springs
Auckland   Bogotá   Caracas   Hamburg   Lisbon   London
Madrid   Mexico   Milan   Montreal   New Delhi   Paris
San Juan   São Paulo   Singapore   Sydney   Tokyo   Toronto

123456789MALMAL96543210

ISBN 0-07-051985-4

The editors were Gail Gavert and Bruce MacGregor.
The production supervisor was Clara B. Stanley. Malloy was printer and binder.
This book was set in Times Roman by Waldman Graphics, Inc.

The Appendix, as well as the figures accompanying questions 158, 172, and 584, has been taken from *Harrison's Principles of Internal Medicine*, 12th ed., with permission.

Library of Congress Cataloging-in-Publication Data

Harrison's principles of internal medicine—PreTest self-assessment
  and review / Richard M. Stone, editor.
      p. cm.
    ''For use with the 12th edition of Harrison's principles of
internal medicine.''
    Includes bibliographical references.
    ISBN 0-07-051985-4 :
    1. Internal medicine—Examinations, questions, etc. I. Harrison,
Tinsley Randolph. II. Stone, Richard M. III. Harrison's
principles of internal medicine. IV. Title: Principles of internal
medicine—PreTest self-assessment and review.
    [DNLM: 1. Internal Medicine—examination questions.   WB 18 H322
Suppl.]
RC46.H333 1991 ‹Suppl.›
616'.0076—dc20
DNLM/DLC
for Library of Congress   90-6614
                                                                   CIP

Contents

Contents

The accuracy, relevance, and clarity of the material in this text benefited from the diligent supervision of the editorial board of Harrison's Principles of Internal Medicine. *My thanks go to Jean D. Wilson, M.D.; Eugene Braunwald, A.B., M.D.; Kurt J. Isselbacher, A.B., M.D.; Robert G. Petersdorf, A.B., M.D.; Joseph B. Martin, M.D., Ph.D.; Anthony S. Fauci, M.D.; and Richard K. Root, M.D.*

Introduction

Harrison's Principles of Internal Medicine: PreTest Self-Assessment and Review has been designed to provide physicians with a comprehensive, relevant, and convenient instrument for self-evaluation and review within the broad area of internal medicine. Although it should be particularly helpful for residents preparing for the American Board of Internal Medicine (ABIM) certification examination and for board-certified internists preparing for recertification, it should also be useful for internists, family practitioners, and other practicing physicians who are simply interested in maintaining a high level of competence in internal medicine. Study of this self-assessment and review book should help to (1) identify areas of relative weakness; (2) confirm areas of expertise; (3) assess knowledge of the sciences fundamental to internal medicine; (4) assess clinical judgment and problem-solving skills; and (5) introduce recent developments in general internal medicine.

This book consists of 835 multiple-choice questions that (1) are representative of the major areas covered in *Harrison's Principles of Internal Medicine,* 12th ed., and (2) parallel the format and degree of difficulty of the questions on the examination of the ABIM. Questions have been appropriately updated and chosen to reflect important recent developments in internal medicine, such as the importance of the AIDS epidemic and the increasing contributions of molecular biology to the understanding, diagnosis, and treatment of many disorders. Each question is accompanied by an answer, a paragraph-length explanation, and a reference to a specific chapter in *Harrison's,* as well as in some cases references to more specialized textbooks and current journal articles. A list of normal values used in the laboratory studies in this book can be found in the Appendix, following a Bibliography listing all the sources used for the questions. As in the current edition of *Harrison's,* the system of international units (SI) appears first in the text and the traditional units follow in parentheses. All color plates referred to in the text are found in the back of the book.

We have assumed that the time available to the reader is limited; therefore, this book has been designed to be used profitably a chapter at a time. By allowing no more than two and a half minutes to answer each question, you can simulate the time constraints of the actual board examinations. When you finish answering all the questions in a chapter, spend as much time as necessary verifying answers and carefully reading the accompanying explanations. If after reading the explanations for a given chapter, you feel a need for a more extensive and definitive discussion, consult the chapter in *Harrison's* or any of the other references listed.

Based on our testing experience, on most medical examinations, examinees who answer half the questions correctly would score around the 50th or 60th percentile. A score of 65 percent would place the examinee above the 80th percentile, whereas a score of 30 percent would rank him or her below the 15th percentile. In other words, if you answer fewer than 30 percent of the questions in a chapter correctly, you are relatively weak in that area. A score of 50 percent would be approximately average, and 70 percent or higher would probably be honors.

We have used three basic question types in accordance with the format of the ABIM certification and recertification examinations. In accordance with the changing format of these examinations, the number of matching questions has been reduced in this edition. Considerable editorial time has been spent trying to ensure that each question is clearly stated and discriminates between those physicians who are well prepared in the subject and those who are less knowledgeable.

This book is a teaching device that provides readers with the opportunity to evaluate and update their clinical expertise, their ability to interpret data, and their ability to diagnose and solve clinical problems.

Harrison's
Principles of Internal Medicine

PreTest® Self-Assessment and Review

Infectious Diseases

DIRECTIONS: Each question below contains five suggested responses. Select the **one best** response to each question.

1. A 14-year-old boy has a history of recurrent respiratory infections with *Staphylococcus aureus* and *Aspergillus fumigatus*. When he was 7 years old he had a hepatic abscess that was drained surgically; no organism was cultured, but the problem responded to drainage and prolonged antibiotic therapy. His parents and two younger siblings are healthy, but an older brother died in infancy of infection.

The laboratory study most likely to assist in establishing the diagnosis is

(A) determination of leukocyte myeloperoxidase level
(B) quantitative determination of serum immunoglobulin levels
(C) T-lymphocyte functional and subpopulation assessment
(D) nitroblue tetrazolium reduction test
(E) bone marrow aspiration and biopsy

2. Which of the following organisms would be LEAST likely to cause infection in a patient with acquired immunodeficiency syndrome (AIDS)?

(A) Cytomegalovirus
(B) *Cryptococcus neoformans*
(C) *Pneumocystis carinii*
(D) *Pseudomonas aeruginosa*
(E) *Mycobacterium avium-intracellulare*

3. A patient is examined for presumed septic arthritis. Joint fluid is aspirated, but the sample inadvertently is left at the bedside for several hours. Culturing which of the following organisms would be most affected by the delay in delivery of the specimen to the laboratory?

(A) *Neisseria gonorrhoeae*
(B) *Staphylococcus aureus*
(C) *Streptococcus pyogenes*
(D) *Haemophilus influenzae*
(E) *Salmonella choleraesuis*

4. A 23-year-old graduate student complains of burning on urination and a vaginal discharge. On physical examination, a bilateral groin rash, generalized vaginal erythema, and a whitish vaginal discharge are observed; the remainder of the physical examination is negative. The laboratory test most likely to detect a specific host-defense defect causing this clinical problem would be

(A) blood glucose concentration
(B) blood urea nitrogen concentration
(C) serum immunoglobulin A concentration
(D) serum immunoglobulin E concentration
(E) serum complement concentration

5. The most common source for bacterial infection of intravenous cannulas is

(A) contamination of fluids during the manufacturing process
(B) contamination of fluids during cannula insertion
(C) contamination at the site of entry through the skin
(D) contamination during injection of medications
(E) seeding from remote sites due to intermittent bacteremia

6. A 73-year-old previously healthy man is hospitalized because of the acute onset of dysuria, urinary frequency, fever, and shaking chills. His temperature is 39.5°C (103.1°F), blood pressure is 100/60 mmHg, pulse is 140 beats per minute, and respiratory rate is 30 breaths per minute. Which of the following interventions would be the most important in the treatment of this acute illness?

(A) Catheterization of the urinary bladder
(B) Initiation of antibiotic therapy
(C) Infusion of Ringer's lactate solution
(D) Infusion of dopamine hydrochloride
(E) Intravenous injection of methylprednisolone

7. Infection with *Pseudomonas* organisms is frequently associated with each of the following EXCEPT

(A) osteomyelitis developing after a nail puncture wound of the foot
(B) ecthyma gangrenosum
(C) both a mild and an invasive form of otitis externa
(D) meningitis in neonatal infants
(E) endocarditis in drug addicts

1

8.   A 17-year-old pregnant girl is hospitalized 2 days after she inserted a metal rod into her uterus during an abortion attempt. She has a temperature of 40.5°C (104.9°F), shaking chills, and a purulent vaginal discharge; blood pressure is normal. Which of the following laboratory results would be LEAST consistent with a diagnosis of septic abortion?

(A)   White blood cell count: 30,000/mm^3 with occasional metamyelocytes, many band neutrophils, and toxic granulation
(B)   Prothrombin time: 16 s (control 12 s)
(C)   Arterial blood gases: pH 7.30; P_{O_2} 90 mmHg; P_{CO_2} 30 mm Hg
(D)   Urinalysis: pH 5.0; glucose negative; protein 2 +; RBC 3 +; many RBC casts
(E)   Serum chemistries: NA$^+$ 138 mmol/L; K$^+$ 4.0 mmol/L; Cl$^-$ 100 mmol/L; HCO$_3^-$ 20 mmol/L; creatinine 88.4 μmol/L (1.0 mg/dL)

9.   Diagnostic accuracy has been enhanced by the ability to detect specific DNA sequences in all the following infecting microorganisms EXCEPT

(A)   cytomegalovirus (CMV)
(B)   *Staphylococcus aureus*
(C)   *Mycoplasma pneumoniae*
(D)   *Legionella*
(E)   human immunodeficiency virus (HIV)

10.   The most common cause of "traveler's diarrhea" ("turista") in Americans traveling abroad is

(A)   *Staphylococcus aureus*
(B)   *Clostridium perfringens*
(C)   *Escherichia coli*
(D)   *Bacillus cereus*
(E)   rotavirus

11.   All the following vaccines are recommended for use in immunocompromised adults EXCEPT

(A)   bacille Calmette-Guerin (BCG) vaccine (against tuberculosis)
(B)   inactivated influenza vaccine for current year
(C)   23-valent pneumococcal vaccine
(D)   quadrivalent meningococcal vaccine
(E)   inactivated polio vaccine

12.   Antibiotic prophylaxis would most likely be of benefit to persons undergoing

(A)   vaginal hysterectomy
(B)   splenectomy
(C)   coronary artery bypass surgery
(D)   ligation of fallopian tubes
(E)   open biopsy of the kidney

13.   Immune globulin postexposure prophylaxis of contacts can be given for each of the following diseases EXCEPT

(A)   hepatitis A
(B)   hepatitis B
(C)   varicella
(D)   polio
(E)   measles

14.   All the following factors are thought to contribute to the pathogenicity of staphylococci EXCEPT

(A)   penicillinase production
(B)   coagulase production
(C)   enterotoxin production
(D)   exotoxin production
(E)   catalase production

15.   Which of the following organisms is most likely to cause infection of a shunt implanted for treatment of hydrocephalus?

(A)   *Staphylococcus epidermidis*
(B)   *Staphylococcus aureus*
(C)   *Corynebacterium diphtheriae*
(D)   *Escherichia coli*
(E)   *Bacteroides fragilis*

16.   A 14-year-old girl has fever, headache, pain on swallowing, and loss of voice. Her cervical lymph nodes are tender to palpation. Of these signs and symptoms, which is LEAST suggestive of a diagnosis of streptococcal pharyngitis?

(A)   Fever
(B)   Headache
(C)   Pain on swallowing
(D)   Loss of voice
(E)   Tender cervical lymph nodes

17.   Meningococcal meningitis can be prevented by the administration of all the following preparations EXCEPT

(A)   group A vaccine
(B)   group B vaccine
(C)   group C vaccine
(D)   sulfonamides
(E)   rifampin

18.   All the following antibiotics require major adjustments of dosage in patients with chronic renal failure EXCEPT

(A)   amikacin
(B)   vancomycin
(C)   ceftazidime
(D)   cefoxitin
(E)   cefotaxime

19.   A 60-year-old insulin-dependent man with diabetes mellitus has had purulent drainage from his left ear for 1 week. Suddenly, fever, increased pain, and vertigo develop. The most likely causative agent is

(A)   *Aspergillus*
(B)   *Mucor*
(C)   *Pseudomonas*
(D)   *Staphylococcus aureus*
(E)   *Haemophilus influenzae*

20.   Typhoid fever can be characterized by all the following statements EXCEPT

(A)   the illness usually is acquired from ingestion of contaminated food, water, or milk
(B)   leukopenia is more common than leukocytosis in acutely ill persons
(C)   rose spots are usually present at the time the fever begins
(D)   chloramphenicol is not effective in preventing relapse
(E)   adults are more likely to become chronic carriers than are children

21.   *Haemophilus influenzae* infections occur with increased frequency in association with all the following conditions EXCEPT

(A)   alcoholism
(B)   sickle cell disease
(C)   splenectomy
(D)   agammaglobulinemia
(E)   chronic granulomatous disease

22.   To determine whether a child with paroxysmal coughing and gasping has whooping cough, a physician would do best to order

(A)   white blood cell count and differential
(B)   Gram stain of the sputum
(C)   blood cultures
(D)   chest x-ray
(E)   lateral x-ray of the neck

23.   Hypersensitivity reactions—such as erythema nodosum, erythema multiforme, arthritis, and arthralgias—are most frequently associated with which of the following infections?

(A)   Histoplasmosis
(B)   Cryptococcosis
(C)   Aspergillosis
(D)   Blastomycosis
(E)   Coccidioidomycosis

24.   Imipenem, a newer antibiotic with a broad antibacterial spectrum, is coadministered with cilastatin because

(A)   the combination of these antibiotics is synergistic against *Pseudomonas* species
(B)   cilastatin aids the gastrointestinal absorption of the active moiety, imipenem
(C)   cilastatin inhibits a β-lactamase that destroys imipenem
(D)   cilastatin inhibits an enzyme in the kidney that destroys imipenem
(E)   cilastatin prevents the hypoprothrombinemic effect of imipenem

25.   All the following are characteristic clinical features of chancroid EXCEPT

(A)   initial presentation as a tender papule
(B)   development of painful genital ulcers
(C)   tender, enlarged inguinal lymph nodes
(D)   *Haemophilus ducreyi* isolated from bacteriologic cultures
(E)   response to ampicillin therapy

26.   A 62-year-old gardener who has chronic lymphocytic leukemia develops lymphangitis and a painless, nodular lesion on his wrist. Subsequently, he becomes severely ill with cavitary right-upper-lobe pneumonia; *Sporothrix schenckii* is isolated. He should be treated with

(A)   chloramphenicol
(B)   potassium iodide
(C)   penicillin
(D)   amphotericin B
(E)   flucytosine

27.   Four days after he and his friends were killing muskrats along a rural creek, a boy becomes ill with headache, fever, and a macular rash. On examination, axillary adenopathy is noted, but otherwise the examination is normal. Which of the following tests would be most helpful in proving that this boy has tularemia?

(A)   Blood culture
(B)   Aspiration and culture of an axillary lymph node
(C)   Determination of serum agglutinins for *Francisella tularensis*
(D)   Bone-marrow culture
(E)   Examination of his friends

28.   A 10-year-old boy is seen in a rural Arizona clinic because of prostration, fever of 40°C (104°F), and severe headache. Examination is negative for rash, stiff neck, joint tenderness, and chest and abdominal abnormalities. However, several tender, enlarged lymph nodes are palpated in the left axilla, which is very edematous. The test most likely to be of greatest help in the immediate management of this boy would be

(A)   blood culture
(B)   examination of a blood smear
(C)   biopsy of an axillary lymph node
(D)   aspiration and Gram stain of an axillary lymph node
(E)   surgical excision of an axillary node

29.   Which of the following organisms often causes diarrhea, confusion, and delirium in conjunction with pneumonia?

(A)   *Legionella pneumophila*
(B)   *Francisella tularensis*
(C)   *Mycoplasma pneumoniae*
(D)   *Haemophilus pneumoniae*
(E)   *Klebsiella pneumoniae*

30.   *Listeria monocytogenes* most frequently causes which of the following infections?

(A)   Endocarditis
(B)   Peritonitis
(C)   Hepatitis
(D)   Meningitis
(E)   Conjunctivitis

31.   Ganciclovir has been shown to be effective in which one of the following manifestations of cytomegalovirus (CMV) infection?

(A)   Hepatitis
(B)   Pneumonitis
(C)   Colitis
(D)   Retinitis
(E)   "Wasting" disease

32.   Which of the following drugs would be LEAST likely to benefit a patient experiencing an acute attack of malaria?

(A)   Quinine
(B)   Chloroquine
(C)   Primaquine
(D)   Hydroxychloroquine
(E)   Mefloquine

33.   Which of the following food- or water-borne bacteria responsible for diarrheal illness has the LONGEST incubation period (time from ingestion to illness)?

(A)   *Clostridium perfringens*
(B)   *Staphylococcus aureus*
(C)   *Bacillus cereus*
(D)   *Campylobacter jejuni*
(E)   *Vibrio parahaemolyticus*

34.   Which of the following pleural-fluid samples is most suggestive of tuberculous pleuritis?

Fluid sample	Color	pH	Protein, g/L	Glucose, mmol/L	LDH, U/mL	WBC Total (per mm³)	% Lymphocytes
(A)	Clear yellow	7.15	35	1.1	600	2,000	95
(B)	Thick green	7.00	40	1.1	600	10,000	50
(C)	Clear yellow	7.30	15	4.4	150	200	50
(D)	Pink-tinged	7.40	30	4.4	600	3,000	50
(E)	Clear yellow	7.30	35	3.3	150	2,000	95

(LDH, lactate dehydrogenase; WBC, white blood cell count)

35. A 27-year-old woman returned from a camping trip in New England. Two weeks later a small red papule developed, which expanded into a large annular lesion. She also had headache, fever, chills, malaise, and fatigue. Which of the following studies would be most useful to confirm the diagnosis of Lyme disease?

(A) Skin biopsy
(B) Giemsa or Wright stain of a blood smear
(C) Culture of skin or blood in Kelly's modified medium
(D) Acute and convalescent serologic studies after several weeks of symptoms
(E) Examination of cerebrospinal fluid

36. A 10-year-old child has malaise, a low-grade fever, and cervical lymphadenopathy. Biopsy of a cervical lymph node reveals granulomatous inflammation; the culture grows *Mycobacterium scrofulaceum*. The best treatment for this child would be

(A) excision of the infected nodes
(B) isoniazid and ethambutol
(C) streptomycin, isoniazid, and ethambutol
(D) rifampin, isoniazid, and ethambutol
(E) observation until the results of sensitivity studies are available

37. A 40-year-old Canadian who operates a tropical fish store sees his physician because of a nonhealing ulcer on his left arm. He is afebrile and gives no history of night sweats, weight loss, or other constitutional symptoms. Biopsy of the lesion shows granulomatous inflammation and rare acid-fast organisms. A tuberculin test is negative. This man most likely has an infection caused by

(A) *Mycobacterium tuberculosis*
(B) *Mycobacterium ulcerans*
(C) *Mycobacterium kansasii*
(D) *Mycobacterium marinum*
(E) *Mycobacterium fortuitum*

38. Legionnaire's disease is characterized by all the following statements EXCEPT

(A) the disease is not spread from person to person
(B) diarrhea, nausea, and vomiting often are prominent early symptoms
(C) chest x-ray usually shows few abnormalities, while chest examination usually is markedly abnormal
(D) fever is usually prolonged
(E) therapy with erythromycin is recommended

39. Which of the following tests is most useful for recognizing infections caused by the "newly discovered" *Legionella* species (e.g., the Pittsburgh pneumonia agent)?

(A) Direct fluorescent antibody staining
(B) DNA probe
(C) Paired serologic testing
(D) Culture of sputum
(E) Culture of a lung biopsy specimen

40. Each of the following diagnostic tests may be indicated in the evaluation of an ulcerative genital lesion EXCEPT

(A) Gram stain
(B) serologic test for syphilis
(C) biopsy
(D) dark-field examination
(E) viral culture

41. The diagnosis of relapsing fever (*Borrelia* infection) usually is made by

(A) serologic testing
(B) blood culture
(C) examination of blood smears
(D) lymph-node aspiration
(E) lumbar puncture

42. The characteristic "sulfur grains" of actinomycosis are composed chiefly of

(A) organisms
(B) neutrophils and monocytes
(C) monocytes and lymphocytes
(D) eosinophils
(E) calcified cellular debris

43. Antigen testing of blood and cerebrospinal fluid is most useful in the diagnosis of

(A) histoplasmosis
(B) blastomycosis
(C) cryptococcosis
(D) coccidioidomycosis
(E) sporotrichosis

44. What is the best therapy for a 23-year-old man with a purulent urethral discharge that contains intracellular gram-negative diplococci?

(A) Benzathine penicillin
(B) Tetracycline (or doxycycline)
(C) Spectinomycin plus tetracycline (or doxycycline)
(D) Ampicillin plus tetracycline (or doxycycline)
(E) Ceftriaxone plus tetracycline (or doxycycline)

Questions 63–64

An 18-year-old, sexually active woman presents with fever, pleuritic pain of the right upper quadrant, and lower abdominal pain. Pelvic examination reveals mucopurulent cervicitis and tenderness upon the production of cervical motion. The right upper quadrant, uterine fundus, and adnexa are slightly tender. The white blood cell count and erythrocyte sedimentation rate are elevated, but the results of the remainder of the laboratory examination, including liver function tests, are normal.

63.   Which of the following agents is the most likely cause of this clinical syndrome?

(A)   Herpes simplex
(B)   Syphilis
(C)   *Neisseria gonorrhoeae*
(D)   *Chlamydia trachomatis*
(E)   *Mycoplasma hominis*

64.   Because the patient appears ill, she is hospitalized. Assuming that pregnancy and appendicitis are excluded, which of the following antibiotic regimens is the best choice?

(A)   Doxycycline plus cefoxitin
(B)   Doxycycline alone
(C)   Acyclovir plus penicillin
(D)   Penicillin alone
(E)   Metronidazole plus gentamicin

65.   A 65-year-old retired banker who spends summers on Nantucket Island off the Massachusetts coast returned to his home in Boston early in September. He noted the gradual onset of a febrile illness with chills, sweats, myalgias, and yellow eyes. His doctor could palpate the spleen and noted a macrocytic anemia, hyperbilirubinemia, and a high serum level of lactic dehydrogenase on laboratory examination.

Which of the following would be the most helpful diagnostic procedure at this point?

(A)   Blood culture
(B)   Examination of leukocytes on blood film
(C)   Examination of erythrocytes on blood film
(D)   Splenic biopsy
(E)   Liver biopsy

66.   All the following represent clinical syndromes produced by *Leishmania* EXCEPT

(A)   fever, pancytopenia, and splenomegaly
(B)   disfiguring facial ulcer
(C)   diffuse skin lesions
(D)   dysphagia, chest pain, and regurgitation
(E)   nasal obstruction and epistaxis

DIRECTIONS: Each question below contains five suggested responses. For **each** of the five responses listed with every question, you are to respond either YES (Y) or NO (N). In a given item **all, some, or none of the alternatives may be correct.**

67. In persons who have endocarditis, which of the following factors would *adversely* affect the prognosis?

(A) The presence of congestive heart failure
(B) Abscess formation
(C) The isolation of organisms resistant to multiple antimicrobial agents
(D) The isolation of *Staphylococcus epidermidis* after cardiac surgery
(E) A delay in instituting therapy

68. Which of the following conditions would warrant antibiotic prophylaxis against infective endocarditis in a patient experiencing invasive dental work?

(A) Atrial septal defect
(B) Ventricular septal defect
(C) Coronary artery bypass grafts
(D) Permanent transvenous pacemaker
(E) Mitral regurgitation associated with mitral valve prolapse

69. True statements regarding right-heart endocarditis include which of the following?

(A) It is unlikely in the absence of murmur
(B) It occurs frequently in drug addicts
(C) Blood cultures are usually negative
(D) Emboli to organs other than the lungs are rare
(E) Prognosis is generally good

70. Correct statements concerning the pathogenesis of fever include

(A) aspirin inhibits the production of endogenous pyrogens
(B) the major endogenous pyrogens in humans are interleukin 1 (IL-1) and tumor necrosis factor (TNF)
(C) endogenous pyrogens are produced by bacteria, protozoa, and fungi
(D) endogenous pyrogens raise body temperature by their effect on skeletal muscle beds
(E) endogenous pyrogens play a role in the cachexia of chronic infections

71. Nosocomial infections can be described by which of the following statements?

(A) Plasmids can readily transfer antibiotic resistance from one gram-negative bacterium to another
(B) Even with the best of care, bladder catheters lead to urinary tract infections in more than 50 percent of cases in which the catheter remains in place for at least 5 days
(C) There is a greater risk of local phlebitis with plastic cannulas than with stainless steel needles
(D) Intravenous cannulas should not be left in place more than 72 h
(E) Surgeons and workers in hemodialysis units are the only two groups of health-care workers for whom hepatitis B vaccine is recommended

72. Correct statements concerning laboratory diagnosis of microbial infections include which of the following?

(A) Infection with *Leishmania* and *Plasmodium vivax* can be recognized by examining Wright-stained blood smears
(B) *Nocardia* and *Mycobacterium* are both acid-fast organisms
(C) *Legionella pneumophila* can be detected in sputum by immunofluorescent staining
(D) A single negative throat culture for *Streptococcus pyogenes* is typically sufficient to exclude the diagnosis of streptococcal pharyngitis
(E) In cases of partially treated meningitis, gram-positive organisms tend to take up the blue dye with increased avidity, so that the organism appears darker than normal

73. A 27-year-old woman treated with combination chemotherapy for diffuse large-cell lymphoma develops fever and chills. Accurate statements concerning her condition include which of the following?

(A) Infections with encapsulated microorganisms (*Haemophilus influenzae, Neisseria meningitidis,* and *Streptococcus pneumoniae*) should be strongly considered
(B) The patient will be at increased risk for staphylococcal infection
(C) Empiric, broad-spectrum antibacterial coverage employing two antibiotics should be instituted
(D) Empiric antifungal therapy should be instituted
(E) *Candida* and *Aspergillus* are the two most common nonbacterial pathogens

74. True statements concerning the pathophysiology of septic shock include which of the following?

(A) Endotoxemia causes thrombocytopenia and granulocytopenia
(B) Reduced C3 levels correlate with a poor outcome
(C) Activation of complement, with the liberation of C5a, increases granulocyte margination
(D) Infusion of prostacyclin, a thromboxane A_2 antagonist, improves the outcome in experimental septic shock
(E) Naloxone, an endorphin antagonist, worsens the outcome in experimental septic shock

75. The carboxyfluoroquinolone ciprofloxacin effectively inhibits which of the following bacterial species?

(A) Methicillin-sensitive staphylococci
(B) *Haemophilus influenzae*
(C) *Bacteroides fragilis*
(D) *Pseudomonas aeruginosa*
(E) *Escherichia coli*

76. Penicillin antibiotic agents can be characterized by which of the following statements?

(A) Penicillin G, procaine penicillin, and benzathine penicillin all differ in the rate of absorption from a site of injection
(B) Amoxicillin is not as well absorbed as ampicillin
(C) Neither ampicillin nor carbenicillin is effective against *Klebsiella*
(D) Ticarcillin is similar to carbenicillin except for its somewhat greater activity against *Pseudomonas*
(E) Methicillin is less nephrotoxic than nafcillin and is used more frequently

77. True statements concerning genitourinary infections include which of the following?

(A) A man who has dysuria, no urethral discharge, and only 1 or 2 leukocytes per high-power field on microscopic examination of material obtained by a urethral swab probably has chlamydial urethritis
(B) A man who has a urethral discharge containing many leukocytes but only extracellular gram-negative diplococci should be treated with tetracycline, pending the results of cultures
(C) A woman who has a watery, malodorous vaginal discharge that does not contain *Candida* or *Trichomonas* on microscopic examination should be treated with a sulfonamide vaginal cream for presumed *Gardnerella vaginalis* infection
(D) A pregnant woman who has mucopurulent cervicitis without gram-negative diplococci on Gram stain or *Neisseria gonorrhoeae* isolated on culture should be treated with tetracycline for 1 to 3 weeks
(E) In the United States, the most common cause of ulcerative genital lesions is herpes simplex virus

78. Correct statements concerning pneumococcal infection include which of the following?

(A) Infections with type 3 pneumococci are associated with a higher mortality rate than infections with any other type of pneumococci
(B) Patients who have had a splenectomy for any reason should receive pneumococcal vaccine
(C) Pneumococcal pharyngitis is the most common precipitating event of pneumococcal meningitis in adults
(D) The occurrence of the "crisis" in pneumococcal pneumonia generally corresponds to the time of maximum leukocytosis
(E) Hypogammaglobulinemia is an important factor contributing to the unfavorable prognosis for pneumococcal pneumonia in alcoholic persons

79. True statements about the pathogenesis of streptococcal infections include which of the following?

(A) Streptococcal strains without M protein in the cell wall are nonpathogenic
(B) Antistreptolysin O (ASO) titers are infrequently elevated in persons with poststreptococcal glomerulonephritis
(C) ASO titers are nearly always elevated in persons with streptococcal pyoderma
(D) Scarlet fever can be caused by group A, C, or G streptococci as well as by certain staphylococci
(E) Streptococcal pyoderma does not lead to acute rheumatic fever

80. Leptospirosis may be characterized by which of the following statements?

(A) Fleas are the most important vector for transmission of *Leptospira* to humans
(B) Leptospirosis usually begins with fever, headache, and myalgias
(C) Leptospiral hepatitis often causes marked hyperbilirubinemia with only moderate transaminasemia
(D) A normal glucose concentration and a moderately elevated white blood cell count (100 to 1000 cells/mm^3) are characteristic cerebrospinal fluid findings in leptospiral meningitis
(E) The best way to diagnose acute leptospirosis is by dark-field microscopic examination of blood smears

81. *Neisseria gonorrhoeae* infections can be described by which of the following statements?

(A) Gonococci with pili tend to be avirulent
(B) Strains of *N. gonorrhoeae* that produce β-lactamase are resistant to penicillin but usually are sensitive to "third generation" cephalosporins, such as ceftriaxone
(C) Gonococcemia frequently occurs during menstruation
(D) The skin lesions of gonococcemia usually appear first on the distal portions of the extremities
(E) Gonococcal arthritis is usually symmetrical in distribution

82. True statements concerning *Acinetobacter* include which of the following?

(A) This organism often is confused with *Neisseria* on Gram stain
(B) This organism often is mistakenly identified as a diphtheroid on Gram stain
(C) This organism can be easily mislabeled as a member of the Enterobacteriaceae family when first isolated on routine laboratory culture media
(D) This organism usually is sensitive to penicillin and ampicillin
(E) Organisms of the genus *Acinetobacter* are rarely isolated from normal patients

83. Correct statements concerning melioidosis include which of the following?

(A) Infection usually is caused by person-to-person transmission
(B) Patients with pneumonia usually have relatively few organisms in the sputum
(C) Diagnosis usually depends on serologic testing
(D) Cavitary lung lesions do not occur
(E) Therapy with a combination of two or three antibiotics is recommended for acutely ill patients

84. Brucellosis can be described by which of the following statements?

(A) Cattle are the most important source of human *Brucella* infections in the United States
(B) Brucellosis is an important cause of abortion in cattle and pigs, but not in humans
(C) Brucellosis should be considered in the differential diagnosis of fever of unknown origin in the United States
(D) *Brucella* cannot be grown in usual blood culture media
(E) A combination of tetracycline and streptomycin is the treatment of choice

85. Cholera can be characterized by which of the following statements?

(A) In endemic areas, it is predominantly a disease of children
(B) The most definitive means of diagnosis is by dark-field microscopy
(C) Oral treatment must include replacement fluids containing glucose and sodium bicarbonate
(D) Treatment with oral tetracycline shortens the duration of diarrhea
(E) Vaccination affords good protection from infection

86. Correct statements regarding treatment of infection by human immunodeficiency virus (HIV) with zidovudine (azidothymidine [AZT]) include

(A) the primary mechanism of action is inhibition of viral DNA polymerase by AZT triphosphate
(B) the chief toxicity of AZT is nausea and vomiting
(C) in the United States AZT is approved for use in all patients with HIV infection
(D) while AZT reduces the number of infections in patients with AIDS, no survival benefit is obvious
(E) most patients on AZT obtain an improvement in their peripheral granulocyte count

87. Syphilis can be described by which of the following statements?

(A) Syphilis acquired by a woman during pregnancy is likely to remain subclinical
(B) All newborn infants of mothers with reactive serologic tests will themselves be reactive
(C) If a person with syphilis goes untreated, the VDRL test will remain reactive indefinitely
(D) Symptomatic neurosyphilis is unlikely in persons treated with at least 6 million units of penicillin G
(E) The major cause of death from untreated syphilis is cardiovascular disease

88. Correct statements regarding antifungal agents include

(A) ketoconazole is effective in the treatment of esophageal candidiasis
(B) the dose of ketoconazole should be altered in the presence of renal failure
(C) amphotericin B is a nephrotoxin that frequently causes dangerously high levels of serum potassium
(D) amphotericin B dosage should be reduced in patients with hepatic insufficiency
(E) flucytosine (5-fluorocytosine) is converted to the antimetabolite 5-fluorouracil (5-FU) inside the fungal cell

89. True statements about mucormycosis include which of the following?

(A) The organism is grown easily from most clinical specimens once an adequate tissue sample is obtained

(B) A characteristic feature of *Mucor* is its tendency to invade blood vessels

(C) In persons with hematologic malignancies, the sinuses are the most frequent site of infection

(D) Diagnosis by serologic testing is not yet clinically practical

(E) The treatment of choice is amphotericin B and surgical debridement

90. True statements about Rocky Mountain spotted fever include which of the following?

(A) Fleas are the characteristic vector of disease spread

(B) The disease is caused by the obligate intracellular organism *Rickettsia rickettsii*

(C) Frank arthritis is a common early manifestation of infection

(D) The initial skin lesions usually appear on the extremities

(E) Treatment of choice consists of early administration of chloramphenicol or tetracycline

91. *Mycoplasma* pneumonia has which of the following characteristics?

(A) The causal organism, *Mycoplasma pneumoniae*, is gram-positive

(B) Persons older than 40 years of age rarely are affected

(C) A fourfold rise in the cold-agglutinin titer within 10 days of the onset of symptoms is specific evidence of this disease

(D) Treatment with tetracycline is effective

(E) Treatment with erythromycin is effective

92. Correct statements concerning toxic shock syndrome include which of the following?

(A) It is associated with a staphylococcal exotoxin

(B) Blood cultures are positive for *S. aureus* in approximately 50 percent of patients

(C) At least 40 percent of cases are nonmenstrual

(D) Involvement of multiple organ systems often occurs

(E) Patients with postoperative staphylococcal wound infections usually have an obvious tissue focus presenting at least 1 week postoperatively

93. Agents elaborated by the patient that are thought to play a role in the manifestations of septic shock due to gram-negative bacillemia include

(A) tumor necrosis factor (TNF)
(B) interleukin 1 (IL-1)
(C) kallikrein
(D) prostaglandin E_2 (PGE_2)
(E) interferon γ

94. For their preventive medical care, which of the following persons should be seriously considered for, if not in fact given, rabies vaccination?

(A) Letter carriers
(B) Cave explorers
(C) Veterinarians
(D) City park-department workers
(E) Children in families owning more than three dogs

95. True statements concerning infectious mononucleosis include which of the following?

(A) The most common symptom of infectious mononucleosis is sore throat

(B) In young adults, the incubation period for infectious mononucleosis is 30 to 50 days

(C) The atypical lymphocytes associated with infectious mononucleosis are T cells

(D) Heterophil antibody titers usually decline within 3 to 6 months from the onset of symptoms

(E) Antibodies to Epstein-Barr virus generally persist longer in the circulation than do heterophil antibodies

96. Cat-scratch disease can be described by which of the following statements?

(A) Only about half of all cases are associated with cat scratches

(B) Lymph node histopathology usually is pathognomonic

(C) Lymph node swelling usually lasts no more than 2 weeks

(D) It is caused by a bacterial pathogen

(E) Treatment with tetracycline is usually effective

97. True statements describing amebiasis include which of the following?

(A) Humans are the principal reservoir
(B) Even in the presence of multiple liver abscesses, abatement of fever usually occurs promptly with medical therapy
(C) In persons who have received metronidazole for liver abscess, the amebic serology usually reverts from positive to negative within 4 to 6 weeks
(D) If the fluid aspirated from a liver cyst identified by liver-spleen scan contains no polymorphonuclear leukocytes or amebas, then amebic abscess is an unlikely diagnosis
(E) The mortality rate for intestinal amebiasis in the United States is less than 5 percent

98. Correct statements regarding liver abscess include which of the following?

(A) The prognosis for patients with multiple small liver abscesses is worse than for those with a single large abscess
(B) Serology is helpful in distinguishing between a pyogenic and an amebic liver abscess
(C) Blood cultures are positive in 50 percent of patients with a bacterial liver abscess
(D) Multiple abscesses tend to present more acutely than does a single lesion
(E) The combination of clindamycin and gentamicin is reasonable empiric therapy for a suspected pyogenic liver abscess

99. Toxoplasmosis can be described by which of the following statements?

(A) A pregnant woman who has acquired *Toxoplasma* any time before pregnancy is unlikely to deliver an infected infant
(B) A woman who develops acute toxoplasmosis during one pregnancy is more likely than other women to give birth to an infected child from a subsequent pregnancy
(C) A woman who acquires toxoplasmosis during the last trimester of pregnancy is more likely to deliver an infected infant than if she acquired the infection during the first trimester
(D) Toxoplasmosis in a person with Hodgkin's disease probably is due to reactivation of a latent infection
(E) Antibody response is not a reliable diagnostic indicator of toxoplasmosis in immunocompromised patients

100. True statements about *Pneumocystis carinii* pneumonia include

(A) fever and marked tachypnea are early signs
(B) pleural effusions are common
(C) pulmonary fibrosis is a common development
(D) systemic dissemination is extremely rare
(E) trimethoprim-sulfamethoxazole is an effective form of treatment

101. A person with liver disease caused by *Schistosoma mansoni* would be likely to have

(A) gynecomastia
(B) jaundice
(C) esophageal varices
(D) ascites
(E) spider nevi

102. True statements regarding *Shigella* and shigellosis include which of the following?

(A) *S. sonnei* is the isolate most frequently found in the United States
(B) Patients who have had gastric surgery or who are taking antacids have an increased susceptibility to infection
(C) There is increased transmission at day-care centers and among male homosexuals
(D) *Shigella* organisms are locally invasive in the bowel, but positive blood cultures are very unusual
(E) Antibiotic therapy should be avoided since it will increase the carrier rate

103. Extrapulmonary tuberculosis can be characterized by which of the following statements?

(A) Pleural effusions associated with tuberculosis usually occur in older patients with reactivation disease developing after an insidious onset
(B) Patients with laryngitis or bronchitis caused by tuberculosis are highly infectious
(C) Pott's disease, with extensive bony involvement of the midthoracic spine and paravertebral cold abscesses, will usually respond well to chemotherapy alone
(D) Cranial nerve findings are frequently associated with tuberculous meningitis because of basilar involvement by infection
(E) The stomach is most likely to be involved in patients with gastrointestinal tuberculosis

104. True statements about Lyme disease include which of the following?

(A) Transmission occurs almost exclusively in the northeastern United States
(B) A typical skin lesion, erythema chronicum migrans, usually occurs within a month of the infected tick bite
(C) Constitutional symptoms are very rare at the time of skin involvement
(D) Meningitis is the only form of neurologic involvement
(E) In patients with frank meningitis or significant cardiac conduction defects, parenteral therapy with 20 million units per day of penicillin G for at least 10 days is indicated

105. Correct statements about clostridial infections include which of the following?

(A) Early antibiotic therapy is important after the isolation of clostridia from any wound to prevent more serious disease
(B) Alpha toxin, a lecithinase, is one of the major clostridial toxins
(C) C. perfringens is one of the most common causes of food poisoning in the United States
(D) The diagnosis of clostridial myonecrosis can be difficult to make because few organisms are present in the skin lesions
(E) Septicemia with C. septicum has been associated with gastrointestinal malignancies

106. Anaerobic organisms should be considered as potential etiologic agents in which of the following patients?

(A) A previously healthy 18-year-old boy with sudden fever, cough, and right lower lobe infiltrate
(B) A 50-year-old man with alcoholism who has marked cellulitis, swelling, and pain of his left lower mandible
(C) A 40-year-old women with a seizure disorder, low-grade fever, malaise, and a right lower lobe infiltrate
(D) A 50-year-old women with fever, hypoxia, and pulmonary infiltrates 4 hours after having general anesthesia for a cholecystectomy
(E) A 38-year-old man with a history of rheumatic fever and severe periodontitis in whom a low-grade fever, malaise, and a new heart murmur develop

107. True statements about varicella-zoster infection include which of the following?

(A) Once dermatomal herpes zoster develops in a patient, repeated recurrences are the rule
(B) Cerebellar ataxia is a serious complication of varicella in children
(C) Chickenpox is very contagious with attack rates estimated at between 70 and 90 percent
(D) Varicella pneumonitis, the most serious complication of chickenpox, occurs more frequently in adults than in children
(E) If available within 72 hours of exposure, varicella-zoster immune globulin should be given to all patients to prevent development of clinical disease

108. Cytomegalovirus (CMV) is accurately described by which of the following statements?

(A) Approximately 60 percent of infants who are breast-fed by seropositive mothers become infected, causing the majority of the cases of cytomegalic inclusion disease in newborn infants
(B) Although 1 percent of newborn infants may be infected with CMV in the United States, less than .05 percent have symptomatic disease
(C) CMV mononucleosis is the most common cause of heterophil-negative mononucleosis
(D) CMV pneumonia, a major cause of morbidity and mortality in bone marrow transplant patients, can be diagnosed only by viral cultures of sputum
(E) Cultures of CMV from urine, saliva, or buffy coat specimens confirm the presence of the virus but do not necessarily imply acute infection

109. Correct statements about viral gastroenteritis caused by rotavirus and Norwalk virus include which of the following?

(A) Both alter cyclic nucleotide levels and cause a secretory diarrhea
(B) Rotaviruses are the most important causes of severe diarrhea in infants
(C) Rotavirus infection can be diagnosed only retrospectively by serologic methods since isolation from stool is very difficult
(D) Norwalk virus has been associated with both food-borne and water-borne epidemics
(E) Both viruses cause a self-limited disease with vomiting and diarrhea

110. True statements about influenza infection include which of the following?

(A) Pandemics are caused by several simultaneous point mutations

(B) Immunity is established by the development of antibodies to the neuraminidase preventing release of replicated viral particles

(C) Outbreaks of influenza B tend to be smaller than those of influenza A because the virus does not undergo extensive antigenic shift as it does in influenza A

(D) In a minority of patients, prolonged weakness and fatigue develop, associated with persistent viral shedding

(E) Amantadine or rimantadine may be useful in prophylaxis or therapy of influenza A if started within 48 hours of infection

111. Tetanus is correctly characterized by which of the following statements?

(A) Neonatal tetanus develops after passage through a contaminated birth canal

(B) If given early enough after exposure, human tetanus immune globulin can significantly modify the course of disease

(C) Tetanus does not recur because lasting immunity develops

(D) Trismus is a common manifestation

(E) In a patient who is uncertain about his or her immunization status, both tetanus toxoid and immune globulin should be given for serious wounds

112. Diphtherial infections are correctly characterized by which of the following statements?

(A) Human infection occurs only with strains producing diphtheria toxin

(B) Serious disease can be prevented by mass immunization with diphtherial cell-wall polysaccharide

(C) A pseudomembrane can be observed in both cutaneous and respiratory forms of infection

(D) A portion of the diphtheria toxin molecule is responsible for specificity; another part inflicts cellular damage by directly inhibiting DNA repair

(E) Cardiac disease is common in those with diphtherial pharyngitis

113. Correct statements concerning non–group A streptococcal disease include which of the following?

(A) Most group B streptococcal infections occur in older, debilitated patients

(B) The terms *group D streptococci* and *enterococci* are synonymous

(C) Some species of viridans streptococci can cause serious pyogenic infections

(D) Ampicillin plus streptomycin is the regimen of choice in the treatment of enterococcal endocarditis

(E) Non–group A streptococci represent the second most common agents responsible for neonatal sepsis

114. True statements concerning *Klebsiella* infections include which of the following?

(A) Most clinical isolates are obtained from the respiratory tract

(B) Predisposing factors for *Klebsiella* pneumonia include alcoholism, diabetes mellitus, and chronic bronchopulmonary disease

(C) *Klebsiella* is closely related to *Enterobacter* and *Serratia*

(D) Finding *Klebsiella* growth from a sputum culture obtained from an intubated patient mandates treatment with an aminoglycoside or a third-generation cephalosporin

(E) At least 2 weeks is often required to successfully treat an established *Klebsiella* infection

115. Which of the following could be part of a reasonable therapeutic strategy for serious *Haemophilus influenzae* infections, including meningitis?

(A) Ampicillin plus chloramphenicol
(B) Chloramphenicol alone
(C) Cefotaxime alone
(D) Ceftriaxone alone
(E) Dexamethasone plus antibiotics

116. Correct statements concerning the diagnosis of tuberculosis include which of the following?

(A) A 30-year-old third-year medical resident with a normal chest x-ray whose tuberculin skin test is positive (no history of prior test) should receive isoniazid for 1 year

(B) Tuberculosis can be ruled out in a 55-year-old alcoholic man with cavitary lung disease and a negative tuberculin skin test

(C) Serologic tests are frequently employed to confirm a diagnosis of tuberculosis

(D) Gastric aspiration yields too high a false-positive rate to be a useful diagnostic test

(E) Tuberculosis is usually a late manifestation of infection by human immunodeficiency virus (HIV)

117. Which of the following parasites will produce pneumonia with significant frequency?

(A) *Enterobius*
(B) *Ascaris*
(C) *Toxocara*
(D) *Taenia*
(E) *Strongyloides*

118. True statements concerning malaria include

(A) malaria caused by each of the four plasmodial species can relapse after initial illness
(B) red cells negative for the Duffy blood group antigen are resistant to *Plasmodium vivax*
(C) renal impairment is a grave prognostic sign in falciparum malaria
(D) *Plasmodium malariae* can cause immune-mediated nephropathy
(E) massive splenomegaly can result from repeated bouts of infection

119. Well-recognized complications of infection with Epstein-Barr virus include

(A) airway obstruction
(B) lymphoma
(C) thrombocytopenia
(D) hemolytic anemia
(E) hepatitis

DIRECTIONS: Each group of questions below consists of lettered headings followed by a set of numbered items. For each numbered item select the **one** lettered heading with which it is **most** closely associated. Each lettered heading may be used **once, more than once, or not at all.**

Questions 120–123

Match each defect in host immunity with the type of infection most commonly associated with it.

(A) Cytomegalovirus
(B) Recurrent *Neisseria gonorrhoeae* infections
(C) Recurrent staphylococcal skin abscesses
(D) *Streptococcus pneumoniae* bacteremia
(E) Gram-negative bacteremia

120. Deficiencies of late complement components

121. Postsplenectomy state

122. Abnormal T-cell suppressor/helper ratio in patients with the acquired immunodeficiency syndrome (AIDS)

123. Chédiak-Higashi syndrome

Questions 124–128

Several preventive measures for viral infections are now at hand. For each of the following viral infections, select the most appropriate method of prevention.

(A) Inactivated virus vaccination
(B) Attenuated virus vaccination
(C) Passive immunization
(D) Prolonged autoclaving of surgical instruments
(E) Chemoprophylaxis

124. Creutzfeldt-Jakob disease

125. Varicella

126. Influenza A

127. Rubella

128. Hepatitis A

Infectious Diseases

Answers

1. The answer is D. *(Wilson, ed 12. chap 81. Malech, N Engl J Med 317:687, 1987.)* This child most likely has chronic granulomatous disease (CGD), a group of inherited disorders that have in common defective oxidative metabolism of neutrophils. This defect results in a heightened susceptibility to infection with catalase-positive organisms such as staphylococci and *Aspergillus*. The diagnosis can be made by demonstrating abnormal neutrophil reduction of nitroblue tetrazolium. Recent studies have suggested that interferon-gamma may be useful in correcting the neutrophil dysfunction characteristic of CGD. Most patients with isolated deficiency of myeloperoxidase are not at increased risk for infection unless another defect is present, in which case infection with *Candida albicans* may be a problem. Decreased serum levels of immunoglobulins predispose to infection with encapsulated organisms such as *Haemophilus* and streptococci, while defects in T-lymphocyte function are manifested as infection with viruses and protozoal pathogens such as *Pneumocystis carinii*.

2. The answer is D. *(Wilson, ed 12. chap 82.)* Acquired immunodeficiency syndrome is characterized by a decreased ratio of helper T cells to suppressor T cells. The commonly associated infections are those requiring a normal T-cell response. Though sepsis can develop in association with marked neutropenia, organisms such as *Pseudomonas aeruginosa* rarely are a problem.

3. The answer is A. *(Wilson, ed 12. chap 80.)* As a rule, all clinical tissue or fluid specimens should be delivered to the appropriate laboratory as quickly as possible, preferably within an hour. In the situation described in the question, the organism most likely to be lost would be *Neisseria*. Such a delay also would adversely affect recovery of *Shigella* from stool samples; thus, in cases of suspected shigellosis, stool should be cultured as quickly as possible.

4. The answer is A. *(Wilson, ed 12. chap 151.)* The physical signs and symptoms listed in the question suggest infection with *Candida albicans*. *C. albicans* infections occur in several clinical settings: diabetes in poor control; broad-spectrum antibiotic therapy; chronic mucocutaneous candidiasis syndrome; and others. Although some of these conditions may be associated with elevated serum levels of immunoglobulins A and E, these are nonspecific findings. On the other hand, a significantly elevated blood glucose concentration would make the diagnosis of diabetes almost certain. In complement deficiency or uremia, the defects in host defense are not characteristically manifested by vaginal candidiasis.

5. The answer is C. *(Wilson, ed 12. chap 83.)* Cannula infections occur most commonly from contamination during cannula insertion or manipulation. Although the daily application of an antibacterial ointment is recommended by some authorities, the best way to prevent these infections is to change the cannula periodically, no less often than every 2 or 3 days. An exception is the use of cuffed catheters, which are inserted surgically into the subclavian vein and can be used for many weeks. Cannula infections occur much less frequently as a result of the other factors listed in the question.

6. The answer is B. *(Wilson, ed 12. chap 89. Bone, N Engl J Med 317:653, 1987.)* In the case presented, the history and physical examination strongly suggest gram-negative sepsis stemming from a urinary-tract infection. In older men, obstruction due to prostatic hypertrophy is usually the cause. Prompt initiation of appropriate antibiotic therapy is most important. The choice of antibiotics can be guided by the history and microscopic examination of a Gram-stained urine specimen. In the absence of definitive laboratory information, initial treatment with broad-spectrum coverage, such as gentamicin or tobramycin plus ampicillin or a cephalosporin, is indicated. Bladder catheterization may be necessary to relieve the obstruction or monitor urine flow. Intravenous infusion of bicarbonate solutions and Ringer's lactate or dextrose-in-saline solutions is needed acutely to correct acidosis, restore vascular volume, and maintain renal perfusion. Corticosteroids may protect against the lethal effects of endotoxin in experimental animals, but recent placebo-controlled trials have failed to support their use in most clinical situations.

7.   The answer is D. *(Wilson, ed 12. chap 111.)* Primary *Pseudomonas* osteomyelitis is very unusual except in intravenous drug addicts, but it should be considered in a nail puncture wound that does not respond to local or oral antibiotic therapy. Ecthyma gangrenosum, an indurated black area approximately 1 cm in diameter with an ulcerated center and surrounding erythema, is highly suggestive of *Pseudomonas* bacteremia. *Pseudomonas* is the most common cause of chronic otitis externa, which usually responds to local measures. In diabetics, however, a rapidly invasive form may develop and require aggressive debridement and antibiotic therapy. *Escherichia coli* is the most frequent cause of gram-negative meningitis in neonatal infants. Development of *Pseudomonas* meningitis usually occurs only after introduction by surgery, trauma, or foreign objects such as shunts. *Pseudomonas* endocarditis usually occurs in intravenous drug users or after open-heart surgery.

8.   The answer is D. *(Wilson, ed 12. chap 89.)* Leukocytosis with a marked shift to immature neutrophils in the blood and prolongation of the prothrombin and partial thromboplastin times frequently occur in persons with sepsis. Metabolic acidosis, reflected by reductions in blood pH and carbon dioxide tension and in serum bicarbonate concentration, is also common. Urinalysis usually shows nonspecific changes; the finding of red-cell casts would be very unusual, unless the patient has another cause for renal injury.

9.   The answer is B. *(Wilson, ed 12. chap 80.)* Recombinant DNA technology has made it possible to identify specific microbial DNA sequences in clinical material. Although specific, this technique may be too sensitive in some cases and blur the distinction between infection and colonization. Probes have been developed for a wide variety of microorganisms, including CMV, EBV, hepatitis B virus, and HIV, as well as mycoplasma, chlamydia, legionella, and gonococci. These probes will become even more sensitive with the use of the polymerase chain reaction to amplify specific sequences.

10.   The answer is C. *(Wilson, ed 12. chap 92.)* Toxigenic *Escherichia coli* is the major cause of diarrhea ("turista") for Americans abroad. *Staphylococcus aureus, Clostridium perfringens,* and *Bacillus cereus* cause various types of acute food poisoning owing to bacterial proliferation and elaboration of toxins in improperly stored food. Children throughout the developing world can suffer acute diarrhea, similar to traveler's diarrhea, caused by rotavirus infection. All five of these agents cause watery diarrhea that generally is without blood, mucus, or fecal leukocytes.

11.   The answer is A. *(Wilson, ed 12. chap 84.)* Since BCG is a live attenuated organism and has been reported to cause disseminated infection in immunocompromised patients, it should not be administered to those with HIV infection or others with suspected immunodeficiency. Though patients with immune dysfunction often do not mount a good response to an administered vaccine, they should still receive certain preparations. Patients about to undergo splenectomy or cancer chemotherapy should, when possible, be vaccinated prior to therapy. Influenza vaccine should be given in autumn to those with any chronic medical illness in addition to those with obvious immune deficiency. The chronically ill, the immunosuppressed, and those at risk for infection with encapsulated microorganisms (anatomic or functional asplenia, multiple myeloma) should receive pneumococcal vaccine. The last group plus those with terminal complement component deficiencies should receive the quad-rivalent meningococcal vaccine. Patients with HIV infection, especially those who are potential household contacts of children who are receiving the oral polio vaccine (attenuated live virus), should receive three doses of the inactivated polio vaccine.

12.   The answer is A. *(Wilson, ed 12. chap 85.)* Antibiotic prophylaxis with a cephalosporin, usually cefa-zolin, is of value in association with vaginal and abdominal hysterectomies. Antibiotic prophylaxis is unlikely to be of value in persons undergoing the other surgical procedures listed in the question. In these operations, the tissues involved are generally sterile, and contamination of the surgical field can be avoided readily.

13.   The answer is D. *(Wilson, ed 12. chap 84.)* Passive immunization via administration of exogenous antibody offers immediate, short-lived protection in certain exposure situations. Immune globulin may offer protection for 3 months to those exposed to hepatitis A, as well as to foreign travelers. Hepatitis B immune globulin should be given to infants of HBsAg-positive mothers and to those who have had sexual or percutaneous contact with the virus; the hepatitis B vaccine should be coadministered. Persons at high risk from disseminated varicella infection should receive varicella-zoster immune globulin if exposed to chickenpox. Immunosuppressed persons, including those with HIV infection, should receive immune globulin if they have been exposed to measles. Immune globulin also offers protection to pregnant women exposed to rubella during the first trimester who do not wish termination of pregnancy. Passive immunization for those exposed to polio is not possible.

14.   The answer is A. *(Wilson, ed 12. chap 100.)* The pathogenicity of staphylococci is related to a number of biologic properties, including the production of coagulase, catalase, exotoxin, and enterotoxin. Coagulase and catalase are thought to protect staphylococci within a host from being destroyed by phagocytes. Some staphylococcal strains produce exotoxins that can cause intraepidermal cleavage and bullae formation, as well as toxic shock syndrome. Other strains elaborate an enterotoxin that produces gastrointestinal disease. The production of penicillinase, though rendering a pathogenic organism harder to destroy pharmacologically, does not contribute to pathogenicity.

15.   The answer is A. *(Wilson, ed 12. chaps 100, 354.)* Probably because of its ubiquity and ability to stick to foreign surfaces, *Staphylococcus epidermidis* is the most frequent cause of infections of central nervous system shunts, as well as an important cause of infection on artificial heart valves and orthopedic prostheses. *Corynebacterium* species (diphtheroids), just like *S. epidermidis,* colonize the skin. When these organisms are isolated from cultures of shunts, it is often difficult to be sure if they are the cause of disease or simply contaminants. Leukocytosis in cerebrospinal fluid, consistent isolation of the same organism, and the character of a patient's symptoms all are helpful in deciding whether treatment for infection is indicated.

16.   The answer is D. *(Wilson, ed 12. chap 101.)* Streptococcal pharyngitis, usually caused by group A streptococci, is an exceedingly common bacterial infection, especially in school-age and adolescent children. Symptoms commonly include sudden sore throat and pain on swallowing, fever, headache, malaise, anorexia, nausea, and abdominal pain; aside from edema, erythema, and lymphoid hyperplasia of the posterior pharynx, physical signs also include tender, enlarged cervical lymph nodes. Because involvement of the larynx does not occur, loss of voice would not be expected.

17.   The answer is B. *(Wilson, ed 12. chap 109.)* Vaccines prepared from high-molecular-weight antigens of *Neisseria meningitidis,* serotypes A and C, have proved effective, but an effective group B vaccine is not available. Although sulfonamide resistance is an important problem in meningococcal epidemics with sulfonamide-sensitive organisms, sulfonamides remain a good choice for prophylaxis. When sulfonamide-resistant strains are isolated but the sensitivity of the organism is not known, rifampin therapy is generally recommended.

18.   The answer is E. *(Wilson, ed 12. chap 85.)* Because of the frequent use of antibiotics in very ill patients subject to compromised renal function, it is important to know which antibiotics are primarily renally excreted. Amikacin and all other aminoglycosides are proximal tubular toxins that accumulate in renal failure, and dosage should be calculated according to blood levels in patients with abnormal renal function. Vancomycin needs to be administered only once a week to treat staphylococcal infections in patients with chronic renal failure. Ceftazidime has excellent antipseudomonal activity and, unlike cefoperazone, does not prolong the prothrombin time; however, it is primarily cleared by glomerular filtration and requires major dosage adjustments in renal failure. Another renally excreted cephalosporin is cefoxitin, which is frequently used in pelvic and anaerobic infections owing to its good activity against the anaerobe *B. fragilis.* On the other hand, cefotaxime, a third-generation cephalosporin used in the treatment of meningitis, has a short half-life in the blood even in patients whose creatinine clearance is below 10 mL/min.

19.   The answer is C. *(Wilson, ed 12. chap 111.)* *Pseudomonas* organisms can cause a rapidly invasive infection resulting in extensive bony erosion in diabetics. Aggressive surgical debridement and parenteral administration of antibiotics are required for treatment. *Aspergillus* organisms can be isolated frequently from external ear swabs but do not cause invasive disease. Mucormycosis must be considered in any seriously ill diabetic patient with sinus or ocular involvement. Infection usually spreads from the nasal cavity and does not involve the ears. Insulin-dependent diabetics are more likely to have their skin colonized by *S. aureus,* but such colonization is not associated with external otitis. *H. influenzae* is a frequent cause of otitis media, especially in children, but not of otitis externa.

20.   The answer is C. *(Wilson, ed 12. chap 113.)* *Salmonella typhi* survives well in food and water and generally causes infection by penetrating the intestinal mucosa and entering the bloodstream. Usually at the time that affected persons present with fever and other signs of an acute illness, the white blood cell count is depressed. In contrast, rose spots usually do not occur until the second week of illness. Therapy with chloramphenicol does not prevent relapses but does alter the course of the acute illness. A chronic carrier state can develop in large part because of the propensity of *S. typhi* to seed and inhabit the gallbladder, especially in adults with gallstones.

21.   The answer is E. *(Wilson, ed 12. chap 115.)* Persons who have sickle-cell disease or agammaglobulinemia and those who have been splenectomized have immune systems that poorly opsonize encapsulated bacteria such as *Haemophilus influenzae. Haemophilus influenzae* infections also are more common in alcoholic persons, in part because of abnormal cellular defense mechanisms. Persons who have chronic granulomatous disease have problems combating infection with *Staphylococcus aureus, Salmonella,* and *Serratia,* but not *Haemophilus influenzae.*

22.   The answer is A. *(Wilson, ed 12. chap 116.)* Because a marked lymphocytosis characteristically is observed in children who have *Haemophilus pertussis* infection (whooping cough) and is rare in other respiratory illnesses, white blood cell count with differential would be useful in making the diagnosis. Blood cultures would be negative, and Gram stain of the sputum and chest and neck x-rays would show nonspecific changes. The diagnosis of pertussis is confirmed in most cases by nasopharyngeal culture.

23.   The answer is E. *(Wilson, ed 12. chap 151.)* Coccidioidomycosis, caused by the inhalation of *Coccidioides immitis,* may present clinically with manifestations of hypersensitivity reactions. Arthralgias and frank arthritis (so-called desert rheumatism) as well as such skin reactions as erythema nodosum and erythema multiforme are associated far more frequently with coccidioidomycosis than with the other mycoses listed in the question. Delayed hypersensitivity to *C. immitis* antigens tends to be a good prognostic sign.

24.   The answer is D. *(Wilson, ed 12. chap 85.)* Imipenem is a novel β-lactam antibiotic in the carbapenem class with activity against most gram-positive organisms, including those that produce β-lactamase. In addition to most strains of *Pseudomonas,* imipenem inhibits the growth of *B. fragilis.* This drug must be given intravenously because of its instability in gastric acid. Since imipenem is hydrolyzed in the renal tubule by dihydropeptidase I, the coadministration of cilastatin, an inhibitor of this enzyme, serves to markedly boost levels of this broad-spectrum antibiotic. Clavulanate is a β-lactamase inhibitor used with partial success when combined with amoxicillin (Augmentin) for treatment of resistant otitis and urinary tract infections.

25.   The answer is E. *(Wilson, ed 12. chap 117.)* *Haemophilus ducreyi* causes painful genital ulcers, which begin as small tender papules. In contrast, syphilitic ulcers are usually painless, and the initial lesions of genital herpes simplex infections are usually vesicular. The organism causing the chancroid can be isolated from both the ulcers and affected lymph nodes; in fact, culturing the lymph nodes may produce a pure culture of this organism. Unlike infection with other members of the genus *Haemophilus,* chancroid is not effectively treated with ampicillin. Trimethoprim-sulfamethoxazole and erythromycin are the antibiotic agents of choice.

26.   The answer is D. *(Wilson, ed 12. chap 151.)* Patients who have localized sporotrichosis can be treated successfully with potassium iodide. However, systemic infections, particularly pneumonia in immunocompromised persons, should be treated with amphotericin B. Untreated persons can develop chronic sporotrichosis.

27.   The answer is B. *(Wilson, ed 12. chap 120.)* Aspiration and culture of an enlarged axillary lymph node would be most helpful in yielding a diagnosis of tularemia in the case described. Blood and bone-marrow cultures rarely are positive for *Francisella (Pasteurella) tularensis.* Agglutinin reactions ordinarily are not positive for at least 1 week after infection. A wide variety of animals and insects can transmit tularemia to humans.

28.   The answer is D. *(Wilson, ed 12. chap 121.)* In the case presented, the diagnosis of plague (*Yersinia pestis* infection) must be considered. To make this diagnosis, affected lymph nodes should be aspirated and the contents Gram-stained. In most cases of bubonic plague, lymph-node aspirates teem with pleomorphic gram-negative bacilli, which can be identified immediately by immunofluorescent staining of the specimen. Blood culture, bone-marrow examination, and lymph-node biopsy might be used to diagnose plague, but with undue delay. In this situation, great care should be exercised in handling the infected materials—there is a significant risk of infection for the laboratory workers.

29.   The answer is A. *(Wilson, ed 12. chap 124.)* Legionnaire's disease is caused by *Legionella pneumophila.* It occurs sporadically or in outbreaks and often begins with myalgias, headache, and fever. Diarrhea and delirium also are early features in many cases. Gastrointestinal symptoms should suggest the possibility of this diagnosis, particularly in persons who have severe pneumonia, scant production of sputum, and other extrapulmonary abnormalities. Of the other organisms listed in the question, all can cause pneumonia; *Mycoplasma pneumoniae* infection is most likely to be confused with Legionnaire's disease.

30. The answer is D. *(Wilson, ed 12. chap 103.)* *Listeria monocytogenes* is a gram-positive motile bacillus that tends to infect infants as well as persons over the age of 55 years. Major illnesses in both groups are meningitis and other forms of central nervous system infection. Many of the older patients are immunosuppressed because of disease (e.g., cancer), immunosuppressive drug therapy, or both. Endocarditis, peritonitis, hepatitis, and conjunctivitis also can be caused by *Listeria* infection.

31. The answer is D. *(Wilson, ed 12. chap 86. Meyers, Am J Med 85:102, 1988.)* Ganciclovir, an analogue of acyclovir, is converted into the triphosphate form and thereby inhibits CMV DNA polymerases. Because of its striking anti-CMV activity, this drug has been extensively used in the HIV-infected population. Unfortunately, it has only been shown to improve the course of CMV retinitis; the effect against hepatitis, colitis, "wasting" disease, and pneumonia is marginal.

32. The answer is C. *(Wilson, ed 12. chap 88.)* Most antimalarial drugs—including quinine, 4-aminoqui-nolines (e.g., chloroquine, hydroxychloroquine), and 4-quinoline-methanols (e.g., mefloquine)—concentrate in erythrocytes, thereby destroying the intracellular schizonts responsible for the acute manifestations of malarial illness. However, these drugs do not readily concentrate in the liver, and they thereby allow survival of hepatic schizonts and reinfection at a later date. In contrast primaquine, an 8-aminoquinoline, can eradicate hepatic parasites, but is not effective in acute illness.

33. The answer is D. *(Wilson, ed 12. chap 92.)* Bacteria that cause diarrhea via toxin elaboration are generally associated with a shorter time from ingestion to illness than are invasive strains. For example, enterotoxigenic *E. coli* (the most common cause of traveler's diarrhea), *C. perfringens* (associated with poorly cooked meat or poultry), *S. aureus* (associated with improperly refrigerated dairy foods), and *B. cereus* (associated with grossly contaminated uncooked rice) all have incubation periods of 24 h or less. Even though the pathogenesis may depend on direct mucosal damage, *V. parahaemolyticus,* which is present in inadequately cooked seafood, can cause a diarrheal illness within 6 to 48 h after consumption of a contaminated food. Resulting from ingestion of water contaminated with the intestinal flora of wild or domestic animals, *C. jejuni* is a frequent cause of acute, sometimes bloody, diarrhea. The incubation period for this invasive bacterium is 2 to 6 days, longer than that associated with other pathogens. Therapy is usually supportive, though erythromycin will shorten the duration of illness.

34. The answer is A. *(Wilson, ed 12. chap 125.)* The diagnosis of a tuberculous pleural effusion is suggested by the following set of pleural-fluid findings: color, clear yellow; pH, < 7.20; protein, > 30 g/L; glucose, < 1.2 mmol/L (25 mg/dL); lactate dehydrogenase (LDH), > 450 U/mL; and a lymphocytosis. Tubercle bacilli rarely are identified on a smear of infected pleural fluid, and cultures are positive in no more than one-quarter of cases. Antituberculous treatment usually should commence as soon as the diagnosis is suspected.

35. The answer is D. *(Wilson, ed 12. chap 132. Steere, N Engl J Med 321:586, 1989.)* In a patient with Lyme disease, biopsy of the typical skin lesion, erythema chronicum migrans, usually shows nondiagnostic perivascular lymphocytic and histiocytic infiltration. Though hematogenous dissemination of the spirochete that causes Lyme disease, *Borrelia burgdorferi,* does occur, it is rarely detected on direct examination. The spirochete has been cultured from blood, skin, and cerebrospinal fluid (CSF), but culture of this organism is not a routine procedure. Frank meningitis with CSF pleocytosis rarely occurs until several weeks or months into the illness. Lymphocytosis and an elevated protein level are typically found but are not diagnostic. The most useful study is a serum determination of IgG antibody titers, which are almost uniformly elevated after several weeks of illness.

36. The answer is A. *(Wilson, ed 12. chap 127.)* Two of the lesser-known species of *Mycobacterium, M. scrofulaceum* and *M. avium-intracellulare,* cause lymphadenitis in children. Usually affected are the lymph nodes that drain the buccal mucosa. Both *M. scrofulaceum* and *M. avium-intracellulare* respond poorly to chemotherapy. Treatment of choice, therefore, is prompt lymph-node excision, before rupture has occurred.

37. The answer is D. *(Wilson, ed 12. chap 127.)* *Mycobacterium marinum* is known as the "swimming pool" or "fishtank" bacillus because ulcerative cutaneous infections can be acquired from contact with contam-inated swimming pools and aquariums. *M. ulcerans* also causes ulcerative skin lesions but characteristically is confined to tropical regions. Other "atypical" mycobacteria that cause cutaneous infections in humans include *M. avium-intracellulare, M. scrofulaceum, M. kansasii,* and *M. fortuitum.*

38.   The answer is C. *(Wilson, ed 12. chap 124.)* Legionnaire's disease is caused by *Legionella pneumophila*. Person-to-person spread of this soil organism has not been documented. Gastrointestinal symptoms preceding pneumonia are sometimes a clue to the diagnosis. In many cases, chest x-ray shows dense infiltrates despite a paucity of physical signs, such as rales or rhonchi; in this regard, the disease resembles *Mycoplasma* pneumonia. Although *L. pneumophila* has been found in vitro to be sensitive to several drugs, erythromycin is the treatment of choice.

39.   The answer is E. *(Wilson, ed 12. chap 124.)* Since the recognition of *Legionella pneumophila*, many other species of *Legionella* have been discovered. These organisms can be detected by silver staining, immunofluorescent staining, and culture of infected materials. It is much better to culture lung tissue or pleural fluid than sputum, because sputum contains a mixture of other organisms that tend to overgrow *Legionella*. Aside from direct methods of diagnosis, serologic tests run on paired serum specimens also are useful. Detecting genomic DNA common to all *Legionella* species can be accomplished with a radiolabeled nucleic acid hybridization kit; false positives have been reported. Direct fluorescent antibody staining is specific, but relatively insensitive.

40.   The answer is A. *(Wilson, ed 12. chap 93. Krockta, Infect Dis Clin North Am 1:217, 1987.)* The presence of vesicles in addition to ulcerative lesions strongly suggests herpes simplex infection. If no vesicles are present, dark-field examination should be performed in order to diagnose syphilis. In all other patients a serologic test for syphilis should be performed. Without a documented etiology after the preceding evaluation, especially with the association of painful lymphadenopathy, additional diagnostic tests are required. Such tests may include a viral culture to define occult herpetic infection, a bacterial culture on special media to isolate *Haemophilus ducreyi* (chancroid), or biopsy to rule out malignancy, lymphogranuloma venereum, and donovanosis (granuloma inguinale).

41.   The answer is C. *(Wilson, ed 12. chap 131.)* Relapsing fever can be diagnosed by finding spirochetal borreliae in a peripheral blood smear. Sometimes it is necessary to examine thick smears or to use phase microscopy to see the organisms. In the western United States, especially in areas in which tick bites are likely to occur, relapsing fever should be suspected in persons with acute febrile illnesses characterized by headache, photophobia, and muscle pains.

42.   The answer is A. *(Wilson, ed 12. chap 152.)* In the examination of purulent material from persons suspected of having actinomycosis, it is important to search the material for the characteristic "sulfur grains" and then to examine the grains for organisms. Actinomycetes are gram-positive, branching organisms. If they are detected in a patient presenting with a suggestive clinical picture, such as a chronic draining sinus in the oropharyngeal area, the gastrointestinal tract, or the pelvic area, then the diagnosis of actinomycosis is ensured.

43.   The answer is C. *(Wilson, ed 12. chap 151.)* Initial diagnosis of cryptococcal meningitis usually is based on finding encapsulated yeast on an India ink preparation. This test, however, is positive in only about half of cases in which the diagnosis is eventually made. Testing of serum and cerebrospinal fluid for cryptococcal antigen is a very helpful adjunctive test because antigen is found in about 90 percent of cases. In pulmonary cryptococcosis, only about one-third of affected persons are antigen-positive.

44.   The answer is E. *(Wilson, ed 12. chap 110.)* Because of the emergence of antibiotic-resistant strains of *Neisseria gonorrhoeae*, the Centers for Disease Control (CDC) published new guidelines for treatment of gonorrhea in 1989. The antibiotic resistance could be on the basis of penicillinase production, plasmid-encoded tetracycline resistance, or chromosomally mediated resistance to both drugs. Also prompting the new guidelines were requirements for effective single-dose therapy and the frequent coexistence of chlamydial infection. Therefore, a single intramuscular dose of ceftriaxone plus a 7-day course of doxycycline (or tetracycline) represents the currently recommended therapy for uncomplicated infection. Erythromycin should be substituted for tetracycline in the pregnant female. Intravenous therapy is probably required in most cases of disseminated gonococcal infection.

45.   The answer is D. *(Wilson, ed 12. chap 151.)* Fungal and yeast infections, predominantly candidiasis, aspergillosis, and mucormycosis, occur frequently in severely immunosuppressed patients, particularly those who have received broad-spectrum antibiotics for a prolonged period. A number of other types of fungal infection occur in these patients. About 75 percent of all cases of *Cryptococcus neoformans* infection occur in persons who have lymphoma, are taking glucocorticosteroids, or are otherwise immunocompromised. The association of cryptococcal meningitis and Hodgkin's disease is important clinically.

46. The answer is D. *(Wilson, ed 12. chap 107.)* *Clostridium difficile* can be isolated on selective agar media, but this method is not dependable for diagnosis. Pseudomembranous colitis (PMC) is caused by the local action of at least two enterotoxins, toxins A and B. Serologic tests are not helpful. The punctate plaques on a hyperemic mucosa are characteristic of PMC, but similar pathologic changes can be seen with ischemic colitis. The best diagnostic test is the demonstration of *C. difficile* cytotoxin, an assay that can be positive in 24 h. Clostridia are part of normal fecal flora, so a Gram stain of the stool would not be helpful.

47. The answer is D. *(Wilson, ed 12. chap 151.)* As primary therapy for dermatophytosis (ringworm), miconazole, clotrimazole, and tolnaftate usually are recommended. In severe cases, griseofulvin generally is used, with ketoconazole recommended for griseofulvin-resistant cases. Amphotericin is not a recommended treatment of dermatophytosis.

48. The answer is E. *(Wilson, ed 12. chap 155.)* Trachoma remains the most important cause of preventable blindness in the world. Blindness occurs primarily because of damage to the cornea and eyelids. Corneal abrasion, scarring of the lids, secondary infections, and loss of lacrimal function are the principal problems.

49. The answer is E. *(Wilson, ed 12. chap 155.)* Fever, chills, headache, cough, and myalgias are the typical presenting signs and symptoms of psittacosis. Gastrointestinal symptoms also may occur but are much less frequent. The diagnosis of psittacosis usually depends on serologic tests or cultures of respiratory secretions. Even a low-titer positive complement fixation antibody test, in conjunction with the clinical setting described, would strongly suggest the diagnosis of psittacosis and warrant the use of tetracycline.

50. The answer is D. *(Wilson, ed 12. chap 146.)* Both mumps and bacterial parotitis produce fever, and both may be associated with elevated serum amylase levels because of the release of salivary amylase into the blood. In persons who have mumps, the parotid glands are usually not as warm and tender as in persons who have bacterial parotitis. Mumps tends to be a disease of children and young adults, whereas bacterial parotitis tends to affect the elderly. The most useful distinguishing feature, however, is probably the nature of the parotid secretions. In bacterial parotitis, significant numbers of leukocytes and bacteria, usually staphylococci, are found in parotid secretions; in mumps, only a small amount of parotid fluid, and no pus, is observed.

51. The answer is C. *(Wilson, ed 12. chap 144.)* As many as 90 percent of the patients with poliovirus are asymptomatic or have only a self-limited febrile illness. Paralytic polio is characterized by an initial febrile illness that resolves and is followed by development of aseptic meningitis and asymmetric paralysis. In contrast to polio, the Guillain-Barré syndrome is characterized by symmetric muscle weakness with frequent paresthesias but normal reflexes. Motor neurons are primarily affected by poliovirus infection resulting in the loss of reflexes and flaccid paralysis. Return of neuronal function may be possible for up to 6 months after infection.

52. The answer is A. *(Wilson, ed 12. chap 139.)* The man described in the question has symptoms suggesting influenza complicated by bacterial pneumonia. Pneumococci and staphylococci are the leading pathogens causing secondary bacterial infection in this situation, and effective therapy would include drugs that act against penicillinase-producing staphylococci. The agent of choice is nafcillin or another semisynthetic penicillinase-resistant penicillin; penicillin G would be an ill-advised choice. Other drugs acceptable as alternative therapies would include vancomycin, clindamycin, and cephalothin.

53. The answer is A. *(Wilson, ed 12. chap 128.)* Lymphadenopathy and papulosquamous rash that includes the palms and soles characteristically accompany secondary syphilis, which appears about 8 weeks after healing of the primary chancre. Lymphadenopathy is not a well-recognized manifestation of late syphilis. The inflammatory lesions of late syphilis are diverse and range from asymptomatic neurosyphilis, characterized only by pleocytosis or elevated protein on CSF examination, to the complex intellectual and functional disturbances caused by parenchymal damage of brain tissue (general paresis). Meningovascular syphilis can lead to middle cerebral artery strokes, which produce hemiparesis and dysphasia. Demyelinization of the posterior columns will lead to the ataxic gait and destroyed joints from loss of position sense characteristic of tabes dorsalis. About

10 percent of patients with late untreated syphilis will experience cardiovascular complications, usually in the form of aneurysms of the ascending aorta. Gummas are nodules of granulomatous inflammation involving the skin and skeleton. Gummas of the skin may take the form of nodules, a papulosquamous eruption, or ulcers.

54.   The answer is D. *(Wilson, ed 12. chap 86.)* Acyclovir is now the drug of choice in the treatment of herpes encephalitis. It has been shown to be more effective than vidarabine and also has fewer side effects. Acyclovir has been shown both to shorten viral shedding in mucocutaneous infections and to prevent outbreaks in immunocompromised patients. Similarly, acyclovir is useful in immunocompromised patients with herpes zoster, but it is not yet indicated in nonimmunocompromised patients in whom the risk of dissemination is very small. Both the frequency and the duration of recurrent episodes of genital herpes are reduced on long-term suppressive therapy. As soon as the drug is discontinued, however, infection recurs.

55.   The answer is E. *(Wilson, ed 12. chap 95.)* Precisely how diabetes mellitus and sickle cell disease predispose to urinary tract infection is unclear. In persons with diabetes, glycosuria and neuropathic changes in bladder function are probably contributory. In association with both diabetes and sickle cell disease, avascular areas in the kidney probably provide sites for bacterial multiplication remote from phagocytic cells. In hyperparathyroidism and gout, stone formation leads to obstruction and infection. Although in Wilson's disease copper is deposited in the kidney and tubular dysfunction occurs, urinary infections generally are not a major problem.

56.   The answer is C. *(Wilson, ed 12. chap 134.)* Retroviruses contain an RNA genome that requires reverse transcription into DNA after entering the host cell. The DNA copy of the viral genome may then integrate into the host genome, enabling transcription of viral genes and ultimately leading to complete viral replication. AIDS, the best known human retroviral disease, is caused by human immunodeficiency virus 1 (HIV-1), which attaches to CD4 molecules on lymphocytes and monocytes and produces lymphopenic immunodeficiency. HIV-2, isolated in Africa, appears to be an infrequent cause of AIDS. The two retroviruses associated with transformation of human cells are human T-lymphotropic viruses I and II (HTLV-I and HTLV-II). The role of HTLV-II in human disease is unclear, although the virus was originally isolated from a patient with a T-cell variant of hairy cell leukemia. One to three percent of those infected with HTLV-I develop a fulminant and refractory malignancy of CD4-positive lymphocytes called *adult T-cell leukemia/lymphoma,* characterized by lymphocytosis, leukemic skin infiltrates, bone lesions, and hypercalcemia. Increased numbers of interleukin 2 receptors can be found on the surface of the malignant cells. A demyelinating disorder termed *tropical spastic paraparesis* and a chronic T-cell leukemia represent other diseases associated with HTLV-I infection. Feline leukemia virus (FeLV), responsible for tumors in cats, does not cause human disease.

57.   The answer is E. *(Wilson, ed 12. chaps 135, 355.)* Among the many viruses that can cause acute encephalitis, the most frequent cause in the United States is herpes simplex. A few years ago, this fact would have been of academic interest only, but with the availability of antiviral chemotherapy, establishment of the specific diagnosis can be fruitful. Brain biopsy and CT scanning are the most helpful procedures for establishing this diagnosis.

58.   The answer is E. *(Wilson, ed 12. chap 166.)* Cryptosporidia, which are protozoa, cannot be cultured from the stool. They stain with iodine but not Gram stain. Investigational serologic tests appear promising but are not readily available. Because of their small size (5 μm) and lack of motility, detection of cysts by wet mounts is very difficult. By using acid-fast stains or rhodamine fluorescence, even a few cysts can be detected easily and the diagnosis of cryptosporidiosis made.

59.   The answer is D. *(Wilson, ed 12. chap 85.)* Methicillin-resistant *Staphylococcus aureus* is becoming a major source of morbidity and mortality. In vitro sensitivity testing may demonstrate sensitivity to cephalosporins, but these tests are unreliable and all strains are resistant in vivo. These strains have an altered penicillin-binding protein and are resistant to all penicillinase-resistant penicillins, alone or in combination with an aminoglycoside. Resistance is not plasmid-mediated, and there is no risk of spread to other bacteria. Administration of vancomycin is the most effective treatment.

60.   The answer is D. *(Wilson, ed 12. chap 126.)* A papular reaction usually develops in patients with tuberculoid leprosy 1 month after injection of killed suspensions of *Mycobacterium leprae,* but it is not diagnostic since positive reactions occur in nearly all adults. Culture of *M. leprae* is exceedingly difficult and can only be accomplished in mice or armadillos. A minimum of 6 months is usually required before the results are available; therefore cultures are not practical for diagnosis. Erythema of existing skin lesions with dapsone therapy usually occurs in borderline patients and is not diagnostic. Demonstration of the organism on microscopic examination of a biopsy specimen is the only definitive way to make the diagnosis of leprosy. A sensitive serologic assay effective in diagnosing lepromatous disease has recently been developed.

61.   The answer is B. *(Wilson, ed 12. chap 165.)* The infective cysts of *G. lamblia* can survive for several months in cold water and have been responsible for large epidemics in communities such as Vail, Colorado. Immunity to giardia is not well understood, but there is no increased incidence in granulocytopenic patients. Intestinal IgA may be important, as deficient patients appear to be at increased risk of infection. Transmission is primarily by the fecal-oral route, resulting in higher incidence in male homosexuals, retarded patients in institutions, and children in day-care centers.

62.   The answer is E. *(Wilson, ed 12. chap 169.)* Adult worms do reside in lymph nodes, but biopsy is relatively contraindicated because of the potential to exacerbate problems with lymphatic drainage. Serologic testing is available at specialized centers using indirect hemagglutination, but cross-reactions with other filariae are common. Intense pruritus and a rash developing after administration of diethylcarbamazine (Mazzotti test) suggest dermal microfilariae; this reaction typically occurs in patients with onchocerciasis. Maintenance of filariae in cultures or animals is extremely difficult. The best animal model is in cats, but this technique plays no role in clinical diagnosis. Diagnosis is best made by demonstrating microfilariae on a Giemsa stain of blood. *W. bancrofti* microfilariae usually maintain a nocturnal periodicity and are found in the bloodstream in greatest number at night. The exact reason for the periodicity is not known, but it may be related to oxygen tension in the pulmonary vessels.

63.   The answer is D. *(Wilson, ed 12. chap 94.)* The findings on pelvic examination coupled with the elevated sedimentation rate in this setting strongly suggest acute pelvic inflammatory disease (PID). About 5 percent of women with PID will have associated perihepatitis, termed the Fitz-Hugh–Curtis syndrome, manifested by pleuritic pain of the right upper quadrant and tenderness on palpation, along with normal liver function tests and ultrasound of the right upper quadrant. Although for many years *N. gonorrhoeae* was considered to be the primary pathogen in this condition, chlamydial salpingitis is now the most common associated finding.

64.   The answer is A. *(Wilson, ed 12. chap 94.)* It is important to pick a well-tolerated regimen with good activity against both *N. gonorrhoeae* (including penicillinase-producing strains) and *C. trachomatis* for the treatment of patients with severe pelvic inflammatory disease. Activity against vaginal anaerobes and members of the Enterobacteriaceae family, which may also play a role in the pathogenesis of this disorder, would also be desirable. A combination of doxycycline and cefoxitin offers the broad-spectrum coverage required for optimal treatment. Clindamycin plus gentamicin acutely, plus a 2-week course of doxycycline to definitively treat *C. trachomatis,* is an acceptable alternative regimen. The combination of metronidazole and gentamicin lacks adequate coverage against both *Chlamydia* and *N. gonorrhoeae* and is therefore not appropriate in this setting.

65.   The answer is C. *(Wilson, ed 12. chap 164.)* This patient was in the right location and has the typical clinical features of a patient infected with *Babesia*, tick-borne protozoa that multiply in red blood cells. Clinical manifestations can be more severe in splenectomized persons. The best way to make the diagnosis is to demonstrate the parasite's presence in erythrocytes in Giemsa-stained peripheral blood smears. Serologic confirmation can also be helpful.

66.   The answer is D. *(Wilson, ed 12. chap 160.)* The four major clinical syndromes of leishmaniasis—visceral (kala azar), cutaneous, diffuse cutaneous, and mucocutaneous—represent sandfly-borne disease caused by members of the protozoal genus *Leishmania*. Kala azar is manifested by fever, cough, diarrhea, splenomegaly, and pancytopenia and may be diagnosed by examination of the buffy coat. A number of species in each hemisphere account for the various cutaneous syndromes. In the Middle East and in the southern Soviet Union, *L. tropica* causes ulcerating facial lesions. Mucocutaneous leishmaniasis, or espundia, is caused by *L. braziliensis,* which can produce (after a long initial quiescent period) excessive destruction of facial soft tissue, including nasal obstruction and epistaxis, as well as systemic signs and symptoms. Massive dissemination of skin lesions without visceral involvement can also occur. This form is refractory to therapy, which usually consists of antimony. Esophageal dysfunction is seen in Chagas' disease, a trypanosomal-mediated infestation.

67. The answer is A-Y, B-Y, C-Y, D-Y, E-Y. *(Wilson, ed 12. chap 90.)* Subacute bacterial endocarditis can be treated quite successfully. However, for persons in whom the offending organisms are highly resistant to standard antimicrobial agents, the prognosis is less favorable. Delay in therapy also compromises the prognosis. The development of congestive heart failure is a most ominous sign. Endocarditis due to *Staphylococcus epidermidis* carries a poor prognosis if acquired at the time of cardiac surgery or if complicated by the adverse factors mentioned above. Valve ring or myocardial abscess is an ominous sign that signals a failure of medical therapy.

68. The answer is A-N, B-Y, C-N, D-N, E-Y. *(Wilson, ed 12. chap 90.)* After transient bacteremia, subacute endocarditis may develop at endocardial sites at which a jet of blood flows from a high-pressure to a low-pressure area. Such lesions include ventricular septal defects and mitral regurgitation. Blood flow velocity across an isolated atrial septal defect is much lower and endocarditis is extremely uncommon in this condition. Similarly, long-standing permanent pacemakers and coronary bypass grafts very rarely result in the degree of turbulent blood flow necessary to incite endocardial infection.

69. The answer is A-N, B-Y, C-N, D-Y, E-Y. *(Wilson, ed 12. chap 90.)* Right-sided endocarditis occurs frequently in persons addicted to parenteral drugs. The usual presentation, aside from such constitutional symptoms as fever, malaise, and anorexia, features septic pulmonary emboli. Blood cultures are positive as frequently in right-heart as in left-heart endocarditis. Heart murmur is often absent. With appropriate treatment the prognosis is generally good.

70. The answer is A-N, B-Y, C-N, D-N, E-Y. *(Wilson, ed 12. chap 20. Dinarello, Rev Infect Dis 10:168, 1988.)* A host of stimuli, including infection with virtually any microorganism, cause macrophages and monocytes to elaborate the key mediators of fever production, TNF and interleukin 1β (the endogenous pyrogens). These 17-kilodalton (kDa) glycoproteins promote the synthesis of E series prostaglandins in the hypothalamus, thereby resetting the central thermostat at a higher level. Aspirin and nonsteroidal anti-inflammatory agents act by inhibiting cyclooxygenase activity so that prostaglandin E_2 (PGE_2) cannot be synthesized; they do not act by reducing TNF and IL-1 production. Glucocorticoids suppress fever both by interfering with arachidonic acid metabolism and down-regulating the production of endogenous pyrogens. TNF and IL-1 also possess diverse effects, including the induction of cachexia by TNF.

71. The answer is A-Y, B-N, C-Y, D-Y, E-N. *(Wilson, ed 12. chap 83.)* Nosocomial infections often are caused by antibiotic-resistant organisms, which acquire their resistance through transfer of R-factor plasmids. Preventive measures are key. For example, if catheter care is good, it should be possible to maintain a sterile urinary tract for at least 5 to 7 days in most patients. Intravenous lines of all types tend to become infected after about 3 days; the danger is somewhat less with needles than with plastic cannulas. There is no good evidence to suggest that persons having hepatitis surface antigen in their blood should be prevented from drawing blood or working directly with patients. All health-care workers who come in contact with blood or body fluids should receive hepatitis B vaccine.

72. The answer is A-Y, B-Y, C-Y, D-Y, E-N. *(Wilson, ed 12. chap 80.)* Each microbial illness is best diagnosed by a specific set of laboratory procedures. For example, although it is difficult to isolate bacteria from the blood in most bacterial infections, the spirochetes causing relapsing fever can be seen in routine blood smears. In malaria, routine Wright staining also is sufficient to recognize the parasites in many cases, although thick smears may be necessary. *Leishmania* can also be identified using a combination of methylene blue and eosin. Both *Nocardia* and *Mycobacterium* are acid-fast organisms, a key to their identification in the laboratory. The early diagnosis of *Legionella* has been facilitated by the development of immunofluorescent staining, but it can only be done reliably in reference laboratories that have highly skilled technologists. Because a single throat swab can detect about 90 percent of patients with streptococcal pharyngitis, a negative result is very helpful in excluding this diagnosis. In persons with partially treated meningitis, gram-positive organisms may fail to stain well and often appear gram-negative.

73. The answer is A-N, B-Y, C-Y, D-N, E-Y. *(Wilson, ed 12. chap 82.)* Cytotoxic chemotherapy invariably reduces granulocyte counts. If the peripheral blood neutrophil count drops below 500 cells per microliter, the risk of infection is markedly increased. Enteric gram-negative bacilli, coagulase-positive and coagulase-negative staphylococci, *Candida,* and *Aspergillus* are the most common pathogens. Defense against encapsulated bacteria, such as *S. pneumoniae* and *H. influenzae*, depends on humoral immunity, which is relatively well preserved after standard cytotoxic chemotherapy. Once fever in the setting of neutropenia is recognized, one should begin broad-spectrum antibacterial antibiotics in combinations that possess synergistic activity against *Pseudomonas* and some antistaphylococcal activity. In the absence of specific indications, antifungal therapy should not be started until the patient fails to respond to several days of antibiotics and neutropenia is persistent.

74.   The answer is A-Y, B-Y, C-Y, D-Y, E-N. *(Wilson, ed 12. chap 89.)* Granulocytopenia and thrombocytopenia are seen in persons with severe septic shock; they are thought to occur because of direct effects of endotoxin on these cells as well as because of changes in the vascular endothelium. In addition, complement activation, with the generation of C5a, appears to increase granulocyte margination and lead to a further reduction in the blood granulocyte count. Sepsis leads to complement activation and increased turnover of complement components in the blood; the lower the C3 level, the worse the outcome. Both prostacyclin and naloxone are beneficial in the treatment of experimental septic shock; both agents improve tissue blood flow and prevent the severe sequelae of hypotension.

75.   The answer is A-Y, B-Y, C-N, D-Y, E-Y. *(Wilson, ed 12. chap 85. Neu, Am J Med 82 (4A):1, 1987.)* The carboxyfluoroquinolones are chemically related to the relatively ineffective quinolones (e.g., nalidixic acid), which bind to bacterial DNA gyrase. These new agents have promise due to their very broad antibacterial spectrum as well as to their favorable bioavailability when given orally. Ciprofloxacin and norfloxacin are the two members of the carboxyfluoroquinolones currently available for use in the United States. Ciprofloxacin inhibits all the Enterobacteriaceae, including *Pseudomonas aeruginosa*, at low serum concentrations. This agent is similarly effective against *Haemophilus, Branhamella*, and methicillin-resistant staphylococci; however, high concentrations are required to inhibit *Bacteroides* and other clostridial species. Ciprofloxacin is well absorbed orally and is widely distributed in most body tissues including the CSF, which it enters at high-enough concentrations to inhibit most meningitis-causing bacteria except *Streptococcus pneumoniae*. The major uses of ciprofloxacin have been for the treatment of *Pseudomonas* infections in patients with cystic fibrosis, in resistant urinary tract infections, and in gastrointestinal disease due to virtually any enteropathogenic bacteria. Except for prolongation of the half-life of theophylline, toxic side effects and adverse reactions due to ciprofloxacin have been unusual.

76.   The answer is A-Y, B-N, C-Y, D-Y, E-N. *(Wilson, ed 12. chap 85.)* Procaine and benzathine penicillins are less painful to administer intramuscularly than is penicillin G (benzyl penicillin) and are more apt to sustain low blood levels of antibiotic because of their slower absorption. Amoxicillin is much better absorbed than ampicillin. Neither ampicillin nor carbenicillin is effective against *Klebsiella;* this organism usually is sensitive to cephalosporin and aminoglycoside antibiotics, such as cephalothin and gentamicin, respectively. Ticarcillin is a semisynthetic penicillin that is two to four times as effective against *Pseudomonas* as is carbenicillin. Clinical evidence has not shown therapeutic superiority for nafcillin and oxacillin over methicillin; nafcillin is used frequently because some data suggest that interstitial nephritis is a more common consequence of methicillin therapy.

77.   The answer is A-N, B-Y, C-N, D-N, E-Y. *(Wilson, ed 12. chap 93.)* A man who has dysuria but no urethral exudate or leukocytes in a urethral swab specimen probably does not have a chlamydial infection. On the other hand, if he has an exudate in which intracellular gram-negative diplococci are not seen, he should be considered to have chlamydial urethritis and treated presumptively with tetracycline, an antibiotic also effective against gonococci. A pregnant woman with presumed chlamydial cervicitis should be treated with erythromycin because tetracycline can produce fetal complications. Sulfa creams are ineffective in the treatment of *Gardnerella vaginalis* (bacterial vaginosis) infections; metronidazole is the preferred form of therapy. Genital ulcers in U.S. residents are due most frequently to herpes simplex virus; elsewhere in the world, syphilis and chancroid are more common.

78.   The answer is A-Y, B-Y, C-N, D-N, E-N. *(Wilson, ed 12. chap 99.)* Type 3 pneumococci cause the most severe of all pneumococcal pneumonias, possibly because such infections occur in debilitated persons. All splenectomized patients, even those without underlying disease, should receive pneumococcal vaccine. The ''crisis'' in pneumococcal pneumonia ordinarily corresponds to the appearance of type-specific antibodies, not maximum leukocytosis. Alcoholic persons who develop pneumococcal pneumonia have a poor prognosis for several reasons: their tendency to aspirate pharyngeal flora, poor functioning of bronchial clearance mechanisms, and impaired leukocyte response (hypogammaglobulinemia generally is not a contributing factor). Pneumococcal pneumonia frequently precedes pneumococcal meningitis. Pneumococci cause pharyngitis extremely rarely.

79.   The answer is A-Y, B-N, C-N, D-Y, E-Y. *(Wilson, ed 12. chap 101.)* Streptococcal M protein is the factor most strongly associated with virulence—strains rich in M protein resist phagocytosis. On the other hand, T protein, which also serves as a basis for typing, is not related to virulence. Titers of antistreptolysin O (ASO) are elevated in many persons who have poststreptococcal glomerulonephritis, particularly those who have had pharyngitis; persons with streptococcal pyoderma generally do not have elevated ASO titers. The erythrogenic toxin causing scarlet fever is produced in bacteria infected with a lysogenic bacteriophage; several types of streptococci as well as staphylococci can be so infected. Streptococcal pyoderma may lead to acute glomerulonephritis but not to acute rheumatic fever. The reason for this phenomenon remains unexplained.

80.   The answer is A-N, B-Y, C-Y, D-Y, E-N. *(Wilson, ed 12. chap 130.)* Leptospirosis can be transferred from infected animals directly to humans who contact contaminated tissue or urine. Leptospirosis often is confused with influenza because of its initial manifestations: fever, headache, and myalgias. It causes hepatitis often associated with very elevated serum bilirubin levels, probably a result of both intravascular hemolysis and impaired bilirubin excretion. Leptospiral meningitis resembles a viral, or aseptic, meningitis; cerebrospinal fluid has a normal glucose concentration, and although a few neutrophils may be present, lymphocytes are the predominant cell type observed. The diagnosis of acute leptospirosis is made best by blood cultures; dark-field microscopy too often gives false-positive or false-negative results.

81.   The answer is A-N, B-Y, C-Y, D-Y, E-N. *(Wilson, ed 12. chap 110.)* Gonococcemia tends to be a problem of menstruating women, although men also are affected. The characteristic skin lesions are small pustules that usually occur first on the fingers and feet. The arthritis associated with gonococcemia is rarely symmetrical, a clinical finding that is often helpful in making the diagnosis. Gonococci producing β-lactamase are resistant to penicillin and ampicillin but are sensitive to the newer cephalosporins, such as ceftriaxone. Treatment with spectinomycin is also effective; this agent usually is recommended as the first choice for treatment failures attributed to penicillinase production by the organism. Gonococci with pili are more virulent than gonococci without pili (pili may help the organism stick to epithelial cells to initiate infection).

82.   The answer is A-Y, B-N, C-Y, D-N, E-N. *(Wilson, ed 12. chap 111.)* *Acinetobacter*, previously called *Mimae herellae* and *Bacterium anitratum*, is a ubiquitous commensal organism that is an important cause of bacteremia, pneumonia, and other serious infections. It is a gram-negative rod that can be confused with *Neisseria* on Gram stain because of its pleomorphic appearance. It is also confused with Enterobacteriaceae species in cultures because of its simple growth requirements. Unlike *Neisseria*, it is resistant to penicillin and ampicillin but sensitive to gentamicin and tobramycin; this difference in antibiotic sensitivity makes it very important to distinguish this organism from *Neisseria* in clinical isolates from patients with serious illnesses.

83.   The answer is A-N, B-N, C-N, D-Y, E-Y. *(Wilson, ed 12. chap 112.)* Melioidosis is caused by *Pseudomonas pseudomallei*, a gram-negative bacillus ubiquitous in many tropical areas of Asia and Africa. Infection occurs from contact with contaminated soil. Pulmonary infections are most frequent; in patients acutely ill with pneumonia, many organisms can be detected in sputum. The organisms can be grown on routine culture media. Serologic tests are used largely for epidemiologic studies. Melioidosis, particularly the chronic form, may be mistaken for tuberculosis; granulomas may develop, but calcification of cavitary lung lesions does not occur. In acute melioidosis, therapy with tetracycline and chloramphenicol or ceftazidime plus trimethoprim-sulfamethoxazole is recommended. Although the organism is usually sensitive to each of these agents, the high fatality rate of this disease (greater than 50 percent) has led to the use of a multiple antibiotic regimen.

84.   The answer is A-Y, B-Y, C-Y, D-N, E-Y. *(Wilson, ed 12. chap 119.)* Brucellosis is an important veterinary disease in those parts of the world from which it has not yet been eradicated. It is still a problem in cattle-raising areas of the United States. The disease usually presents with low-grade fever and constitutional symptoms; affected persons have lymphadenopathy, splenomegaly, and, sometimes, hepatomegaly. During the early bacteremic phase of the illness, *Brucella* can be isolated using routine cultures, provided they are kept long enough (i.e., up to 4 weeks). The diagnosis also is made using agglutination tests. Therapy with streptomycin and tetracycline still is best.

85.   The answer is A-Y, B-N, C-Y, D-Y, E-N. *(Wilson, ed 12. chap 122.) Vibrio cholerae* enterotoxin causes a diffuse, noninflammatory secretion of isotonic intestinal fluid without injury to the absorptive surface. Early diagnosis is aided by dark-field microscopy or immobilization of organisms with type-specific antisera; definitive diagnosis, however, depends on culturing the organisms. Oral therapy with solutions containing sodium bicarbonate and either glucose or sucrose is recommended. This therapy usually is begun on the basis of a presumptive diagnosis in endemic areas. Oral tetracycline also is useful because it can shorten the symptomatic period, but it is not recommended for children under age 8. Infection confers some immunity, so that, in endemic areas, children are usually the ones affected. Cholera vaccine is not particularly effective and is now not ordinarily recommended for travelers to endemic areas.

86.   The answer is A-N, B-N, C-N, D-N, E-N. *(Wilson, ed 12. chap 86. Fischel, N Engl J Med 317:185, 1987.)* AZT is converted to AZT triphosphate in infected cells. AZT triphosphate is a competitive inhibitor of HIV reverse transcriptase, the enzyme responsible for converting retroviral RNA into DNA so the viral genome may be replicated. Administration of AZT to patients with AIDS or AIDS-related complex was associated with a decreased frequency of infections and prolonged survival compared with a control group given placebo. AZT is now approved for use in patients with AIDS or AIDS-related complex whose CD4 (T4) lymphocyte count is < 200 cells per microliter. Ongoing trials are attempting to define the role of this agent in patients with asymptomatic HIV infection. The major problem with AZT is its bone marrow toxicity. In fact, hematopoietic growth factors such as erythropoietin and granulocyte macrophage-colony stimulating factor are being evaluated for their ability to ameliorate the anemia and granulocytopenia associated with AZT administration.

87.   The answer is A-Y, B-Y, C-N, D-Y, E-Y. *(Wilson, ed 12. chap 128.)* Syphilis causes few symptoms in its earliest phases, especially in pregnant women. The newborn infants of infected women will be reactive serologically, because maternal IgG antibodies cross the placenta and circulate in the fetal blood. In untreated syphilis, the VDRL test often becomes nonreactive; however, the more sensitive fluorescent *Treponema pallidum* antibody-absorption (FTA-ABS) test remains reactive. Untreated persons are more likely to die of a ruptured aortic aneurysm or other cardiovascular event than from neurosyphilis or any other cause. Treatment with at least 6 million units of penicillin G is usually sufficient to prevent the development of symptomatic neurosyphilis.

88.   The answer is A-Y, B-N, C-N, D-N, E-Y. *(Wilson, ed 12. chap 87.)* Until the recent approval of fluconazole, ketoconazole was the only orally available antifungal drug with activity against certain invasive fungal infections, including mucocutaneous and esophageal candidiasis. Unaffected by renal disease, ketoconazole is metabolized hepatically (occasionally resulting in serious liver failure) and can lead to elevated blood levels of warfarin and cyclosporine. Amphotericin B is the only effective therapy for many deep mycoses; however, it is difficult to tolerate because of frequent side effects, including fever, chills, phlebitis, and nausea. Although amphotericin B can be given at standard doses in patients with hepatic insufficiency, this agent can lead to azotemia as well as massive renal tubular wasting of potassium and magnesium. In patients suffering from severe candidiasis and cryptococcosis, flucytosine (5-fluorocytosine) can be used orally in addition to intravenous amphotericin B. In the fungal cell, flucytosine is converted to the antimetabolite 5-fluorouracil, a thymidine synthase inhibitor employed in cancer chemotherapy. Elevated levels of flucytosine in the blood are associated with thrombocytopenia and granulocytopenia.

89.   The answer is A-N, B-Y, C-N, D-Y, E-Y. *(Wilson, ed 12. chap 151.)* The molds *Mucor* and *Rhizopus,* the main causes of mucormycosis, are more often seen in than grown from pathologic specimens. The reasons they are so hard to grow have not been identified. Fungal hyphae tend to invade blood vessels, which leads to hemorrhagic necrosis. Sinusitis is the predominant illness in infected persons who have diabetes mellitus; in persons with hematologic malignancies, pulmonary disease is more common. Diagnosis is best accomplished by biopsy and histologic examination (serology is still in the investigative stages). Amphotericin is the only known nonsurgical treatment of mucormycosis.

90.   The answer is A-N, B-Y, C-N, D-Y, E-Y. *(Wilson, ed 12. chap 153.)* Rocky Mountain spotted fever is a tick-borne disease caused by *Rickettsia rickettsii,* an obligate intracellular organism. The disease is associated with severe headache, myalgias, and arthralgias, but not frank arthritis. The characteristic rash is at first macular and confined to the extremities; after several days, the rash spreads to involve the buttocks, trunk, axilla, neck, and face and becomes maculopapular, then hemorrhagic, and finally ulcerative. Treatment with chloramphenicol or tetracycline, which are rickettsiostatic agents, is most effective if begun before the rash has become hemorrhagic. Ticks found on household pets should be removed carefully with tweezers, and not by hand, in order to prevent infection through minor skin abrasions.

91.   The answer is A-N, B-Y, C-N, D-Y, E-Y. *(Wilson, ed 12. chap 154.)* *Mycoplasma pneumoniae* is an important cause of pneumonia, particularly in young adults. The organism cannot be seen by Gram stain, because it does not retain the dye-iodine complex. The cold-agglutinin test is nonspecific; firm serologic evidence of mycoplasma infection usually comes from a complement-fixation test (other specific serologic tests also are available). Treatment with either tetracycline or erythromycin is effective. In nonepidemic situations in which it is often difficult to know whether a person has a pneumococcal or *Mycoplasma* infection, erythromycin is the better choice of treatment.

92.   The answer is A-Y, B-N, C-Y, D-Y, E-N. *(Wilson, ed 12. chap 100. Arbuthnot, Rev Infect Dis 11 (suppl 1):51, 1989.)* Toxic shock syndrome (TSS) is a toxin-mediated disorder that has been linked to the ability of hyperabsorbent tampons to provide the surface area required to promote *S. aureus* growth and toxin (TSST-1) production. Though the patients may appear to be in shock, with refractory hypotension, blood cultures are almost uniformly negative. With the increased recognition and prevention of menstruation-associated TSS, the relative frequency in nonmenstruating women and in men is increasing. In the severe form of the syndrome, gastrointestinal, hepatic, renal, muscular, and CNS involvement occurs not infrequently. The diagnosis of TSS in a postsurgical patient may be a clinical challenge since the signs of infection are usually minimal and occur as soon as 2 days after the operation. Treatment includes antistaphylococcal antibiotics, drainage of focal collections, and supportive care.

93.   The answer is A-Y, B-Y, C-Y, D-Y, E-Y. *(Wilson, ed 12. chap 89. Girardin, N Engl J Med 319:397, 1988.)* The lipid A component of lipopolysaccharide (LPS) present in the cell wall of gram-negative bacteria sets in motion a complex array of host responses that are together responsible for the dramatic manifestations of septic shock. In addition to activating the complement system, LPS can directly activate the coagulation and kinin systems by leading to activation of Hageman factor. Activation of Hageman factor in turn leads to the elaboration of kallikrein from its precursor, prekallikrein. Kallikrein generates kinins, which cause vasodilation and enhance capillary permeability. LPS has been shown to induce the formation of both IL-1 and TNF by endothelial cells and macrophages. These cytokines produce many of the cardinal manifestations of sepsis, such as fever, myalgias, and leukocytosis. Interferon γ, which is also present in high serum levels during sepsis, may augment the effects of TNF. Arachidonic acid metabolites are also involved in producing the clinical picture of sepsis. Prostaglandin E$_2$, a cyclooxygenase metabolite of arachidonic acid, is believed to be the centrally active mediator of fever induced by TNF and IL-1. Both leukotrienes, which are 5-lipoxygenase metabolites of arachidonic acid and may be involved in the characteristic pulmonary capillary leak of sepsis, and the vasodilatory platelet activating factor (PAF) are released as a result of the effect of LPS on hematopoietically derived cells.

94.   The answer is A-N, B-Y, C-Y, D-N, E-N. *(Wilson, ed 12. chap 147.)* With the development of progressively less toxic rabies vaccines, such as the currently available human diploid cell vaccine (HDCV), the indications for prophylactic vaccination are widening. Spelunkers (cave explorers), in addition to veterinarians, animal pathologists, and laboratory technicians who work with potential sources of rabies virus, should be considered for vaccination. With HDCV, preexposure prophylaxis would consist of three intramuscular injections on days 0, 7, and 21 to 28. Antibody titers should be checked periodically to ensure that an adequate level of immunity persists.

95.   The answer is A-Y, B-Y, C-Y, D-Y, E-Y. *(Wilson, ed 12. chap 137.)* The most common features of infectious mononucleosis are fever, sore throat, and lymphadenopathy. Sore throat, the most commonly described symptom, is observed in about 80 percent of young adults with this infection. Atypical lymphocytes, identified as T cells with suppressor and cytotoxic action, appear in the peripheral blood during the first week of illness. Heterophil antibodies, which are sheep red-cell agglutinins associated with the immunoglobulin M serum fraction, usually persist in the serum for a few months. On the other hand, antibodies to Epstein-Barr virus, especially to EBV nuclear antigens, often can be detected for years in the serum of persons who have had infectious mononucleosis. The incubation period in young adults is thought to be 30 to 50 days; in children, the incubation period is much shorter.

96.   The answer is A-N, B-N, C-N, D-Y, E-N. *(Wilson, ed 12. chap 98. Hainer, J Fam Pract 25:497, 1987.)* Cat-scratch disease, as the name implies, is transmitted to humans chiefly by cat scratches. Other animal vectors have not been definitively recognized. Lymphadenopathy often persists for weeks; examination of a lymph-node biopsy specimen may show the granulomatous inflammation also noted in lymphogranuloma venereum, tularemia, brucellosis, tuberculosis, and some lymphomas. Splenomegaly generally does not develop. Antibiotics are ineffective in treating persons with cat-scratch disease, although it is now recognized that the etiologic agent is a bacterium with a defective cell wall.

97.   The answer is A-Y, B-Y, C-N, D-N, E-Y. *(Wilson, ed 12. chap 158.)* Although *Entamoeba histolytica* can infect some animals, the principal hosts are humans. Even in the presence of large or multiple amebic liver abscesses, defervescence usually occurs in 1 to 3 days with appropriate medical therapy. The abscess cavity in amebic liver abscess usually contains no neutrophils or amebas; the infection does not evoke a typical acute inflammatory response, and amebas are found only at the edge of the advancing infection. Amebic serologic tests stay positive for months to years despite therapy. Deaths from amebiasis are uncommon; however, failure to make the diagnosis in a timely fashion is among the most important causes of these deaths.

98.   The answer is A-Y, B-Y, C-Y, D-Y, E-Y. *(Wilson, ed 12. chap 91. Barnes, Medicine 66:472, 1987.)* Unlike liver abscesses caused by bacteria, amebic abscesses rarely need to be drained. A positive serology for *Entamoeba histolytica,* which indicates prior exposure to this organism, is a most helpful differential point in deciding between the two causes. Bacterial hepatic abscesses may be caused by ascending cholangitis, bacteremia, direct extension (including peritoneal infection), or trauma. In the former two cases, especially in the instance of complete biliary obstruction, the presentation is more likely to be acute and the abscesses are more likely to be multiple; multiple abscesses carry a poorer prognosis than does a solitary abscess. Blood cultures enable noninvasive, specific diagnosis (although not all organisms in the abscess may grow in the blood) about half the time. Given the preponderance of anaerobic (including the penicillin-resistant *B. fragilis*) and gramnegative bacterial forms in the biliary and GI tracts, empiric therapy, if required, should include an aminoglycoside and clindamycin.

99.   The answer is A-Y, B-N, C-Y, D-Y, E-Y. *(Wilson, ed 12. chap 162.)* Toxoplasmosis is a relatively common infection; serologic data indicate that possibly as many as two-thirds of the U.S. adult population have had some form of the infection. The most serious manifestations appear to arise when the disease is acquired during pregnancy. Infection during the first trimester can result in spontaneous abortion, stillbirth, prematurity, or severe disease in any of several organ systems; infection during the third trimester more commonly leads to neonatal disease, which, however, tends to be asymptomatic. Infections acquired before pregnancy generally are of little consequence to the offspring. Immunocompromised persons usually have recrudescent disease. Diagnosis in these patients is often difficult to make, in part because the serologic responses are blunted by the underlying disease process. Serologic screening of asymptomatic immunocompromised patients may be helpful for recognizing toxoplasmosis at a later date.

100.   The answer is A-Y, B-N, C-N, D-Y, E-Y. *(Wilson, ed 12. chap 163.)* The onset of *Pneumocystis carinii* pneumonia is characterized by a paucity of physical findings. Sputum, which is produced in scant amounts, usually contains normal flora and very few, if any, leukocytes. Pleural effusions are rare, and because there is little cellular reaction the lung usually is not damaged permanently. However, fully developed *P. carinii* pneumonia can lead to marked tachypnea and dyspnea, massive consolidation, and extensive changes on chest x-ray. Systemic dissemination is rare but may be increasing. The infection generally arises as a result of a serious underlying disease; consequently, the prognosis is poor. Trimethoprim-sulfamethoxazole and pentamidine are equally efficacious; however, trimethoprim-sulfamethoxazole is preferred because it can be given orally and has fewer side effects.

101.   The answer is A-N, B-N, C-Y, D-N, E-N. *(Wilson, ed 12. chap 170.)* *Schistosoma mansoni* infection of the liver causes cirrhosis from vascular obstruction but relatively little hepatocellular injury. Hepatosplenomegaly, hypersplenism, and esophageal varices develop quite commonly, and schistosomiasis usually is associated with eosinophilia. Spider nevi, gynecomastia, jaundice, and ascites are uncommon.

102.   The answer is A-Y, B-N, C-Y, D-Y, E-N. *(Wilson, ed 12. chap 114.)* *Shigella sonnei* is the most common isolate in developed countries, while *S. dysenteriae* and *S. flexneri* predominate in tropical areas. Fewer than 100 organisms can cause disease irrespective of gastric acidity. Transmission by the fecal-oral route is the most important and occurs most frequently in areas of crowding and poor sanitation. Bacteremia with *Shigella* organisms is distinctly unusual, probably because the organism is sensitive to complement-mediated lysis. Unlike such therapy for infection with *Salmonella* organisms, antibiotic therapy of shigellosis can shorten both symptoms and fecal shedding.

103. The answer is A-N, B-Y, C-Y, D-Y, E-N. *(Wilson, ed 12. chap 125.)* Pleural effusions occur most frequently in young patients with primary infection associated with an abrupt onset of symptoms. Effusions are being noted more frequently in older patients with reactivation disease, but they still account for less than one-third of patients in North America with pleurisy. Laryngeal and bronchitic tuberculosis are very infectious because the bacilli are readily aerosolized. Response to therapy is usually good. In the absence of neurologic abnormalities, extensive bony involvement by tuberculosis usually requires chemotherapy alone. Involvement of the basilar meninges is very common in meningeal tuberculosis and results in cranial nerve abnormalities. Gastrointestinal infection usually occurs in association with cavitary disease with large numbers of organisms. The terminal ileum and cecum are the most common sites, which results in disease that can be difficult to differentiate from Crohn's disease. The stomach is very resistant to infection.

104. The answer is A-N, B-Y, C-N, D-N, E-Y. *(Wilson, ed 12. chap 132.)* The complete clinical spectrum of Lyme disease was first identified in the northeastern United States, but it is now recognized to have a worldwide distribution. Erythema chronicum migrans usually starts as an erythematous macule at the site of the tick bite and eventually forms a characteristic annular lesion with central clearing, which is present in approximately 90 percent of patients within a month. Constitutional symptoms including headache, fever, chills, and fatigue are common at the time of onset of skin lesions. Approximately 10 to 15 percent of patients have neurologic involvement with Lyme disease, which can be manifested as meningitis (with a lymphocytic pleocytosis), cranial neuritis, chorea, mononeuritis multiplex, or motor and sensory radiculoneuritis. Parenteral therapy with penicillin or ceftriaxone is recommended for patients with significant neurologic or cardiac involvement.

105. The answer is A-N, B-Y, C-Y, D-N, E-Y. *(Wilson, ed 12. chap 107.)* *Clostridium* species are present in high numbers in normal intestinal flora and soil, and it is not surprising that they are frequent isolates from wound cultures. The presence of necrotic tissue and a low oxidation reduction potential are necessary to establish severe disease. Treatment is based on the clinical setting, and a culture positive for clostridia alone does not warrant therapy. *Clostridium perfringens* produces at least 12 toxins, one of the most important of which is the alpha toxin. It has been associated with hemolysis and capillary and platelet damage. *C. perfringens* is a common cause of food poisoning associated with contaminated meats and poultry. The serous discharge from the overlying skin in a patient with gas gangrene has many gram-positive rods but few inflammatory cells, emphasizing the importance of an early Gram stain when the diagnosis is suspected. More than 70 percent of cases of *C. septicum* septicemia reported in the literature are associated with malignant neoplasms, especially of the gastrointestinal tract.

106. The answer is A-N, B-Y, C-Y, D-N, E-N. *(Wilson, ed 12. chap 108.)* Anaerobic pulmonary infections most often develop in the setting of aspiration. The sudden development of a bacterial pneumonia in a healthy teenager would most likely be caused by *Streptococcus pneumoniae*. Both anaerobic and aerobic organisms are implicated in Ludwig's angina, an infection originating from the third molar which can rapidly spread through soft tissues of the mandible and pharynx. Pharyngeal anaerobic bacteria, including *Bacteroides melaninogenicus, Fusobacterium* sp., and anaerobic cocci, cause bacterial aspiration pneumonia in a patient who has a diminished gag reflex, such as with a seizure disorder. It is important to differentiate bacterial aspiration, which requires antibiotic therapy, from aspiration of stomach contents, which usually occurs after general anesthesia and resolves with symptomatic therapy. Anaerobic bacteria are a very unusual cause of endocarditis, which—as is the case with aerobic gram-negative organisms—may in part be explained by a failure to adhere to damaged valves.

107. The answer is A-N, B-Y, C-Y, D-Y, E-N. *(Wilson, ed 12. chap 136.)* Less than 5 percent of patients will have a second recurrence of herpes zoster unless they are immunosuppressed. Acute cerebellar ataxia is the most common form of neurologic involvement in children. This benign condition usually develops 3 weeks after the rash and resolves spontaneously. Chickenpox is one of the most contagious diseases, infecting up to 90 percent of seronegative persons, presumably via the respiratory route. Varicella pneumonia can cause fever and severe hypoxia, complicating the course of chickenpox infection in up to 20 percent of adults. Varicella-zoster immune globulin is recommended only for immunodeficient patients under the age of 15 years who have been exposed to varicella.

108. The answer is A-N, B-Y, C-Y, D-N, E-Y. *(Wilson, ed 12. chap 138. Drew, Rev Infect Dis 10:S468, 1988.)* Perinatal transmission of CMV occurs by passage through an infected birth canal or through the breast milk of a seropositive mother. Though such transmission is very common, symptomatic infection is distinctly unusual except in premature infants in whom interstitial pneumonitis may develop. Congenital infection with CMV occurs in approximately 1 percent of births in the United States, but detectable disease develops in less than 0.05 percent of births, almost exclusively in association with primary maternal infections. CMV produces a syndrome very similar to mononucleosis with Epstein-Barr virus. Cervical lymphadenopathy and exudative pharyngitis are usually not present, however, and heterophil antibodies are absent. CMV pneumonia can prove fatal in greater than 80 percent of bone marrow transplant patients. Salivary excretion of the virus or positive sputum cultures do not implicate CMV as the cause of pulmonary infiltrates. Definitive diagnosis rests on the demonstration of the characteristic pathologic findings—intranuclear inclusions in enlarged epithelial cells—on lung biopsy. Diagnosis of CMV infection rests on characteristic pathologic findings, a fourfold rise in serology titer, or culture of CMV, usually from urine, saliva, or buffy coat. Because viral excretion can continue for weeks to months, isolation of CMV does not always implicate acute infection.

109. The answer is A-N, B-Y, C-N, D-Y, E-Y. *(Wilson, ed 12. chap 145.)* Both Norwalk virus and rotavirus infect the small intestinal epithelium and cause malabsorption and osmotic diarrhea. Worldwide, rotavirus is the most important cause of dehydrating diarrhea in infants. Rotavirus is shed in large quantities in the stool allowing for easy diagnosis by culture or immunoassays to detect viral antigens. Norwalk virus is presumably spread by the fecal-oral route and has also been implicated in food-borne and water-borne epidemics. The clinical manifestations of infection by both viruses are characterized by vomiting, diarrhea, and, occasionally, low-grade fever. Rotavirus is a major cause of diarrhea in children under 3 years of age, while Norwalk virus causes disease more often in older children and adults.

110. The answer is A-N, B-N, C-Y, D-N, E-Y. *(Wilson, ed 12. chap 139.)* Major epidemics are associated only with influenza A and have been attributed to ''antigenic shifts'' or reassortment of genomic segments possibly with animal strains. Between pandemics, minor antigenic variations occur through point mutations. Antibodies against the hemagglutinin are most important, presumably preventing viral attachment. Influenza B tends to cause smaller outbreaks, with less severe disease, because there is no animal reservoir and major antigenic shifts do not occur. Prolonged fatigue or ''postinfluenzal asthenia'' may occur, but the etiology is not known. Viral shedding usually stops 2 to 5 days after symptoms in uncomplicated influenza. Both amantadine and rimantadine can either prevent or attenuate infection with influenza A. In major outbreaks, therapy may be useful until immunity can be established by immunization.

111. The answer is A-N, B-Y, C-N, D-Y, E-Y. *(Wilson, ed 12. chap 105.)* Neonatal tetanus is associated with a more than 60 percent mortality rate. It is caused by infections of the umbilical stump. In third world countries the infection is often associated with practices of applying dirt or feces to the umbilical stump to speed sloughing. Human immune globulin cannot affect tetanus toxin that is already bound in the central nervous system, but it can be helpful if given early to bind any free toxin. Such small amounts of tetanospasmin are present that no immunity develops and active immunization must be initiated. Trismus or lockjaw is the most common manifestation of tetanus; it is caused by neuromuscular blockade and central disinhibition of motor neurons. Immune globulin provides protective antibody levels for up to 4 weeks and should be given along with toxoid for serious wounds if fewer than two previous doses of toxoid have been given.

112. The answer is A-N, B-N, C-Y, D-N, E-Y. *(Wilson, ed 12. chap 102.)* The gram-positive rod *Corynebacterium diphtheriae* may produce human disease upon infection of skin or mucous membranes. Specific viruses, termed *corynephages,* must infect *C. diphtheriae* to convert the bacterium to a toxin-producing strain. Disease can occur as a result of infection with toxin-producing or toxin-negative strains, but the serious manifestations of carditis and neuritis occur as a result of toxins. The toxin, elaborated as a single polypeptide chain by the lysogenized bacteria, is proteolytically cleaved into an A portion, which binds to cell membranes, and a B portion, which catalyzes the adenosine diphosphate ribosylation and inactivation of elongation factor 2, a vital element in ribosome-mediated protein synthesis. Most unimmunized patients with diphtherial pharyngitis experience myocardial abnormalities with manifestations ranging from an abnormal electrocardiogram to congestive heart failure and ventricular fibrillation. Formaldehyde-treated diphtheria toxin creates toxoid, a vaccine component that can provide 10 years of protection against serious disease. Pharyngeal and cutaneous infections with toxigenic strains produce edema, hyperemia, and a dense, fibrinopurulent exudate (termed a *pseudomembrane*) teeming with *C. diphtheriae*. Formation of the pseudomembrane can lead to obstruction of the upper airway. Administration of antitoxin is the primary specific modality of treatment for those with suspected infections.

113. The answer is A-N, B-N, C-Y, D-N, E-Y. *(Wilson, ed 12. chap 101.)* Differences in cell-wall carbohydrates account for the alphabetized classification system used to describe streptococcal strains. Group A streptococcal infection is usually associated with pharyngitis or pyoderma and is notable for the incidence of poststreptococcal nonsuppurative complications (acute rheumatic fever and acute glomerulonephritis). The beta-hemolytic and bacitracin-resistant group B streptococci colonize the female genital tract and are the second most common cause, after *E. coli,* of neonatal sepsis and meningitis. Systemic disease, including urinary tract infections and endocarditis, in debilitated adults may also be caused by group B streptococci. Group D streptococci include both enterococcal and nonenterococcal forms. Unlike most streptococci, which are exquisitely penicillin-sensitive, enterococci are relatively resistant. Enterococcal endocarditis should be treated with the synergistic combination of ampicillin plus an aminoglycoside. The aminoglycoside of choice is gentamicin, since many strains are now highly resistant to the formerly administered streptomycin. Nonenterococcal group D strains, typified by *Streptococcus bovis,* which tends to cause bacteremia in patients with colonic neoplasia, can be identified by their ability to grow in 6.5% NaCl. Viridans streptococci inhabit the mouth and are the organisms most frequently associated with subacute bacterial endocarditis. Certain subtypes of viridans streptococci, including *Streptococcus milleri,* can cause major suppurative disease, such as liver abscesses and empyema.

114. The answer is A-N, B-Y, C-Y, D-N, E-Y. *(Wilson, ed 12. chap 111.)* *Klebsiella* and the related *Serratia* and *Enterobacter* are the most important enteric organisms other than *E. coli* to infect humans. Although respiratory disease is important (*Klebsiella* accounts for 1 percent or less of community-acquired pneumonia), most clinical isolates now come from the urinary tract. All three genera are important pulmonary nosocomial pathogens. However, merely finding these organisms growing in the sputum of a very ill hospitalized patient does not necessarily implicate the bacteria as pathogenic in that particular circumstance and may indicate colonization rather than infection. Clinical context and procurement of the sample in a sterile fashion (transtracheal aspiration, bronchoscopy) will aid in diagnosis. Chronic alcoholics, diabetics, and those with chronic lung disease are at increased risk for *Klebsiella* pneumonia, a difficult disease to treat because of the frequency of suppurative complications (empyema and abscess) with the associated requirement for prolonged ($>$2 weeks) therapy.

115. The answer is A-Y, B-N, C-Y, D-Y, E-Y. *(Wilson, ed 12. chap 115. Lebel, N Engl J Med 319:964, 1988.)* Recent isolation of increased numbers of β-lactamase–producing (15 to 50 percent) and chloramphenicol-resistant ($<$10 percent) strains has led to the development of new protocols for treating those with serious *H. influenzae* infection. Ampicillin plus chloramphenicol is still perfectly reasonable therapy until the results of susceptibility tests are available. Chloramphenicol is a bacteriostatic, not bactericidal antibiotic and has no role as a single agent. However, either ceftriaxone or cefotaxime, which are β-lactamase–stable third-generation cephalosporins that enter the CSF at bactericidal concentrations, is as effective as ampicillin and chloramphenicol. Recent data suggest that long-term benefit is associated with administering intravenous dexamethasone early in the course of *H. influenzae* meningitis, in addition to supportive care, especially airway maintenance.

116. The answer is A-Y, B-N, C-N, D-N, E-N. *(Wilson, ed 12. chap 125. Chaisson, Am Rev Respir Dis 136:570, 1987.)* Persons previously infected with *Mycobacterium tuberculosis* who thereafter acquire infection with human immunodeficiency virus (HIV) have a 50 percent chance of developing clinical tuberculosis, although the radiographic manifestations may be atypical. In this setting, tuberculosis often precedes any other infectious manifestation of HIV infection. The diagnosis of tuberculosis is best established by documenting acid-fast bacilli in the relevant human specimen. In the case of suspected pulmonary tuberculosis, if expectorated sputum is not available, nasotracheal aspiration, bronchoscopy, or examination of early morning gastric aspirates can be helpful. In the last case, the presence of a few nontuberculous mycobacteria in gastric secretions generally does not yield a false-positive result. Although at least 2 weeks is required, sputum culture will confirm the diagnosis made by examination of stained tissues or secretions. Serologic tests are experimental and not routinely useful or available. About 15 percent of patients with active pulmonary disease will be anergic, i.e., unable to respond to the tuberculin or other skin tests. Therefore, a negative skin test does not rule out the disease. However, a positive skin test strongly supports the diagnosis of prior infection. In order to prevent subsequent reactivation tuberculosis, all patients under age 35 with a positive skin test and a chest x-ray not consistent with active disease should receive 1 year of isoniazid. Despite an increased risk of hepatitis, many older patients who have long life expectancies as well as those at high risk for reactivation (i.e., patients who are medically immuno-suppressed or HIV-infected or who have renal failure) are candidates for chemoprophylaxis.

117. The answer is A-N, B-Y, C-Y, D-N, E-Y. *(Wilson, ed 12. chap 171.)* Certain nematodes have a life-cycle phase wherein larvae migrate through the lungs of the human host. In such cases, pneumonia and pulmonary symptoms are possible. The most frequent complaint associated with enterobiasis (pinworm) is pruritus ani; the worms rarely leave the distal end of the gastrointestinal tract. Both *Toxocara* (visceral larva migrans) and *Ascaris* larvae are capable of diffuse migration and may cause bronchopneumonia with migratory pulmonary infiltrates as the organisms migrate through the lung. *Strongyloides* larvae enter through the skin, float through the blood stream into the lungs, are coughed into the oropharynx, and swallowed into the gastrointestinal tract, where they live and cause problems. Cough, dyspnea, and gross hemoptysis accompany the passage through the lungs. The intestinal cestode *Taenia saginata* remains in the jejunum to cause marked gastrointestinal symptoms. *Taenia solium,* the pork tapeworm, can cause cystic disease of the brain, as well as bothersome stomach symptoms.

118. The answer is A-N, B-Y, C-N, D-Y, E-Y. *(Wilson, ed 12. chap 159.)* Only in *P. vivax* and *P. ovale* infections may relapses occur because a portion of the intrahepatic forms remain dormant. *P. vivax* depends upon the Duffy antigen to enter red cells; patients who lack this antigen are resistant. *P. falciparum* produces a form of disease that can lead to coma and death. Seizures and hypoglycemia, grave prognostic signs, may also be present. Renal failure in falciparum malaria seems to occur on the basis of tubular sequestration of parasitized erythrocytes and tends to abate. Renal failure with *P. malariae* infection may be due to deposition of soluble immune complexes in glomeruli. Repeated malarial infections can result in massive splenomegaly.

119. The answer is A-Y, B-Y, C-Y, D-Y, E-Y. *(Wilson, ed 12. chap 137.)* Serious complications of infectious mononucleosis (IM) due to infection with Epstein-Barr virus (EBV) are uncommon. Mild hepatitis occurs in 90 percent of patients. Airway obstruction, which is sensitive to glucocorticoid therapy, is sometimes a result of the massive pharyngeal adenopathy accompanying IM. IgM antibodies elicited by EBV may be directed against the i antigen on red blood cell membranes, thereby causing a transient autoimmune hemolytic anemia. Mild antibody-mediated thrombocytopenia is common, but a serious drop in the platelet count is unusual. Some patients develop cranial nerve palsies and encephalitis as the result of EBV infection. There is growing recognition of the association between EBV infection and B-cell lymphoproliferative disorders in immunocompromised patients.

120–123. The answers are: 120-B, 121-D, 122-A, 123-C. *(Wilson, ed 12. chap 82.)* Several distinct infectious syndromes have been linked to specific deficits in host defenses. Complement appears to be critical in the defense against neisserial infections since patients with deficiencies in the late components have recurrent *N. gonorrhoeae* and *meningitidis* infections. The spleen is one of the most important sites for phagocytosis of opsonized organisms. After splenectomy, whether surgical or functional as in sickle cell diseases, patients are at risk for development of bacteremia with organisms for which antibody forms the major host defense, such as *S. pneumoniae* and *Haemophilus influenzae*. Patients with AIDS are susceptible to multiple infections against which intact cellular immunity is required. *Pneumocystis carinii* is the most frequent infection, but cytomegalovirus, *Mycobacterium avium-intracellulare,* and cryptococcal infections are also common. In Chédiak-Higashi syndrome, a defect in neutrophil chemotaxis and phagocytosis results in recurrent staphylococcal infections.

124–128. The answers are: 124-D, 125-C, 126-A, 127-B, 128-C. *(Wilson, ed 12. chaps 84, 85.)* Steady progress is being made in the prevention and treatment of viral infections. Inactivated virus vaccines are available for influenza, rabies, polio, and several arboviruses causing encephalitis. Attenuated virus vaccines are available for rubella, mumps, measles, polio, and yellow fever. A recombinant hepatitis B vaccine is now available and recommended for those at high risk. Passive immunization is used for hepatitis A and varicella; broader application is hampered because the procedure is cumbersome and expensive. Transfer of the slow virus that causes Creutzfeldt-Jakob disease is prevented by careful sterilization of surgical equipment used for neurosurgical procedures. Chemoprophylaxis with amantadine for influenza has been useful; however, vaccination is a more effective preventive measure.

Disorders of the Heart and Vascular System

DIRECTIONS: Each question below contains five suggested responses. Choose the **one best** response to each question.

129. A 48-year-old man is admitted to the coronary care unit with an acute inferior myocardial infarction. Two hours after admission, his blood pressure is 86/52 mmHg; his heart rate is 40 beats per minute with sinus rhythm. Which of the following would be the most appropriate initial therapy?

(A) Immediate insertion of a temporary transvenous pacemaker
(B) Intravenous administration of atropine sulfate, 0.6 mg
(C) Administration of normal saline, 300 mL over 15 min
(D) Intravenous administration of dobutamine, 0.35 mg/min
(E) Intravenous administration of isoproterenol, 5.0 μg/min

130. All the following are features of captopril EXCEPT that it

(A) decreases plasma renin activity
(B) retards the degradation of circulating bradykinin
(C) inhibits formation of angiotensin II
(D) can be used safely in combination with a beta blocking agent
(E) is contraindicated in patients with bilateral renal artery stenosis

131. All the following statements regarding beta blocking agents are true EXCEPT

(A) pindolol has partial beta-agonist activity
(B) metoprolol is a selective beta$_1$ antagonist
(C) labetelol is both an alpha- and a beta-receptor blocking agent
(D) atenolol can be administered safely in large doses to asthmatic patients
(E) nadolol can be administered effectively once a day

132. Which of the following physical findings is associated with the chest x-ray shown below?

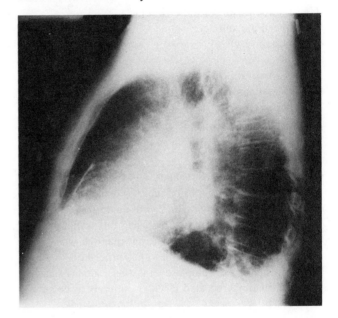

(A) Wide splitting of the second heart sound
(B) Opening snap and diastolic rumble
(C) Pericardial knock
(D) Late-peaking systolic ejection murmur
(E) Central cyanosis

133. Combined echocardiographic and Doppler echocardiographic studies are useful in the evaluation of all the following disorders EXCEPT

(A) aortic stenosis
(B) atrial septal defect
(C) tricuspid regurgitation
(D) mitral stenosis
(E) calcification of the left coronary artery

134. A 73-year-old man recently began having frequent syncopal episodes upon rising from recumbency. Associated complaints include constipation, difficulty voiding, and dry skin. Evaluation reveals orthostatic hypotension in the absence of compensatory tachycardia while the man is standing, but no evidence of degeneration of the central nervous system, including the extrapyramidal tracts and basal ganglia. Glucocorticoid and mineralocorticoid secretion is normal; plasma norepinephrine concentration, measured while the man is supine, is low. The treatment LEAST likely to benefit this man is

(A) high salt intake
(B) elastic supportive hose
(C) fludrocortisone acetate (Florinef)
(D) ephedrine sulfate
(E) tyramine

135. All the following statements regarding percutaneous transluminal coronary angioplasty (PTCA) are true EXCEPT

(A) restenosis resulting after successful dilation develops in approximately 20 percent of patients within 6 months
(B) stenoses within saphenous vein bypass grafts can be dilated using this technique
(C) a recent complete *occlusion* of a coronary artery can be successfully dilated using this technique
(D) a 65 percent stenosis of the left main coronary artery is a contraindication to this procedure
(E) if restenosis develops several weeks after a successful dilation, repeated PTCA is unlikely to be successful

136. A 42-year-old woman has bilateral ankle edema of recent onset. On examination, her jugular venous pulse is 5 cmH₂O and the hepatojugular reflux is negative. All the following should be considered in the differential diagnosis of the woman's ankle edema EXCEPT

(A) pelvic thrombophlebitis
(B) venous varicosities
(C) cyclic edema
(D) hypoalbuminemia
(E) right heart failure

137. All the following causes of congestive heart failure are associated with a widened arterial–mixed venous oxygen difference EXCEPT

(A) tricuspid stenosis
(B) alcoholic cardiomyopathy
(C) Paget's disease
(D) constrictive pericarditis
(E) right ventricular infarction

138. Digitalis glycosides enhance myocardial contractility primarily by which of the following mechanisms?

(A) Opening of calcium channels
(B) Release of calcium from the sarcoplasmic reticulum
(C) Stimulation of myosin ATPase
(D) Stimulation of membrane phospholipase C
(E) Inhibition of membrane Na⁺-K⁺-ATPase

139. An elderly person who has been taking digitalis for heart failure is brought to the hospital because of anorexia and nausea. On examination, ventricular bigeminy is noted. Digoxin level is 1.5 pg/L. All the following factors would be expected to contribute to digitalis intoxication EXCEPT

(A) chronic obstructive lung disease with hypoxemia
(B) addition of quinidine to the therapeutic regimen
(C) diuretic therapy with loop diuretics
(D) hyperthyroidism
(E) hyperparathyroidism

140. Clues to the presence of atrioventricular nodal block (as opposed to trifascicular block) would include all the following EXCEPT

(A) clinical evidence of inferior myocardial infarction
(B) Wenckebach periodicity to conduction
(C) escape-focus rate faster than 50 beats per minute
(D) a narrow QRS complex at the escape focus
(E) unresponsiveness of the escape focus to atropine

141. A 79-year-old woman has daily episodes of lightheadedness. A rhythm strip shows sinus bradycardia at 52 beats per minute and 2.5-second sinus pause that produces no symptoms. The next step in this woman's management should be

(A) implantation of a permanent demand ventricular pacemaker
(B) trial of a temporary transvenous pacemaker
(C) institution of sublingual isoproterenol therapy
(D) continuous 24-hour Holter monitoring
(E) exercise tolerance testing

142. A 60-year-old man is admitted to a hospital because of respiratory failure and tachycardia. His rectal temperature is 38.3°C (101°F), respiratory rate 32 breaths per minute, and blood pressure 100/60 mmHg. His admission electrocardiogram is shown below. Which of the following measures would constitute the most appropriate management for this man?

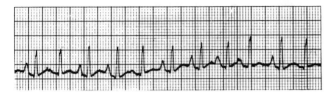

(A) Electrical cardioversion after the blood pressure is raised
(B) Supplemental oxygenation or mechanical ventilation
(C) Administration of digitalis
(D) Administration of quinidine
(E) Administration of verapamil

143. A 57-year-old previously healthy woman develops atrial flutter, 2:1 atrioventricular conduction, and a ventricular rate of 150 beats per minute. Her ventricular rate could be decreased safely with the use of all the following EXCEPT

(A) digoxin
(B) verapamil
(C) propranolol
(D) quinidine
(E) carotid sinus massage

144. All the following statements regarding secundum atrial septal defect are true EXCEPT

(A) surgical correction is advisable when the pulmonary-to-systemic flow ratio has reached 2.0
(B) affected persons are usually asymptomatic in childhood
(C) electrocardiography shows a leftward axis
(D) echocardiography shows abnormal ventricular septal motion
(E) atrial arrhythmias are common

145. A 64-year-old man is examined because of episodes of exertional chest pain. An M-mode echocardiogram is shown below. A continuous-wave Doppler signal across the aortic valve showed a peak systolic velocity of 5 m/s; no diastolic turbulence was detected. Which of the following statements concerning this patient is true?

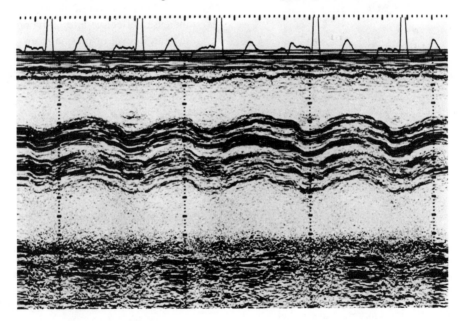

(A) Significant aortic regurgitation is most likely present
(B) The peak gradient across the aortic valve is approximately 100 mmHg
(C) The gradient across the aortic valve cannot be determined from the information given
(D) Coronary arteriography is unnecessary in this patient; immediate aortic valve replacement is indicated
(E) The Doppler findings rule out important aortic stenosis; an exercise test should be performed to evaluate this man's chest pain

146. The chest x-rays below would likely have been taken of which of the following persons?

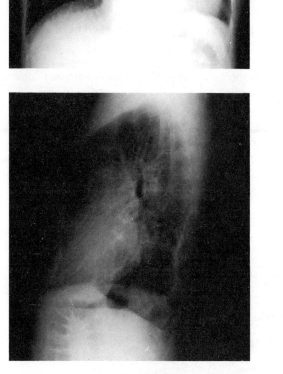

(A)   A 38-year-old woman who has hemoptysis, dyspnea on exertion, and fatigability
(B)   A 36-year-old woman who has a heart murmur but is asymptomatic
(C)   A 32-year-old woman who has a continuous murmur, widened systemic pulse pressure, and dyspnea on exertion
(D)   A 40-year-old woman who has a loud first heart sound, a diastolic rumble, a large *v* wave in her jugular pulse, and ascites
(E)   None of the above

147. A 20-year-old woman has mild pulmonic stenosis (transvalvular gradient is 20 mmHg). All the following statements regarding this situation are true EXCEPT

(A)   heart size on chest x-ray is likely to be normal
(B)   electrocardiogram is likely to be normal
(C)   her jugular *a* wave is likely to be prominent
(D)   compared to other valvular defects, the risk of endocarditis is relatively low
(E)   frequent monitoring for progression of the stenosis is indicated

148. All the following findings would be expected in a person with coarctation of the aorta EXCEPT

(A)   a systolic murmur across the anterior chest and back and a high-pitched diastolic murmur along the left sternal border
(B)   a higher blood pressure in the right arm than in the left arm
(C)   inability to augment cardiac output with exercise
(D)   rib notching on chest x-ray
(E)   persistent hypertension despite complete surgical repair

149. Factors accounting for the pedal edema associated with congestive heart failure include all the following EXCEPT

(A)   increased secretion of aldosterone
(B)   increased effective arterial blood volume
(C)   increased level of plasma renin
(D)   decreased atrial natriuretic peptide
(E)   sympathetic nervous system–mediated renal vasoconstriction

150. Embolism to the lower extremities most commonly arises from

(A)   an abdominal aortic aneurysm
(B)   an ulcerated plaque along the thoracic aorta
(C)   the heart
(D)   localized femoral artery thrombosis
(E)   none of the above

151. Which of the following statements best describes long-acting nitrate preparations?

(A)   Tolerance often develops
(B)   Their effect can be blocked by high doses of beta$_2$ selective inhibitors
(C)   Nitroglycerin ointment is most effective pharmacologically when applied to the anterior chest
(D)   Oral preparations are more effective than sublingual ones
(E)   Oral administration of isosorbide should not exceed 15 mg every 3 to 4 h

152. A 62-year-old woman was started on a regimen of quinidine sulfate because of asymptomatic ventricular couplets. One week later, she was admitted to the hospital after a syncopal episode. Serum electrolyte concentrations were normal. The arrhythmia shown below appeared transiently on her cardiac monitor. The recommended course at this time is to

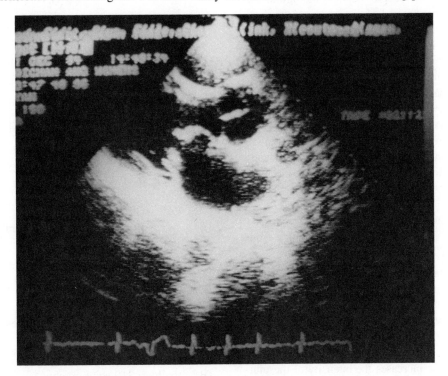

(A)   increase the quinidine dose
(B)   discontinue administration of quinidine and observe
(C)   begin intravenous administration of procainamide 2 mg/min
(D)   administer sodium bicarbonate, 70 meq, intravenously
(E)   administer potassium chloride, 10 meq, intravenously over 1 h

153. This two-dimensional echocardiogram was most likely recorded in which of the following patients?

(A)   A 54-year-old man with syncopal episodes when bending forward
(B)   A previously healthy 68-year-old man with sudden onset of pulmonary edema and a new holosystolic murmur
(C)   A 17-year-old girl with atypical chest pain and a midsystolic click
(D)   A 42-year-old woman with palpitations, exertional dyspnea, and episodes of hemoptysis
(E)   An asymptomatic 32-year-old cardiologist

154. A previously healthy 58-year-old man is admitted to the hospital because of an acute inferior myocardial infarction. Within several hours, he becomes oliguric and hypotensive (blood pressure is 90/60 mmHg). Insertion of a pulmonary artery (Swan-Ganz) catheter reveals the following pressures: pulmonary capillary wedge, 4 mmHg; pulmonary artery, 22/4 mmHg; and mean right atrial, 11 mmHg. This man would best be treated with

(A) fluids
(B) digoxin
(C) norepinephrine
(D) dopamine
(E) intraaortic balloon counterpulsation

155. All the following statements regarding myocardial hypertrophy are true EXCEPT

(A) the beta$_2$-adrenergic receptor bears homology to the c-*mas* proto-oncogene
(B) the proto-oncogenes c-*sis*, c-*myc*, c-*ras*, and c-*fos* are all induced in myocardial tissue during hypertrophy
(C) a gene responsible for familial hypertrophic cardiomyopathy has been mapped to chromosome 14
(D) angiotensin II can stimulate hypertrophy by direct effects on smooth muscle
(E) hypertrophy due to hemodynamic overload is accompanied by a similar synthetic induction of fetal myosin forms to that observed in the hypertrophy associated with hyperthyroidism

156. All the following statements regarding physiologic maneuvers used to distinguish one cardiac condition from another are true EXCEPT

(A) the Valsalva maneuver results in a decreased length and intensity for most systolic murmurs, except those due to mitral valve prolapse and hypertrophic cardiomyopathy
(B) in the case of mitral valve prolapse, squatting results in increased intensity of the systolic murmur
(C) handgrip exercise increases the intensity of the murmurs of mitral stenosis and mitral regurgitation
(D) murmurs of tricuspid regurgitation and tricuspid stenosis increase during inspiration
(E) the murmur of aortic stenosis increases following a ventricular premature beat

157. A 68-year-old man who has had a recent syncopal episode is hospitalized with congestive heart failure. His blood pressure is 160/80 mmHg, his pulse rate is 80 beats per minute, and there is a grade III/VI harsh systolic murmur. An echocardiogram shows a disproportionately thickened ventricular septum and systolic anterior motion of the mitral valve. Which of the following findings would most likely be present in this man?

(A) Radiation of the murmur to the carotid arteries
(B) Decrease of the murmur with hand grip
(C) Delayed carotid upstroke
(D) Reduced left ventricular ejection fraction
(E) Signs of mitral stenosis

158. Which factor accounts for the prolonged QRS complex depicted in this figure?

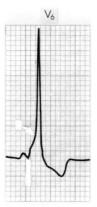

(A) Left ventricular hypertrophy
(B) Accessory conducting fibers parallel to the AV junction
(C) Right ventricular infarction
(D) Left bundle branch block
(E) Right bundle branch block

159. Each of the following techniques can detect nonviable myocardium EXCEPT

(A) positron emission tomography
(B) thallium 210 scintigraphy
(C) technetium 99m stannous pyrophosphate scintigraphy
(D) standard computed tomography
(E) echocardiography

160. For the last 6 h, a 33-year-old man has had sharp, pleuritic, substernal chest pain that is relieved when he sits upright. His electrocardiogram shows diffuse ST-segment elevation. Which of the following observations would LEAST support a diagnosis of acute pericarditis?

(A) Frequent atrial premature beats
(B) PR-segment depression
(C) Diffuse T-wave inversion with ST-segment elevation
(D) Twice-normal serum creatine phosphokinase concentration
(E) No rub

161. All the following can help prevent abrupt closure or thrombus formation in a coronary artery dilated by percutaneous transluminal coronary angioplasty (PTCA) EXCEPT

(A) nitrates
(B) aspirin
(C) heparin
(D) calcium channel antagonists
(E) beta blockers

162. All the following electrocardiographic findings may represent manifestations of digitalis intoxication EXCEPT

(A) bigeminy
(B) junctional tachycardia
(C) atrial flutter
(D) atrial tachycardia with variable block
(E) sinus arrest

163. All the following are indications for surgical intervention in the treatment of dissection of the aorta EXCEPT

(A) compromised femoral pulse
(B) new murmur of aortic regurgitation
(C) persistent chest pain
(D) involvement of the ascending aorta
(E) involvement of the descending aorta

164. All the following congenital cardiac disorders will lead to a left-to-right shunt, generally without cyanosis, EXCEPT

(A) anomalous origin of the left coronary artery from the pulmonary trunk
(B) patent ductus arteriosus without pulmonary hypertension
(C) total anomalous pulmonary venous connection
(D) ventricular septal defect
(E) sinus venosus atrial septal defect

165. Each of the following may represent a MAJOR feature (according to the revised Jones criteria) of acute rheumatic fever EXCEPT

(A) arthritis in both knees
(B) pericardial friction rub
(C) prolonged PR interval
(D) a pink rash with serpiginous margins
(E) painless swellings over bony prominences

166. True statements describing dissection of the aorta include all the following EXCEPT

(A) nearly all cases involve medial necrosis
(B) coexisting hypertension is present in more than two-thirds of the patients
(C) all false aneurysms begin with rupture of the aorta
(D) dissection associated with Marfan's syndrome (type II dissection) stops before the great vessels arising from the aortic arch
(E) appropriate medical management could consist of labetolol or a combination of nitroprusside and a beta blocker

167. Clear contraindications to the use of thrombolytic agents in the setting of an acute anterior myocardial infarction include all the following EXCEPT

(A) left carotid artery occlusion with hemiparesis 1 month ago
(B) transurethral resection of the prostate 1 week ago
(C) diastolic blood pressure of 110 mmHg during chest pain
(D) patient age greater than 70
(E) epigastric pain and melena 1 week ago treated with histamine receptor antagonists

168. Which of the following situations in the periinfarction period would suggest the presence of ventricular septal perforation?

(A) Systolic murmur, large v waves in pulmonary capillary wedge tracing; P_{O_2} in right atrium equals that in right ventricle
(B) Systolic murmur, large v waves in pulmonary capillary wedge tracing; P_{O_2} in right atrium is greater than that in the right ventricle
(C) Systolic murmur, large v waves in pulmonary capillary wedge tracing; P_{O_2} in right atrium is less than that in the right ventricle
(D) Diastolic murmur, large v waves in the pulmonary capillary wedge tracing; P_{O_2} in the right atrium is less than in the right ventricle
(E) Diastolic murmur, large v waves in the pulmonary capillary wedge tracing; P_{O_2} in the right atrium is greater than in the right ventricle

169. A 50-year-old man with a history of smoking, hypertension, and chronic exertional angina develops several daily episodes of chest pain at rest compatible with cardiac ischemia. The patient is hospitalized. All the following would be part of an appropriate management plan EXCEPT

(A) intravenous heparin
(B) aspirin
(C) intravenous nitroglycerin
(D) lidocaine by bolus infusion
(E) diltiazem

170. Cardiac catheterization disclosing decreased cardiac output, elevation of right and left end-diastolic pressures, and a dip and plateau configuration during the diastolic portion of the ventricular pressure trace could be seen in all the following conditions EXCEPT

(A) Duchenne's muscular dystrophy
(B) amyloidosis
(C) hemochromatosis
(D) hypereosinophilic syndrome
(E) endomyocardial fibrosis

171. All the following patients are at increased risk for the development of deep venous thrombosis EXCEPT

(A) a 35-year-old woman with systemic lupus erythematosus and a prolonged partial thromboplastin time
(B) a 75-year-old woman with a Colles fracture of the wrist
(C) a normotensive 18-year-old woman taking an oral contraceptive
(D) a 55-year-old man 3 days after an uncomplicated inferior myocardial infarction
(E) a 55-year-old man 5 days after complete resection of a squamous cell carcinoma of 2 cm in diameter in the periphery of the right lung

172. Which of the following statements regarding thrombolytic therapy in the treatment of acute myocardial infarction is true?

(A) If treatment begins within 8 h of the onset of chest discomfort, it is likely that benefit will occur
(B) In comparison with streptokinase, tissue plasminogen activator (tPA) reduces mortality
(C) Reelevation of ST segments 24 h after the administration of streptokinase indicates reperfusion
(D) Aspirin and heparin should be administered after thrombolytic therapy
(E) None of the above

173. This figure most likely represents the pulmonary capillary wedge and left ventricular pressure tracing from which of the following patients?

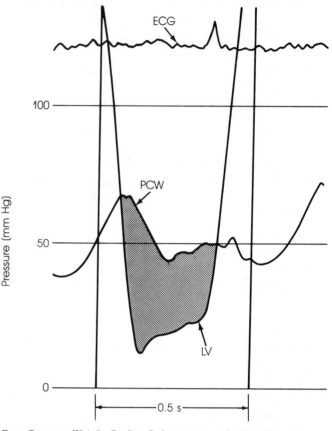

From Grossman W (ed): *Cardiac Catheterization and Angiography*, 3d ed. Philadelphia, Lea & Febiger, 1986, with permission.

(A) A 40-year-old woman with a history of rheumatic fever, orthopnea and hemoptysis
(B) A 24-year-old intravenous drug abuser with fever, holosystolic murmur, and large mitral valve vegetation
(C) A 26-year-old man with long arms, abnormal lenses, and a diastolic murmur
(D) A 72-year-old man with left ventricular hypertrophy, syncope, and a systolic murmur
(E) A 35-year-old woman with elevated neck veins and a large mediastinal mass due to non-Hodgkin's lymphoma

DIRECTIONS: Each question below contains five suggested responses. For **each** of the five responses of **each** item, you are to respond either YES (Y) or NO (N). In a given item **all, some, or none** of the responses may be correct.

174. A 62-year-old man loses consciousness in the street, and resuscitative efforts are undertaken. In the emergency room an electrocardiogram is obtained, part of which is shown below. Which of the following disorders could account for this man's presentation?

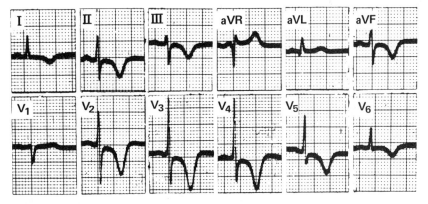

From Marriott HJL: *Practical Electrocardiography.* Baltimore, Williams & Wilkins, 7th ed, 1983, p. 400, with permission.

(A) Subendocardial infarction
(B) Hyperkalemia
(C) Intracerebral hemorrhage
(D) Myocardial ischemia
(E) Hypocalcemic tetany

175. Ebstein's anomaly is correctly described by which of the following statements?

(A) Most affected persons die in infancy
(B) A systolic murmur varying with respiration is frequent
(C) Giant P waves on electrocardiography are typical
(D) The right ventricle is characteristically dilated and hypertrophied
(E) The tricuspid valve is redundant

176. A loud first heart sound is associated frequently with

(A) hypothyroidism
(B) Lown-Ganong-Levine syndrome
(C) mitral stenosis
(D) mitral regurgitation
(E) fever

177. Acute hyperkalemia is associated with which of the following electrocardiographic changes?

(A) QRS widening
(B) Prolongation of the ST segment
(C) Decrease in the P wave
(D) Prominent U waves
(E) Peaked T waves

178. Bifascicular block commonly is associated with

(A) anteroseptal myocardial infarction
(B) inferior myocardial infarction
(C) prolonged HV interval on a His bundle electrogram
(D) calcific aortic stenosis
(E) mitral valve surgery

179. True statements regarding exercise tolerance tests include which of the following?

(A) Requiring ≥ 2.0 mm of ST depression to define a test as positive enhances the sensitivity of the test compared with a situation in which only 0.5 mm of ST depression is required to count as positive
(B) Given a specificity of 90 percent and a sensitivity of 80 percent, a positive test in a patient whose prior probability of having coronary artery disease (based on clinical factors) is 10 percent suggests a greater than 80 percent likelihood that the patient actually has coronary artery disease
(C) Thallium 201 exercise scanning increases both the sensitivity and specificity for detecting ischemic heart disease
(D) A thallium 201 scan done at peak exercise that reveals a nonperfused area of myocardium indicates that the patient has suffered a prior myocardial infarction
(E) A marked increase in blood pressure during the test suggests poor conditioning and will likely cause the test to be nondiagnostic

180. The rhythm shown on the electrocardiogram below can be associated with

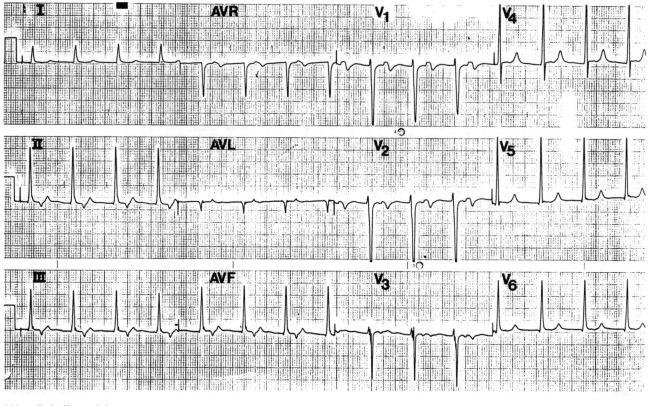

(A) digitalis toxicity
(B) acute myocarditis
(C) anterior myocardial infarction
(D) mitral valve surgery
(E) hypercalcemia

---

181. Features of chest pain that increase the probability that the patient has myocardial ischemia include which of the following?

(A) Radiation of pain to the forehead
(B) Abrupt, sharp pain in the substernal area radiating to the back
(C) Relief of pain 2 min after the administration of sublingual nitroglycerin
(D) Relief of pain seconds after recumbency
(E) Radiation of pain to the teeth

182. Mild heart failure due to left ventricular dysfunction is accurately described by which of the following statements?

(A) Cardiac output would be depressed at rest
(B) Plasma norepinephrine levels would be higher than in normal controls during exercise
(C) Myocardial norepinephrine content would be high
(D) Left ventricular end-diastolic pressure would rise more during exercise than in normal controls
(E) Cardiac output would fail to rise appropriately when oxygen consumption is increased during exercise

183. Sudden cardiac death is accurately described by which of the following statements?

(A) Ventricular tachycardia or ventricular fibrillation during the convalescent phase (3 days to 8 weeks) after a myocardial infarction is a risk factor for subsequent sudden cardiac death

(B) A patient convalescing from a myocardial infarction displaying a salvo of three ventricular premature beats is at greater risk than a similar patient who has 35 unifocal premature beats per hour

(C) If only one person is present to provide basic life support, chest compressions should be performed at a rate of 80 per minute and breaths at a rate of 4 per minute

(D) Assuming there is no spontaneous pulse, a 400-joule shock should be delivered immediately upon recognition of ventricular tachycardia or ventricular fibrillation

(E) Intravenous sodium bicarbonate should be given approximately every 5 min during cardiac arrest

184. Drugs that would *antagonize* the interaction of catecholamines with adrenergic receptors include

(A) prazosin
(B) clonidine
(C) phenylephrine
(D) yohimbine
(E) isoproterenol

185. A 40-year-old woman with asthma has been taking terbutaline and aminophylline. She comes to the emergency room with palpitations, light-headedness, and shortness of breath. The electrocardiogram shown below is obtained. The rhythm disturbance evident on the ECG can be described by which of the following statements?

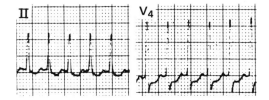

Reprinted with permission from Marriott HJL: *Practical Electrocardiography*. Baltimore, Williams & Wilkins, 7th ed, 1983, p. 164.

(A) It arises from sustained reentry, probably through the atrioventricular (AV) junction

(B) It is dependent upon delayed conduction and unidirectional block

(C) It involves concealed conduction within the AV junction

(D) It may be reliably terminated by administration of nifedipine

(E) Intravenous edrophonium (Tensilon), 10 mg, would be appropriate therapy

186. A 37-year-old man with Wolff-Parkinson-White syndrome develops a broad-complex tachycardia at a rate of 200 beats per minute. He appears comfortable and has little hemodynamic impairment. Useful treatment at this point might include

(A) digoxin
(B) quinidine
(C) propranolol
(D) verapamil
(E) direct-current cardioversion

187. A 17-year-old girl has an atrial septal defect of the sinus venosus type, with a 3:1 pulmonary-to-systemic blood flow ratio. True statements concerning her condition include which of the following?

(A) She is probably asymptomatic

(B) She probably has partial anomalous connection of the pulmonary veins

(C) The magnitude of the shunt is a function of the amount of total blood flow

(D) A systolic murmur would likely be due to flow across the defect

(E) A diastolic rumble would strongly suggest coexistence of mitral stenosis (Lutembacher's syndrome)

188. For which of the following patients would cardiac surgery be appropriately recommended?

(A) An asymptomatic 18-year-old woman who has an atrial septal defect with a 2:1 pulmonary-to-systemic flow ratio

(B) An asymptomatic 19-year-old man who has a loud murmur and ventricular septal defect with a 1.5:1 pulmonary-to-systemic flow ratio

(C) A 33-year-old man who has chest pain, fatigue, cyanosis, a large ventricular septal defect, a 2:1 right-to-left shunt, and a normal pulmonary outflow tract and pulmonic valve

(D) A 52-year-old man who has chronic mitral regurgitation and has recently developed pulmonary edema associated with the onset of rapid atrial fibrillation

(E) A 54-year-old man who has aortic stenosis and has chest pain on moderate-to-strenuous exertion

189. Substances involved in endothelial cell-mediated vasodilation include

(A) prostacyclin (PGI$_2$)
(B) cyclic AMP
(C) nitric oxide
(D) endothelin
(E) cyclic GMP

190. The initial positive deflection in the jugular venous pulse (*a* wave) can be accentuated in which of the following conditions?

(A) Junctional rhythm
(B) Tricuspid stenosis
(C) Atrial fibrillation
(D) Multiple pulmonary emboli
(E) Complete heart block

191. Accurate descriptions of acute rheumatic fever include which of the following?

(A) Group A streptococcal skin infections can initiate an attack
(B) Recurrent rheumatic fever occurs more frequently in persons with preexisting rheumatic heart disease than in others
(C) Large numbers of macrophages are found commonly in the first drop of blood extracted from the earlobe
(D) Diagnosis of acute rheumatic fever in a young person presenting with migratory arthritis and congestive heart failure is unlikely if group A streptococci cannot be isolated from a throat culture
(E) All affected persons, even those without carditis, should receive antibiotic prophylaxis for at least 5 years

192. A 64-year-old man with aortic stenosis is admitted to the hospital because of the recent onset of congestive heart failure. True statements characterizing his condition include which of the following?

(A) The development of atrial fibrillation (ventricular response of 70 beats per minute) could explain the deterioration of his condition
(B) The absence of left ventricular hypertrophy on the electrocardiogram excludes severe obstruction
(C) Absence of aortic valve calcification on echocardiography rules out severe aortic stenosis
(D) Once his congestive heart failure is treated, he may do well for several more years
(E) If an echocardiogram shows cusp calcification, then his aortic stenosis is likely to be severe

193. True statements regarding balloon valvuloplasty include

(A) balloon dilation of a stenotic pulmonary valve is not feasible because of the danger of rupture of the thin-walled pulmonary artery
(B) mitral valvuloplasty increases the effective diastolic valve area to normal size
(C) balloon aortic valvuloplasty is contraindicated in calcific aortic stenosis because the fracture of calcium deposits on the leaflets leads to cerebral emboli
(D) the restenosis rate after aortic valvuloplasty is 40 percent during the first year after the procedure
(E) aortic valvuloplasty results in symptomatic improvement for most patients

194. True statements regarding hemodynamic changes occurring during exercise include which of the following?

(A) Venous return is augmented by the pumping action of skeletal muscles
(B) The increased adrenergic nerve impulses to the heart as well as an increased concentration of circulating catecholamines help to augment the contractile state of the myocardium
(C) Venoconstriction in exercising muscles as well as increased cardiac output leads to marked increases in systemic blood pressure
(D) End-diastolic volume increases in the failing heart during exercise
(E) Stroke volume and heart rate increase

195. A 32-year-old woman who has rheumatic mitral valve disease but has been relatively free of symptoms now presents with pulmonary edema. Conditions that could have been responsible for this woman's clinical presentation include

(A) pregnancy
(B) atrial fibrillation
(C) anemia
(D) hypoxia
(E) bacterial endocarditis

196. A 34-year-old woman is bothered by palpitations and chest pain. On auscultation, the first heart sound is normal, but there is a midsystolic click and a late systolic murmur. Her electrocardiogram shows T-wave inversions in leads II, III, and aVF. True statements concerning her condition include which of the following?

(A) An exercise stress test would most likely be positive

(B) An echocardiogram may show abrupt posterior displacement of both mitral leaflets

(C) The woman's chest pain could be due to excessive stress on the papillary muscles

(D) The click and murmur would be expected to occur later in systole when the woman stands

(E) Prophylactic measures should be taken to prevent subacute bacterial endocarditis

197. A permanent atrioventricular sequential pacemaker (DDD) would be preferred to a standard ventricular pacemaker (VVI) in which of the following patients?

(A) A 64-year-old woman with atrial fibrillation and a ventricular rate of 40 beats per minute

(B) A 56-year-old man with complete heart block and a global left ventricular ejection fraction of 36 percent

(C) An active 46-year-old man with high-grade atrioventricular block

(D) An 80-year-old woman with symptomatic bradyarrhythmias and normal left ventricular function

(E) A 50-year-old man with hypertrophic cardiomyopathy and infranodal second-degree atrioventricular block

198. A 58-year-old man with a history of severe hypertension, three prior myocardial infarctions, and a left ventricular ejection fraction of 15 percent, presents with a 30-pound weight loss. Workup for malignancy is negative. Which of the following factors could explain the patient's cachexia and weight loss?

(A) Digitalis intoxication

(B) Protein loss in the gastrointestinal tract due to high right-sided pressures

(C) Elevation of the metabolic rate

(D) Malabsorption of nutrients

(E) Incomplete gastric filling

199. Correct statements regarding cardiac transplantation include

(A) the 5-year survival is greater than 90 percent

(B) two P waves are typically evident on the electrocardiogram of patients with a transplanted heart

(C) risk factors for accelerated coronary vascular disease include the number of rejection episodes and hyperlipidemia

(D) rejection accounts for the majority of late ($>$ 1 year after transplant) deaths

(E) immunosuppressive drugs can be discontinued after 5 years since the risk of rejection after that point is extremely low

200. A 70-year-old man with a history of the "bradytachy syndrome" treated by insertion of a ventricular demand pacemaker (VVI) develops fatigue, dizziness, and syncope. Assuming no deterioration in his intrinsic cardiac function, which of the following factors could account for his symptoms?

(A) Pacemaker-mediated triggering of tachyarrhythmias due to ventriculoatrial conduction

(B) Loss of atrial contribution to ventricular systole

(C) Large a waves on the jugular venous pulse

(D) Systemic and pulmonary venous regurgitation due to atrial contraction against a closed AV valve

(E) Intermittent ventricular tachycardia induced by chronic irritation of the right ventricular wall by the pacemaker lead

201. A 50-year-old woman with a history of hypertension (but who is taking no medication currently) presents to the emergency ward with a complaint of sudden palpitations and faintness. Her pulse is 120 and the 12-lead ECG discloses a wide-complex tachycardia. Which of the following characteristics would suggest a ventricular origin for her tachycardia rather than supraventricular tachycardia with aberrant conduction?

(A) A QRS complex of 0.12 s

(B) A QRS complex of 0.22 s

(C) Retrograde P waves with the same beat-to-beat association with each QRS complex

(D) A positive QRS direction in each precordial lead

(E) A Q wave in lead V_6 and a broad R wave in V_1

202. Correct statements regarding coronary artery bypass grafting (CABG) include which of the following?

(A) Between 10 and 20 percent of saphenous venous grafts occlude in the first postoperative year
(B) Approximately 85 percent of patients will have an improvement in angina
(C) CABG is contraindicated in patients with severe three-vessel coronary disease and an ejection fraction of 35 percent
(D) Saphenous venous coronary grafts to the left anterior descending artery have a higher patency rate than internal mammary artery grafts
(E) In a patient with normal ventricular function, the surgical mortality is approximately 5 percent

203. True statements about the side effects of antiarrhythmic drugs include which of the following?

(A) Verapamil can cause hemodynamic collapse if administered to patients with sustained ventricular tachycardia
(B) Blue-gray skin pigmentation, thyroid abnormalities, and corneal deposits are seen with prolonged use of flecainide
(C) Thrombocytopenia is a well-recognized, occasional consequence of procainamide
(D) Glaucoma can develop after the institution of disopyramide for ventricular tachycardia
(E) Quinidine can precipitate digitalis toxicity

204. Blood levels of high-density lipoprotein are increased by

(A) estrogens
(B) androgens
(C) cigarette smoking
(D) alcohol
(E) jogging

205. True statements regarding the cardiac effects of hyperthyroidism include which of the following?

(A) Cardiac symptoms of angina and congestive heart failure are resistant to treatment
(B) Pericardial effusion is frequent
(C) Atrial fibrillation is frequent
(D) Density of myocardial beta receptors is increased
(E) Voltage typically is low on electrocardiography

206. A 23-year-old man has had recent onset of exertional dyspnea. A grade III/VI systolic murmur is heard at the left sternal border. Electrocardiography shows apical and lateral Q waves and left ventricular hypertrophy. Echocardiography reveals asymmetrical septal hypertrophy without evidence of obstruction. Correct statements regarding this clinical situation include which of the following?

(A) The man's dyspnea is best explained by lateral wall infarction
(B) First-degree relatives should be evaluated
(C) The risk of sudden death is low
(D) Calcium-channel blockers may relieve symptoms
(E) The man's heart is normal histologically, aside from changes of infarction

207. Aortic regurgitation is accurately characterized by which of the following statements?

(A) Most cases of aortic regurgitation (with or without associated lesions) are due to congenital (including Marfan's syndrome), syphilitic, or spondylitic causes
(B) Quincke's pulse refers to the pistol-shot sound audible over the femoral arteries
(C) The Graham Steell murmur of pulmonary regurgitation is frequently associated
(D) The echocardiogram frequently reveals fluttering of the anterior leaflet of the mitral valve
(E) Surgical correction can be delayed if the patient is asymptomatic and retains normal left ventricular function

208. True statements with respect to the use of vasodilator drugs in the treatment of chronic congestive heart failure include which of the following?

(A) Reflex tachycardia is expected with administration of afterload reducing agents
(B) Afterload reducing agents reduce left ventricular end-diastolic pressure and stroke volume
(C) Nitrates are more potent afterload reducing agents than hydralazine
(D) Captopril dilates both the venous and arterial beds, resulting in elevation of cardiac output and reduction in left ventricular filling pressure
(E) Despite the ability of angiotensin-converting enzyme (ACE) inhibitors to result in symptomatic improvement, there is no proven survival benefit in patients with chronic congestive heart failure

209. Correct statements regarding the laboratory evaluation of suspected myocardial infarction include which of the following?

(A) Creatine phosphokinase usually rises 4 h after a myocardial infarction
(B) A rise in lactic dehydrogenase (LDH) following the death of myocardium may persist for 14 days
(C) Increased LDH isoenzyme 1 (LDH$_1$) is a more sensitive indicator of myocardial infarction than is total LDH
(D) In hypothyroid patients, serum creatine phosphokinase levels will not rise even after a myocardial infarction
(E) The opening of a coronary occlusion after an infarction will lead to a delayed and blunted elevation of creatine phosphokinase

210. In which of the following patients would drug therapy of a known or potential infarction-associated ventricular arrhythmia be appropriate initial management?

(A) A 48-year-old man with precordial ST elevations and 100 unifocal ventricular premature beats per hour
(B) A 60-year-old man with inferior infarction and three consecutive ventricular premature beats in the first hour of observation in the CCU
(C) A 60-year-old woman with subendocardial ischemia, ventricular tachycardia, and a blood pressure falling from 120 to 80 mmHg
(D) A 40-year-old man with precordial ST elevations and a single ventricular ectopic beat, which occurred early in diastole
(E) A 50-year-old woman with an inferoposterior myocardial infarction who is sustaining 30 min of ventricular tachycardia despite lidocaine bolus therapy; she is alert and has a blood pressure of 120 and clear lungs

211. Which of the following findings would likely be present in a patient who sustained recurrent pulmonary emboli?

(A) Decreased lung volumes on spirometric testing
(B) Enlarged P waves on electrocardiographic examination
(C) Tricuspid regurgitant flow on Doppler echocardiography
(D) Positive right ventricular uptake on thallium 201 scintigraphy
(E) Prominent *a* waves on physical examination of jugular venous pulsation

212. True statements regarding the effect of alcohol on the heart include which of the following?

(A) Chronic ingestion of alcohol will lead to a restrictive cardiomyopathy
(B) Once heart failure develops, discontinuing consumption of alcohol will not appreciably affect the natural history of the disease
(C) If thiamine deficiency is present in the alcoholic, high output failure is noted
(D) If the patient with heart failure due to ethanol continues to drink, he or she is unlikely to be alive in 3 years
(E) The most common arrhythmia associated with a drinking binge is ventricular tachycardia

213. A 45-year-old woman with a history of metastatic breast cancer develops shortness of breath, cardiomegaly, and elevated neck veins. Findings consistent with pericardial involvement by tumor include

(A) a right ventricular free-wall collapse during left ventricular systole on the echocardiogram
(B) a 15 mmHg decrease in systolic arterial pressure during inspiration
(C) a prominent *x* descent on jugular venous pressure tracing
(D) pericardial pressure equal to right atrial pressure
(E) left ventricular systolic pressure equal to right ventricular end-systolic pressure

214. True statements regarding cardiac neoplasms include

(A) lymphoma is the most common malignant neoplasm to primarily involve the heart
(B) the most common site for a myxoma is the left atrium
(C) myxomas may arise as part of a familial syndrome that also includes pigmented skin lesions and endocrine abnormalities
(D) a midsystolic "plop" typically indicates the presence of a cardiac myxoma
(E) weight loss and fever are frequent presenting manifestations of cardiac myxoma

215. True statements regarding risk factors for accelerated atherosclerosis include which of the following?

(A) Increasing risk for the development of premature heart disease can be detected at serum cholesterol levels higher than 5.2 mmol/L (200 mg/dL)

(B) Hypertriglyceridemia without a concomitant increase in cholesterol level is an independent risk factor for premature ischemic heart disease

(C) All adults should have at least one lipoprotein electrophoresis as part of routine health care screening

(D) Hyperlipidemia may be exacerbated by any of the following conditions: hypothyroidism, uremia, diabetes mellitus, and multiple myeloma

(E) Reduction of serum glucose levels in a patient with diabetes mellitus will lower the risk of development of premature atherosclerosis

216. For the purpose of diagnosing secondary causes of high blood pressure, which of the following patients with hypertension should have workup beyond routine laboratory studies (blood urea nitrogen, glucose, creatinine, calcium, uric acid, potassium, cholesterol, triglycerides, electrocardiogram, and chest x-ray)?

(A) A 35-year-old man with a prior history of normotension who presents with a blood pressure of 160/105, but otherwise normal physical examination

(B) A 35-year-old woman with a prior history of normotension who presents with a blood pressure of 160/105 and an abdominal bruit

(C) A 60-year-old man with a prior history of normotension who presents with a blood pressure of 160/100

(D) A 40-year-old woman with a prior history of normotension who presents with a blood pressure of 160/105 unresponsive to enalapril and hydrochlorothiazide

(E) A 45-year-old man with an unknown prior history who presents with a blood pressure of 160/100 and left ventricular heave on physical examination

217. True statements regarding the pharmacologic treatment of hypertension include which of the following?

(A) Side effects of thiazide diuretics include hypokalemia, hyperuricemia, hyperglycemia, hypercalcemia, and hyperlipidemia

(B) Clonidine is a centrally acting alpha agonist

(C) Continuous infusion of diazoxide can be useful in the treatment of malignant hypertension only in conjunction with monitoring of arterial blood pressure

(D) Prazosin, like hydralazine, is a direct vasodilator that can cause reflex tachycardia

(E) Angiotensin-converting enzyme inhibitors, because of their effect on serum renin levels, are the drugs of choice for patients with renal insufficiency

218. Peripheral arterial insufficiency is correctly characterized by which of the following statements?

(A) Pentoxifylline is useful in the treatment of patients with claudication

(B) At least 70 percent of femoral occlusions treated with a saphenous vein bypass graft remain open at 5 years

(C) Patients with claudication should be advised to stay off their feet until a definitive treatment plan is outlined

(D) A ratio of ankle to brachial artery pressures of 1.2:1 indicates arterial occlusive disease

(E) Pain at rest due to arterial insufficiency mandates either angioplasty or arterial reconstruction

DIRECTIONS: Each group of questions below consists of lettered headings followed by a set of numbered items. For each numbered item select the **one** lettered heading with which it is **most** closely associated. Each lettered heading may be used **once, more than once, or not at all.**

Questions 219–223

For each of the disorders below, select the characteristic hemodynamic pattern.

(A)   Equalization of diastolic pressures
(B)   Dip-and-plateau pattern
(C)   Slow *y* descent
(D)   Tall *v* wave
(E)   None of the above

219. Pericardial tamponade

220. Amyloidosis

221. Mitral stenosis

222. Acute mitral regurgitation

223. Acute septal rupture

Questions 224–227

For each syndrome below, select the associated cardiovascular abnormality.

(A)   Coarctation of the aorta
(B)   Pulmonic stenosis
(C)   Mitral regurgitation
(D)   Endocardial cushion defect
(E)   Cor pulmonale

224. Marfan's syndrome

225. Turner's syndrome

226. Congenital rubella

227. Cystic fibrosis

Questions 228–231

Match each of the causes of right heart failure below with the most characteristic set of hemodynamic measurements.

	Right atrial pressure, mmHg	Pulmonary arterial pressure, mmHg	Pulmonary capillary wedge pressure, mmHg
(A)	16	75/30	11
(B)	16	35/17	16
(C)	16	100/30	28
(D)	16	45/22	20
(E)	16	22/12	10
Normal values	0–5	12–28/3–13	3–11

228. Right ventricular infarction

229. Cor pulmonale from bronchitis

230. Mitral stenosis

231. Constrictive pericarditis

Disorders of the Heart and Vascular System

Answers

129. The answer is B. *(Wilson, ed 12. chap 189.)* The combination of hypotension and bradycardia suggests a vagal response in the setting of an acute myocardial infarction. Administration of the anticholinergic agent atropine is the treatment of choice. If the bradyarrhythmia and hypotension persist after 2.0 mg of atropine has been administered in divided doses, insertion of a temporary pacemaker is indicated. Isoproterenol should be avoided in patients with acute myocardial infarction since it may greatly increase myocardial oxygen consumption and thereby intensify ischemia. Volume replacement or inotropic support may be required if hypotension persists after correction of the bradyarrhythmia, but they are not indicated as initial therapies.

130. The answer is A. *(Wilson, ed 12. chap 196.)* Captopril is an inhibitor of angiotensin-converting enzyme, and thus it impairs the production of angiotensin II, a potent vasoconstrictor. Through removal of feedback inhibition, renin secretion is *increased*. Additional antihypertension effects of captopril result from a reduction of bradykinin degradation and stimulation of vasodilating prostaglandin production. Converting enzyme inhibitors can be added to a regimen of beta blockade for an additional antihypertensive effect. Captopril is contraindicated in patients with bilateral renal artery stenosis, since reduction in systemic arterial pressure may lead to progressive renal hypoperfusion.

131. The answer is D. *(Wilson, ed 12. chap 196.)* The beta blocking agents are effective antihypertensive and antianginal agents. Beta₁ cardioselective agents include metoprolol and atenolol. Although these two drugs may be safer than the other agents for patients with bronchospasm, selectivity is lost with larger doses, and they are relatively contraindicated in those with lung disease. Nadolol and atenolol can be administered on a once-a-day regimen by virtue of their long half-lives. Pindolol is a nonselective beta blocking agent with partial agonist activity, resulting in less bradycardia than the other agents. Labetolol has both beta- and alpha-receptor antagonist actions.

132. The answer is C. *(Wilson, ed 12. chap 193.)* The lateral-view chest film demonstrates calcification of the anterior pericardium, consistent with constrictive pericarditis. This pattern is seen in approximately one-half of patients with long-standing constriction, and pericardial thickening can often be confirmed by echocardiography. In patients with this disease, a pericardial knock is often heard 0.06 to 0.12 s after aortic valve closure, corresponding to the sudden cessation of ventricular filling. Murmurs are typically absent.

133. The answer is E. *(Wilson, ed 12. chap 177.)* Two-dimensional and M-mode echocardiograms directly image the intracardiac valves and are extremely useful in the detection of valvular stenosis. Doppler echocardiography permits the calculation of the pressure gradient across the intracardiac valves. Regurgitant lesions, such as those of the tricuspid valve, can be detected and the severity estimated by this technique. Although the echocardiographic findings of atrial septal defect are nonspecific (right ventricular volume overload pattern), Doppler studies can determine the presence of the transatrial shunt. Coronary calcification cannot at present be imaged with a high degree of sensitivity.

134. The answer is E. *(Wilson, ed 12. chap 21.)* Chronic idiopathic orthostatic hypotension, most common among elderly men, is characterized by orthostatic hypotension in the absence of reflex tachycardia. Other autonomic disturbances typically are present, including anhidrosis, difficulty with urination, and constipation. In this condition, peripheral norepinephrine synthesis is deficient and plasma norepinephrine levels are low. Treatment consists of increasing intravascular volume and venous return and administering directly acting sympathomimetic agents. Tyramine and other indirectly acting sympathomimetic agents are not helpful. In central preganglionic autonomic insufficiency, a condition related to chronic idiopathic orthostatic hypotension, peripheral norepinephrine stores and plasma levels are normal but release of norepinephrine is deficient; this condition, which has a variety of central nervous system manifestations, may respond to tyramine.

135. The answer is E. *(Wilson, ed 12. chap 190.)* PTCA is now widely used to revascularize suitable coronary lesions. Although adequate dilation is achieved in more than 85 percent of patients, recurrent stenosis develops in approximately 20 percent within 6 months. Angioplasty has been successfully performed on obstructive lesions within bypass grafts and in patients with recent total occlusion (within 3 months) of native coronaries. Significant left main artery disease ordinarily remains a contraindication to the procedure; coronary artery bypass grafting appears to be safer at present. The success rate of repeated PTCA is actually *better* than that of the first procedure.

136. The answer is E. *(Wilson, ed 12. chap 182.)* Many persons who have ankle edema are inappropriately diagnosed as having heart failure. In particular, the diagnosis of right heart failure should not be made in the absence of jugular venous distention. Venous varicosities, cyclic edema, thrombophlebitis, and hypoalbuminemia all cause ankle edema and should be considered in the differential diagnosis.

137. The answer is C. *(Wilson, ed 12. chap 182.)* Congestive heart failure associated with pulmonary and systemic venous congestion may occur either with low cardiac output and widened arterial–mixed venous oxygen difference or with high output and normal or narrowed arterial–mixed venous oxygen difference. High-output states are associated with unusually low systemic vascular resistance and peripheral shunting. If Paget's disease is widespread, increased bony vascularity and overlying cutaneous vasodilation can lead to shunting and a high-output state. Venous congestion occurs when the ventricles are unable to handle the increased venous return.

138. The answer is E. *(Wilson, ed 12. chap 182.)* Digitalis glycosides augment contractility of the heart and slow atrioventricular conduction and heart rate. The primary mechanism of action is inhibition of Na^+-K^+-ATPase, which is located in the sarcolemmal membrane. This action leads to intracellular accumulation of sodium and, subsequently, calcium by way of a sodium-calcium exchange mechanism.

139. The answer is D. *(Wilson, ed 12. chap 182.)* Elderly persons are particularly prone to develop digitalis intoxication at relatively low doses and apparently normal serum levels (<2.0 pg/L). Exacerbating factors in the development of toxicity are hypoxemia and hypercalcemia. Potassium wasting and, perhaps, hypomagnesemia from potent loop diuretics also can foster toxicity. By mechanisms not yet elucidated, quinidine can increase the serum levels of digoxin, thereby inducing toxicity. Hyperthyroidism tends to decrease the efficacy of digitalis, while hypothyroidism enhances the likelihood of toxicity.

140. The answer is E. *(Wilson, ed 12. chap 184.)* The escape focus in atrioventricular nodal block is relatively high in the conduction system, in an area of vagal innervation. Thus, a beneficial response to vagolytic drugs, such as atropine, is usually apparent. The rate at the escape focus is relatively rapid, and the QRS complex is narrow. Unless complete heart block persists, some Wenckebach periodicity can be observed. Inferior myocardial infarction, mitral valve surgery, and digitalis toxicity can lead to atrioventricular nodal block.

141. The answer is D. *(Wilson, ed 12. chap 184.)* Sinus bradycardia and a long sinus pause raise the possibility of sick sinus syndrome, which is not an infrequent cause of lightheadedness among the elderly. It is important that the relationship between symptoms and the arrhythmias documented by Holter monitoring be clarified before implantation of a permanent pacemaker is considered. An exercise tolerance test, though it may strengthen the suspicion of sick sinus syndrome by showing an inadequate heart rate response, cannot prove that the condition is responsible for the patient's symptoms. Sublingual isoproterenol has little usefulness in the management of chronic bradyarrhythmias.

142. The answer is B. *(Wilson, ed 12. chap 185.)* The rhythm demonstrated in the electrocardiogram presented is multifocal atrial tachycardia, which is characterized by variable P-wave morphology and PR and RR intervals. Control of multifocal atrial tachycardia, usually associated with severe pulmonary disease, comes with improved ventilation and oxygenation. Carotid sinus massage, electrical cardioversion, and administration of digitalis, verapamil, or quinidine are of little benefit, although verapamil may temporarily slow the ventricular rate.

143. The answer is D. *(Wilson, ed 12. chap 185.)* The ventricular rate in atrial flutter can be decreased by interfering with atrioventricular conduction and slowing the atrial rate. Quinidine slows the rate but enhances conduction; the net result is 1:1 conduction at a somewhat slower atrial rate and a more rapid ventricular rate. Quinidine thus should not be used to treat atrial flutter without the addition of digoxin, verapamil, or propranolol to block atrioventricular conduction.

144. The answer is C. *(Wilson, ed 12. chap 186.)* Atrial septal defect (ASD) is usually asymptomatic in childhood. Clinical presentation occurs in the third or fourth decade of life and results from atrial arrhythmias and pulmonary hypertension. A frequent cause of symptoms and of right heart failure is coexistent left ventricular dysfunction—even mild left atrial pressure elevation is not tolerated well when transmitted into the systemic venous circulation. Secundum atrial septal defect is associated with a rightward axis on electrocardiography; the axis is leftward in primum defects. Echocardiography also reveals evidence of right ventricular volume overload, including abnormal motion of the ventricular septum (i.e., right-to-left movement) during diastole. Though small shunts are well tolerated, operative repair is usually indicated when the pulmonary flow is at least 1.5 times the systemic flow.

145. The answer is B. *(Wilson, ed 12. chaps 178, 188.)* The echocardiographic studies demonstrate thickening and calcification of the aortic valve, with minimal leaflet separation in systole—findings consistent with aortic stenosis. Doppler echocardiography can be useful in estimating the severity of the aortic disease as follows: Peak gradient across the valve $= 4 \times$ (peak velocity)^2. In this case, the peak velocity distal to the valve is 5 m/s, yielding a peak gradient of 100 mmHg, which suggests significant aortic stenosis. No diastolic turbulence was detected, which rules against aortic regurgitation. Although severe aortic stenosis may be the cause of this patient's exertional chest pain, coronary arteriography is indicated to rule out significant coronory arterial disease, which may require coronary artery bypass grafting along with aortic valve replacement.

146. The answer is B. *(Wilson, ed 12. chaps 186, 188.)* The chest x-rays presented in the question show enlargement of the right ventricle and main pulmonary artery and pulmonary vascular plethora, or "shunt" vasculature—classic findings for an atrial septal defect, which could well be asymptomatic in a 36-year-old woman. The chest x-ray of a patient with mitral stenosis and hemoptysis and dyspnea would show left atrial enlargement, even in the presence of primary or secondary tricuspid regurgitation, ascites, and a large jugular venous *v* wave. Continuous murmur, widened systemic pulse pressure, and dyspnea on exertion combine to suggest patent ductus arteriosus, which would produce x-ray evidence of left ventricular and perhaps left atrial enlargement and shunt vasculature without right ventricular enlargement.

147. The answer is E. *(Wilson, ed 12. chap 186.)* Adults with mild pulmonic stenosis are generally asymptomatic. Unlike congenital aortic stenosis, this condition usually does not progress; thus, followup need not be frequent. The risk of endocarditis is somewhat lower for pulmonic valves than for the other heart valves, whether normal or stenotic. Clinical signs of mild pulmonic stenosis include prominent *a* wave on jugular venous pulse, normal electrocardiogram, and normal cardiac size on chest x-ray.

148. The answer is C. *(Wilson, ed 12. chap 186.)* Coarctation of the aorta usually occurs just distal to the origin of the left subclavian artery; if it arises above the left subclavian, blood pressure elevation may only be evident in the right arm. The associated murmur is continuous only if obstruction is severe; otherwise, a systolic ejection murmur is heard anteriorly and over the back. Coarctation of the aorta commonly is accompanied by a bicuspid aortic valve, which can produce the diastolic murmur of aortic regurgitation. X-ray findings include the "3" sign, caused by aortic dilation just proximal and distal to the area of stenosis, and rib notching, caused by increased collateral circulation through dilated intercostal arteries. Hypertension is the major clinical problem and may persist even after complete surgical correction. Unless hypertension is very severe, or left ventricular failure has ensued, cardiac output responds normally to exercise.

149. The answer is B. *(Wilson, ed 12. chap 38.)* A fall in cardiac output from any cause leads to a decrease in effective arterial blood volume. Increased release of renin from juxtaglomerular cells in the kidney leads to the release of angiotensin I from its hepatically synthesized substrate, angiotensinogen. The decapeptide angiotensin I is proteolytically cleaved to angiotensin II, a vasoconstrictor and secretagogue for aldosterone. After release from the adrenal gland, aldosterone leads to renal proximal tubular salt and water retention. Renal vasoconstriction, which also causes proximal sodium absorption by increasing the filtration fraction, is also caused by the augmented sympathetic nervous system activity associated with a diminished cardiac output.

150. The answer is C. *(Wilson, ed 12. chap 198.)* Although each of the items listed is a potential source of peripheral embolism, the most common source is the heart. The lesions that predispose to this development include mural left ventricular thrombus (associated with recent myocardial infarction or cardiomyopathy), left atrial thrombus associated with atrial fibrillation or mitral valve disease, and valvular thrombus, especially of a prosthetic valve.

151. The answer is A. *(Wilson, ed 12. chap 190.)* Nitrates are generalized smooth-muscle dilators whose direct effect on the vasculature is not blocked by any agents presently available. Long-acting preparations of nitroglycerin may be completely degraded by the liver in some patients and thus are generally less effective than sublingual forms. Because individual variability in metabolism is considerable, dosages should be titrated against side effects and should not conform to a rigidly standardized regimen. Tolerance is common and must be considered if a patient fails to respond to a previously efficacious dose. Nitroglycerin ointment is absorbed well through any noncornified skin; application to the chest only adds a placebo effect to the therapeutic one.

152. The answer is B. *(Wilson, ed 12. chap 185.)* The rhythm strip shows polymorphic ventricular tachycardia characteristic of torsades de pointes ("twisting of the points"). This life-threatening rhythm is associated with prolongation of the QT interval, resulting, in this case, from the administration of quinidine. The appropriate therapy is to discontinue the offending agent and to withhold other agents that prolong the QT interval, such as procainamide. Hypokalemia can also prolong the QT interval and result in this rhythm; however, this patient had normal serum electrolyte concentrations.

153. The answer is D. *(Wilson, ed 12. chap 188.)* The echocardiogram shows that the left atrium is enlarged, and there is calcification and thickening of the mitral valve and chordal apparatus. The mitral leaflets show diastolic doming, resulting from fusion of the valve commissures. These are the typical findings of rheumatic mitral stenosis, exemplified by this 42-year-old woman. The aortic leaflets are also mildly thickened, consistent with rheumatic disease. The symptoms of the patient described in Option A are suggestive of a left atrial myxoma. The patient in Option B has acute mitral regurgitation. The patient in Option C has mitral valve prolapse.

154. The answer is A. *(Wilson, ed 12. chap 189.)* The man described in the question probably has a right ventricular infarction complicating his inferior myocardial infarction, because right atrial pressure is elevated out of proportion to the left atrial (pulmonary capillary wedge) pressure. Cardiac output is probably depressed, given the low left-heart filling pressure. The best treatment consists of administration of fluids.

155. The answer is E. *(Wilson, ed 12. chap 173. Jarcho, N Engl J Med 321:1372, 1989.)* Thyroid hormone acts directly on nuclear receptors to regulate myosin heavy chain gene transcription, thus increasing the level of myosin enzyme V1 (fast myosin), whereas in response to pressure load on the heart, fetal forms of myosin such as V3 (slow myosin) are induced. The c-*sis* proto-oncogene, which encodes for the B chain of platelet-derived growth factor; c-*myc* and c-*fos*, which code for nuclear proteins involved in regulation of the cell cycle; and c-*ras*, which encodes for guanosine-binding proteins are all induced in myocardial tissue undergoing hypertrophy. Lineage analysis through the use of restriction-fragment length polymorphisms has allowed mapping of a gene associated with familial hypertrophic cardiomyopathy to chromosome 14. Angiotensin II binds to the c-*mas* proto-oncogene product, which bears homology to the beta$_2$-adrenergic receptor, thereby leading to hypertrophy of smooth muscle.

156. The answer is B. *(Wilson, ed 12. chap 175.)* Inspiration, which augments systemic venous return because of negative intrathoracic pressure, will cause accentuation of right-sided murmurs. Prolonged expiratory pressure against a closed glottis (Valsalva maneuver) reduces the intensity of most murmurs by diminishing both right and left ventricular filling. By reducing filling, and thereby reducing chamber size, the murmurs of hypertrophic cardiomyopathy and mitral valve prolapse will increase. The cycle following a premature ventricular beat will have a larger stroke volume so the gradient across an obstructed semilunar valve (aortic or pulmonary) will increase, thereby leading to a louder murmur. Squatting, which increases both venous return and chamber size as well as systemic arterial resistance, increases most murmurs except those due to hypertrophic cardiomyopathy and mitral valve prolapse. Sustained handgrip, which increases heart rate and systemic arterial pressure, often accentuates the murmurs of mitral stenosis and mitral regurgitation by impeding outflow and by decreasing diastolic filling.

157. The answer is B. *(Wilson, ed 12. chap 192.)* Echocardiographic evidence of a disproportionately thickened ventricular septum and systolic anterior motion of the mitral valve strongly suggests idiopathic hypertrophic subaortic stenosis (IHSS). The typical harsh systolic murmur does not usually radiate to the carotid arteries and decreases when ventricular volume enlarges with isometric exercise (e.g., hand grip). The carotid upstroke is brisk, often bifid. Congestive failure often occurs because of reduced ventricular compliance despite normal ventricular systolic function. Malposition of the mitral apparatus, a result of the distorted septum, often leads to some degree of mitral regurgitation.

158. The answer is B. *(Wilson, ed 12. chap 176.)* A delta wave or slowed QRS upstroke is depicted. This finding occurs in the Wolff-Parkinson-White syndrome in which accessory Kent bundles result in an apparently short PR interval caused by the bypassed AV node and early onset of the QRS complex. Left bundle branch block could result in marked initial delay, whereas right bundle branch block results in late delay. Left ventricular hypertrophy causes minor uniform QRS prolongation. Right ventricular infarction has little effect on QRS duration in the absence of right bundle branch block.

159. The answer is D. *(Wilson, ed 12. chaps 177, 178.)* Lack of motion (akinesis) in a segment of myocardium visualized by echo indicates tissue death, as does an area of reduced thallium accumulation during exercise that fails to "fill in" at rest. Since pyrophosphate appears to bind calcium and macromolecules in irreversibly damaged myocardial cells, an area of increased uptake indicates myocardial infarction if the injection is performed between 48 and 72 h after suspected transmural infarction. Using a combination of $[^{13}N]H_3$ (blood flow marker) and $[^{18}F]$deoxyglucose (glucose uptake), positron emission tomography can identify nonviable myocardium if there is a defect in the uptake of both isotopes. Standard computed tomography cannot detect global or regional left ventricular function, although fast, or cine, CT may be able to detect infarction by monitoring changes in ventricular volume and wall thickness.

160. The answer is C. *(Wilson, ed 12. chap 193.)* Acute pericarditis is associated with ST-segment elevation and, frequently, PR-segment depression. Usually, reciprocal ST-segment depression is not present. T waves begin to invert only *after* the ST segment becomes isoelectric. Elevations in serum creatine phosphokinase levels to twice normal may be associated with uncomplicated pericarditis.

161. The answer is E. *(Wilson, ed 12. chap 180.)* While some degree of local vascular dissection occurs in virtually all PTCA procedures, more extensive dissection can lead to abrupt closure of the dilated segment soon after withdrawal of the balloon catheter. Vasodilators such as nitrates and calcium channel antagonists, anticoagulation (heparin), and antiplatelet therapy can help prevent early vessel closure caused by spasm or thrombus formation. If closure does occur, repeat PTCA may be helpful. Emergency coronary artery bypass surgery is required in only 2 percent of all PTCA attempts.

162. The answer is C. *(Wilson, ed 12. chap 182.)* Digitalis glycosides are effective in increasing myocardial contractility and in treatment of certain atrial tachyarrhythmias. However, digoxin actually increases myocardial automaticity (increase in premature beats) and facilitates reentry (atrial tachycardias). Digoxin also slows conduction through AV nodal tissue and has central effects that can mimic vagal influence on the heart and may thus produce sinus arrest. Paroxysmal atrial tachycardia with variable block represents the classic rhythm of digitalis intoxication. Digoxin is profibrillatory, but its administration should not lead to atrial flutter.

163. The answer is E. *(Wilson, ed 12. chap 197.)* Complications of dissection of the aorta include loss of a major pulse, dissection into the pericardial or pleural space, and acute aortic regurgitation. When these events occur, surgical intervention is required. Because the risk of these complications is higher in persons with dissection of the ascending aorta, these persons usually are treated surgically. In contrast, persons with dissection of the descending aorta often can be treated medically. Persistence of pain, which suggests that dissection is continuing, is another indication for surgery.

164. The answer is C. *(Wilson, ed 12. chap 186.)* Left-to-right shunts occur in all types of atrial and ventricular septal defects, but generally do not result in cyanosis, whereas large right-to-left shunts frequently do. The magnitude of the shunt depends on the size of the defect, the diastolic properties of both ventricles, and the relative impedance of the pulmonary and systemic circulations. Defects of the sinus venosus type occur high in the atrial septum near the entry of the superior vena cava or lower near the orifice of the inferior vena cava and may be associated with anomalous connection of the right inferior pulmonary vein to the right atrium. In the case of anomalous origin of the left coronary artery from the pulmonary artery, as pulmonary vascular resistance declines immediately after birth, perfusion of the left coronary artery from the pulmonary trunk ceases and the direction of flow in the anomalous vessel reverses. Twenty percent of patients with this defect can survive to adulthood owing to myocardial blood supply totally through the right coronary artery. In the absence of pulmonary hypertension, blood will flow from the aorta to the pulmonary artery throughout the cardiac cycle, which results in a "continuous" murmur at the left sternal border. In total anomalous pulmonary venous connection, all the venous blood returns to the right atrium; therefore, an interatrial communication is required and right-to-left shunts with cyanosis are common.

165. The answer is C. *(Wilson, ed 12. chap 187.)* Two major criteria or one major and two minor criteria indicate a high probability of rheumatic fever in the presence of evidence of preceding streptococcal infection (history of scarlet fever, elevated ASO titer, or positive throat culture). The major criteria include carditis (new heart murmur, increase in heart size, pericardial friction rub, or CHF), polyarthritis, chorea (usually a delayed manifestation), erythema marginatum, and subcutaneous nodules. The minor criteria, which are relatively common and nonspecific, include fever, arthralgia, previous rheumatic fever or rheumatic heart disease, elevated erythrocyte sedimentation rate (ESR), or prolonged PR interval.

166. The answer is D. *(Wilson, ed 12. chap 197.)* Factors predisposing to aortic dissection include hypertension (present in at least 70 percent of cases), cystic medial necrosis, Marfan's syndrome, coarctation, bicuspid aortic valve, and third trimester of pregnancy. Dissection of the aorta is a disease of the media, either from arteriosclerosis or cystic medial necrosis. The associated intimal tear that initiates the dissection almost always begins in the ascending aorta (2 to 5 cm above the valve) or just distal to the left subclavian artery; at these two points the aorta is relatively fixed, so that shear forces are increased. Type I dissections extend around the aortic arch and can affect the abdominal aorta; most type II dissections proceed variably into the arch or reach the left subclavian artery. Dissection can result in aortic rupture, which can result in a false aneurysm (an "aneurysm" contained within the adventitia or a clot) or, if the dissection is of the ascending aorta, in hemopericardium. Medical therapy should be aimed at reducing both cardiac contractility and systemic arterial pressure in order to reduce shear stress on the aortic wall. This can be accomplished either by labetolol, a combined alpha and beta blocker, or by simultaneous administration of nitroprusside and a beta blocker.

167. The answer is D. *(Wilson, ed 12. chap 189.)* While prompt initiation of thrombolytic therapy during an acute myocardial infarction is associated with improvement in mortality and limitation of the size of infarct, all thrombolytic agents, including tissue plasminogen activator, are associated with an increased risk of major bleeding. These agents should not be given if there is a history of a cerebrovascular accident, a surgical procedure within 2 weeks, active peptic ulcer disease, or marked hypertension during acute presentation (systolic pressure greater than 180 or diastolic pressure greater than 100 mmHg). Other situations in which the risk of bleeding might be higher (such as advanced age) are not absolute contraindications, but the potential benefit of administration of thrombolytic therapy should be carefully considered in each case.

168. The answer is C. *(Wilson, ed 12. chap 189.)* Apical systolic murmurs associated with a myocardial infarction may represent either mitral regurgitation (on the basis of papillary muscle rupture or newly dilated heart size) or ventricular septal defect. In both conditions large *v* waves may be recorded in the pulmonary capillary wedge position. In the case of ventricular septal defect, but not mitral regurgitation, there will be an increase in the partial pressure of oxygen as a catheter is advanced from the right atrium to the right ventricle.

169. The answer is D. *(Wilson, ed 12. chap 190.)* Any patient with recent onset of severe and frequent angina, accelerating angina, or angina at rest is considered to have unstable angina. Such patients are likely to have one or more stenoses in major coronary arteries and require emergent management. Hospitalization with identification and treatment of predisposing conditions (heart failure, fever, thyrotoxicosis) is indicated. Since thrombus formation frequently complicates this condition, intravenous heparin followed by oral aspirin should be given. Beta blockers and calcium channel blocking drugs should be administered if possible. Antiarrhythmics are only required in the presence of specific arrhythmias. Intravenous nitroglycerin is effective, but requires continuous blood pressure monitoring.

170. The answer is A. *(Wilson, ed 12. chap 192.)* The cardiac catheterization findings described are consistent with increased impedance to ventricular filling as may be seen in either restrictive cardiomyopathies or constrictive pericarditis. Restrictive cardiomyopathies often are due to myocardial infiltration with neoplastic cells, eosinophils, iron, amyloid, or fibrous tissue. The transmural necrosis noted in patients with Duchenne's muscular dystrophy can lead to a dilated cardiomyopathy.

171. The answer is B. *(Wilson, ed 12. chap 198.)* Conditions associated with stasis, vascular damage, or hypercoagulability lead to an increased risk for deep venous thrombosis. Risk is increased by any condition leading to immobility, such as recuperation after a myocardial infarction (of any severity), a major thoracic resection (even if the cancer was completely resected), and trauma or operation involving the hip or leg. A wrist fracture in an elderly woman would probably not lead to any increased risk if her baseline mobility was present. Hypercoagulable states include systemic cancers; pregnancy; exogenous or endogenous estrogens; deficiencies of antithrombin III, protein C, and protein S; circulating lupus anticoagulant (manifested by elevated partial thromboplastin time); or myeloproliferative disease.

172. The answer is D. *(Wilson, ed 12. chap 190. Muller, Ann Intern Med 108:1, 1988. TIMI Study Group, N Engl J Med 320:618, 1989.)* The sooner thrombolytic therapy is started after the onset of symptoms, the greater the likelihood of benefit. Patients treated within 1 to 3 h will benefit most. Though tPA is more effective than streptokinase in restoring patency of vessels, a difference in mortality has not been demonstrated. Although the optimum adjunctive anticoagulant and antiplatelet regimen has not yet been established, up to 325 mg of aspirin and 5000 units of heparin should be given on the day of treatment and continued for up to 5 days. Any evidence for reocclusion, such as recurrent chest pain or ST elevation, should be met with emergent angioplasty, readministration of thrombolytic therapy, or surgical revascularization, depending on circumstances.

173. The answer is A. *(Wilson, ed 12. chap 179.)* A gradient between the left atrium (as measured by the pulmonary capillary wedge tracing) and the left ventricle in diastole indicates mitral stenosis as exemplified by the woman with a history of rheumatic fever and hemoptysis. The intravenous drug abuser with mitral regurgitation caused by a mitral valve vegetation would exhibit large *v* waves on the pulmonary capillary wedge tracing. The aortic regurgitation associated with Marfan's syndrome would cause an equilibration between left ventricular and peripheral pressures. A feature of severe aortic regurgitation occurs when left ventricular pressure exceeds pulmonary capillary wedge (i.e., left atrial) pressure during early diastole, which results in premature mitral valve closure. In aortic stenosis, as exemplified by the elderly man with left ventricular hypertrophy, the left ventricular pressure is higher than aortic pressure during systole. In pericardial tamponade, as might be seen in the patient with lymphoma, there is equalization of right and left diastolic pressures.

174. The answer is A-Y, B-N, C-Y, D-Y, E-N. *(Wilson, ed 12. chap 176.)* The electrocardiographic T wave represents myocardial repolarization, and its configuration can be altered nonspecifically by metabolic abnormalities, drugs, neural activity, and ischemia by a dispersion effect on the activation or repolarization of action potentials. Although myocardial ischemia and subendocardial infarction can produce deep, symmetric T-wave inversions, which would result in tachyarrhythmias and syncope, such noncardiac phenomena as intracerebral hemorrhage can similarly affect ventricular repolarization. Hyperkalemia is manifested by tall, peaked T waves, not inverted ones. Hypocalcemia is manifested by prolonged QT intervals.

175. The answer is A-N, B-Y, C-Y, D-N, E-Y. *(Wilson, ed 12. chap 186.)* In Ebstein's anomaly, the tricuspid leaflets are redundant and positioned lower and further into the right ventricle than usual. Hence, the right atrium appears giant, while the right ventricle is small and hypoplastic. Tricuspid regurgitation is frequent. Most affected persons survive to middle age.

176. The answer is A-N, B-Y, C-Y, D-N, E-Y. *(Wilson, ed 12. chap 175.)* The intensity of S_1 is determined by the contractility of the left ventricle ("slamming the door shut"), the degree of separation of mitral leaflets at the onset of contraction, and the thickness and pliability of the mitral leaflets. Contractility increases with fever but is diminished in hypothyroidism. Lown-Ganong-Levine syndrome is associated with a short PR interval, so that atrial contraction just precedes ventricular contraction; S_1 tends to be loud. Mitral regurgitation may lead to poor leaflet apposition and a soft S_1; on the other hand, mitral stenosis is associated with a loud S_1, unless the thickened valve leaflets are restricted in motion by heavy calcification.

177. The answer is A-Y, B-N, C-Y, D-N, E-Y. *(Wilson, ed 12. chap 176.)* Hyperkalemia leads to partial depolarization of cardiac cells. As a result, there is slowing of the upstroke of the action potential as well as reduced duration of repolarization. The T wave becomes peaked, the QRS complex widens and may merge with the T wave (giving a sine-wave appearance), and the P wave becomes shallow or disappears. Prominent U waves are associated with hypokalemia; ST-segment prolongation is associated with hypocalcemia.

178. The answer is A-Y, B-N, C-N, D-Y, E-N. *(Wilson, ed 12. chap 184.)* Anterior myocardial infarction and calcification arising from the aortic valve ring may damage the fascicular conduction system and thus lead to bifascicular block. Inferior myocardial infarction and mitral valve surgery are more likely to interfere with conduction at the level of the atrioventricular node. On a His bundle electrogram, prolongation of the HV interval (i.e., the time in which an impulse is conducted from the common His bundle to the ventricular myocardium) occurs only when all three fascicles are damaged.

179. The answer is A-N, B-N, C-Y, D-N, E-N. *(Wilson, ed 12. chaps 2, 177, 190.)* Making a test's cutoff point for positivity more stringent (i.e., > 2.0 mm of ST depression rather than 0.5 mm) will enhance specificity (there will be fewer false positives) at the expense of sensitivity (there will be more false negatives). Bayesian analysis dictates that low prior probability (e.g., 10 percent—odds 1:9) can only be enhanced to a 50 percent posttest (or posterior) probability for a test with the given operating characteristics [1:9 × sensitivity/(1 − specificity)], where sensitivity is defined as the probability of a positive test in a patient with the disease and specificity is defined as the probability of a negative test result in a patient without the disease. Thallium scans can increase the sensitivity for detecting coronary artery disease by about 20 percent and increase specificity by 10 percent. Such scans are most useful in patients with an uninterpretable or nondiagnostic electrocardiogram due to failure to achieve 85 percent of predicted maximal heart rate, left ventricular hypertrophy, left bundle branch block, or drug effects. A prior myocardial infarction can be inferred if a defect on thallium scintigraphy noted during exercise also fails to be perfused at rest. Blood pressure and heart rate should rise during a normal exercise tolerance test. Failure of the blood pressure to rise or an actual decrease may suggest global left ventricular dysfunction.

180. The answer is A-Y, B-Y, C-N, D-Y, E-N. *(Wilson, ed 12. chap 185.)* The electrocardiogram presented in the question demonstrates nonparoxysmal junctional tachycardia. The junctional rhythm is at a rate of 82 beats per minute, which is faster than the usual escape nodal rhythm. Retrograde P waves can be seen. This rhythm can occur following mitral valve surgery and in association with digitalis toxicity, acute myocarditis, and inferior myocardial infarction. These processes all can irritate the atrioventricular node and accelerate its action.

181. The answer is A-N, B-N, C-Y, D-N, E-Y. *(Wilson, ed 12. chap 16.)* Angina is usually described as a vague substernal pain that is precipitated by exercise or emotion and may radiate into the left arm or jaw. The discomfort may radiate into the teeth, but rarely above the maxilla. A sharp pain radiating to the back, particularly if long-lasting, suggests aortic dissection. Relief of pain at rest (but not by change of position) or within 5 min of sublingual nitroglycerin is highly suggestive of pain due to coronary ischemia.

182. The answer is A-N, B-Y, C-N, D-Y, E-Y. *(Wilson, ed 12. chap 181. Cohn, N Engl J Med 311:819, 1984.)* Stroke volume and cardiac output at rest are not sensitive indexes of myocardial dysfunction. Stroke volume is often normal, though at the expense of higher end-diastolic volume (Frank-Starling mechanism). Even when stroke volume begins to diminish, cardiac output can be maintained by increases in heart rate. However, when the heart is stressed by exercise, cardiac output does not rise proportionately to oxygen consumption, and left ventricular end-diastolic pressure rises more than in normal controls. Although plasma norepinephrine levels are elevated in persons with left ventricular dysfunction, myocardial levels are typically low.

183. The answer is A-Y, B-Y, C-Y, D-N, E-N. *(Wilson, ed 12. chap 40.)* Frequent premature ventricular complexes (defined as > 30 per minute), salvos or nonsustained ventricular tachycardia, and a low ejection fraction (<20 percent) are associated with an increased risk of sudden cardiac death. Advanced forms (triplets or longer) are more predictive of risk than even a high density of unifocal premature beats. It is unclear whether suppressing ectopic activity can reduce risk. Conventional techniques of cardiopulmonary resuscitation require lung inflation every 15 s and chest compressions 80 times per minute if only one provider is present. In the case of ventricular fibrillation or ventricular tachycardia in a pulseless patient, the first shock should be delivered at 200 joules, followed by additional higher energy shocks (up to 360 joules in the absence of response). Intravenous sodium bicarbonate, formerly recommended, is no longer considered routinely necessary and may be dangerous (unless pH monitoring indicates profound acidosis).

184. The answer is A-Y, B-N, C-N, D-Y, E-N. *(Wilson, ed 12. chap 67.)* The antihypertensive agent prazosin blocks alpha$_1$ receptors that mediate vasoconstriction. Clonidine is also an antihypertensive agent, but works by stimulating alpha$_2$ receptors in the brainstem, thereby reducing sympathetic outflow. Phenylephrine is an alpha$_1$ agonist with pressor effects that is frequently employed in over-the-counter nasal decongestants. By antagonizing presynaptic alpha$_2$ receptors, yohimbine increases parasympathetic activity that may augment penile blood flow and may be useful in the treatment of erectile impotence. Isoproterenol stimulates beta$_1$ and beta$_2$ receptors and can increase chronotropy in the setting of heart block.

185. The answer is A-Y, B-Y, C-N, D-N, E-N. *(Wilson, ed 12. chap 188.)* The rhythm demonstrated in the electrocardiogram presented in the question is supraventricular tachycardia, a reentry tachycardia probably involving longitudinal stratification in the atrioventricular (AV) junction. Delayed conduction in one limb of the reentry pathway with unidirectional block allows perpetuation of the arrhythmia. Vagal stimuli and carotid sinus massage often terminate the arrhythmia. Although some calcium-channel antagonists (e.g., verapamil) would terminate the arrhythmia predictably by decreasing AV nodal conduction, nifedipine is only rarely effective. Edrophonium (Tensilon), a parasympathomimetic drug, is also useful in treating supraventricular tachycardia but is contraindicated in patients who have asthma.

186. The answer is A-N, B-Y, C-N, D-N, E-Y. *(Wilson, ed 12. chap 185.)* Persons who have Wolff-Parkinson-White syndrome are predisposed to developing two major types of atrial tachyarrhythmias. The first, which resembles paroxysmal supraventricular tachycardia (SVT) with reentry, involves the atrioventricular node in anterograde conduction and the bypass tract in retrograde conduction. This tachycardia typically has a narrow QRS complex and can be treated similarly to other forms of SVT. The other, more dangerous tachyarrhythmia (present in the man described in the question) is atrial fibrillation, which usually is conducted anterograde down the bypass tract and has a wide QRS configuration. The ventricular rate is quite rapid, and cardiovascular collapse or ventricular fibrillation may result. Usual treatment is direct-current cardioversion, though quinidine may also be of use in slowing conduction through the bypass tract. Verapamil and propranolol have little effect on the bypass tract and may further depress ventricular function, which already is compromised by the rapid rate. Digoxin may accelerate conduction down the bypass tract and lead to ventricular fibrillation.

187. The answer is A-Y, B-Y, C-N, D-N, E-N. *(Wilson, ed 12. chap 186.)* Atrial septal defects (ASD) of the sinus venosus type are located high in the atrial septum and commonly are associated with anomalous pulmonary venous return. The magnitude of the shunt depends upon defect size, relative ventricular compliance, and the relative resistances in the pulmonary and systemic circuits, but *not* upon total blood flow. The systolic ejection murmur associated with ASD arises from increased flow across the pulmonic valve; a diastolic rumble due to increased flow across the tricuspid valve is common and should not necessarily be attributed to mitral stenosis, which is associated with ASD in a disorder known as Lutembacher's syndrome. Most persons even with a large ASD are asymptomatic until late in adult life.

188. The answer is A-Y, B-N, C-N, D-N, E-Y. *(Wilson, ed 12. chaps 186, 188.)* The risks of cardiac surgery always must be weighed against the potential benefits. The risk is extremely low in the correction of atrial septal defects, and surgery may prevent the development of atrial arrhythmia and pulmonary hypertension, complications that can arise later in life. Small ventricular septal defects, on the other hand, almost never cause hemodynamic problems later in life. The presence of Eisenmenger's reaction—cyanosis and a right-to-left shunt from pulmonary hypertension—is a contraindication to surgery, regardless of the underlying lesion. Persons with symptomatic aortic stenosis warrant consideration for surgery because hemodynamic deterioration can ensue quickly. Chronic mitral regurgitation, however, is far more indolent, and mild symptoms or acute decompensation from a correctable cause does not necessarily require surgical intervention.

189. The answer is A-Y, B-Y, C-Y, D-N, E-Y. *(Wilson, ed 12. chap 173. Vanhoutte, Circulation 80:1, 1989.)* Endothelial-derived relaxing factor (nitric oxide), a potent vasodilator due to its effect on vascular smooth muscle, increases cGMP levels via activation of guanylate cyclase. Prostacyclin (PGI$_2$) is another vasodilator released from endothelial cells, but its effects depend on adenylate cyclase–mediated elevations in cAMP. A 21-amino-acid peptide termed *endothelin* is a potent vasoconstrictor.

190. The answer is A-Y, B-Y, C-N, D-Y, E-Y. *(Wilson, ed 12. chap 175.)* Large *a* waves indicate contraction of the right atrium against increased resistance, such as might occur with obstruction at the tricuspid valve (tricuspid stenosis) or more commonly with increased resistance to right ventricular filling. Right ventricular filling could be impaired in pulmonary stenosis or any condition that causes pulmonary hypertension, such as multiple pulmonary emboli. The *a* wave will also be pronounced if the right atrium contracts while the tricuspid valve is closed by right ventricular systole, as would be the case in atrioventricular dissociation, complete heart block, or junctional rhythm. The *a* wave is absent in patients with atrial fibrillation, since no organized atrial contraction occurs.

191. The answer is A-N, B-Y, C-N, D-N, E-Y. *(Wilson, ed 12. chap 187.)* Acute rheumatic fever is a later complication of pharyngeal streptococcal infections. It is often difficult to isolate group A streptococci by a throat culture at the onset of acute rheumatic fever, though past streptococcal infection can be documented by serologic studies. Recurrences, which are common after the initial episode, are most common in persons who have rheumatic heart involvement. As a result, all affected persons should receive prophylactic antibiotic treatment for at least 5 years. Earlobe macrophages are associated with subacute bacterial endocarditis, not acute rheumatic fever.

192. The answer is A-Y, B-N, C-Y, D-N, E-N. *(Wilson, ed 12. chap 188.)* Although aortic stenosis may be present in affected persons for several decades, survival for more than 2 years is unlikely once symptoms of heart failure occur. Atrial fibrillation with the loss of synchronized atrial systole can precipitate clinical deterioration. Stenosis of the aortic valve becomes of critical importance when the effective orifice is reduced to less than 0.7 cm^2/m^2 body surface area. Absence of calcification in aortic valve cusps studied by fluoroscopy or echocardiography essentially rules out severe aortic stenosis in adults; this relationship, however, does not apply to plain chest x-ray. Normal boxlike separation of the aortic cusps on echocardiography excludes the presence of severe aortic stenosis; however, cusp calcification and poor mobility may not necessarily indicate significant valvular stenosis. While in advanced cases a strain pattern on the electrocardiogram is present, there is no close correlation between the electrocardiogram and the hemodynamic severity of the lesion.

193. The answer is A-N, B-N, C-N, D-Y, E-Y. *(Wilson, ed 12. chap 180. Safian, N Engl J Med 919:125, 1987.)* Safe and effective (it reduces gradients from 75 to 15 mmHg), balloon valvuloplasty is the preferred treatment for pulmonary stenosis. Rheumatic mitral stenosis secondary to commissural fusion with associated leaflet thickening is the mitral lesion most amenable to treatment with balloon dilation. Such dilation can increase valve size to 2.0 cm^2 or more, but usually not to the normal 3.5 to 5.0 cm^2 area. The indications for balloon aortic valvuloplasty in patients who are poor operative risks include congenital, rheumatic, or acquired calcific aortic stenosis. In the last group, valvuloplasty fractures leaflet calcium and provides new hinge points along which leaflets may open. Surprisingly, stroke is an uncommon complication of this procedure and most patients experience a reduction in symptoms. Restenosis is common, but can be treated with repeat aortic valvuloplasty.

194. The answer is A-Y, B-Y, C-N, D-Y, E-Y. *(Wilson, ed 12. chap 181.)* The cardiac output must increase during exercise since oxygen demand is greater. This increase is accomplished by a physiologic augmentation in stroke volume and heart rate. The pumping action of hyperventilation increases ventricular filling and thereby stroke volume rises. Catecholamine synthesis and secretion increase, which leads to faster heart rate and greater stroke volume through augmented myocardial contractility. Since blood pressure is determined by cardiac output and resistance, once cardiac output increases, blood pressure would also tend to rise. However, vasodilation in muscle beds counteracts this tendency somewhat. In the normal heart, catecholamine-mediated changes in the force-volume curve lead to decreased or similar end-diastolic volumes (filling pressure) during exercise; heart failure is characterized by marked, and sometimes dangerous, rises in end-diastolic volume, possibly even to the point of pulmonary edema.

195. The answer is A-Y, B-Y, C-Y, D-Y, E-Y. *(Wilson, ed 12. chap 188.)* A precipitating cause in the presence of an underlying structural heart disorder should be sought in all patients who present with congestive heart failure. The increased demand for cardiac output associated with such processes as fever, anemia, pregnancy, hypoxia, and infection can overburden a heart that has a limited reserve but operates well when not stressed. Arrhythmias such as atrial fibrillation reduce ventricular filling time while depriving the ventricle of the usual augmentation to filling provided by atrial systole. Persons with valvular disease are at risk for endocarditis, which can exacerbate heart failure. If the precipitating factor is reversible and preventable, affected persons may not require valvular surgery.

196. The answer is A-N, B-Y, C-Y, D-N, E-Y. *(Wilson, ed 12. chap 188.)* The systolic click-murmur syndrome is associated with mitral valve prolapse, which can place excessive stress on the papillary muscles and lead to ischemia and chest pain. Although often associated with inferior T-wave changes, the systolic click-murmur syndrome only occasionally results in an ischemic response to exercise. On standing or during a Valsalva's maneuver, as ventricular volume gets smaller the click and murmur move earlier into systole. Echocardiography reveals midsystolic prolapse of the posterior mitral leaflet, or on occasion both mitral leaflets, into the left atrium. Persons with mitral regurgitation from prolapse are at risk for developing subacute bacterial endocarditis and should be treated accordingly.

197. The answer is A-N, B-Y, C-Y, D-N, E-Y. *(Wilson, ed 12. chap 184.)* The choice of a permanent pacemaker type depends on the underlying conduction disease and the patient's clinical profile. DDD pacing preserves the normal relationship between atrial and ventricular contraction, and physiologic atrial sensing with ventricular pacing improves exercise tolerance in young, active persons. As this form of pacing preserves the normal atrial contribution to cardiac output, it is desired in patients with decreased left ventricular function or hypertrophied ("stiff") left ventricular chambers. DDD pacing is contraindicated in atrial fibrillation or flutter since the ventricular rate response is unpredictable.

198. The answer is A-Y, B-Y, C-Y, D-Y, E-Y. *(Wilson, ed 12. chap 182.)* With severe chronic heart failure from any cause there may be severe weight loss due to (1) elevation of the metabolic rate, which results from extra respiratory muscle work; (2) anorexia, nausea, and vomiting due to central causes, digitalis intoxication, or congestive hepatomegaly and abdominal fullness (including ascites with impairment of gastric filling and early satiety); (3) impaired intestinal absorption due to intestinal venular congestion; and (4) a protein-losing enteropathy.

199. The answer is A-N, B-Y, C-Y, D-N, E-N. *(Wilson, ed 12. chap 183.)* A 5-year survival rate of between 60 and 70 percent suggests that cardiac transplantation is the therapy of choice for patients with end-stage heart disease. Because the posterior walls of the host's atria are left in place at the time of transplantation, the recipient's sinus node remains innervated and under the influence of the autonomic nervous system, but the donor sinus node controls the rate of the transplanted heart (and has a regular PR interval in contrast to the dissociated P waves generated by the residual host atria). Accelerated coronary vascular disease and infection, not rejection, are the major factors limiting long-term survival. The vascular disease is a consequence of fibrointimal hyperplasia brought on by injury during rejection episodes and high serum lipids. The high serum lipids are a side effect of the immunosuppressive medicines that must be administered. Immunosuppression must continue for a lifetime. Recent reports have warned of a drug-drug interaction between lipid-lowering drugs, such as lovastatin and gemfibrozil, and certain immunosuppressive drugs, such as azathioprine; the interaction has been noted to lead to rhabdomyolysis.

200. The answer is A-N, B-Y, C-Y, D-Y, E-N. *(Wilson, ed 12. chap 184.)* The standard VVI pacemaker paces the ventricle, senses the ventricle, and is inhibited by spontaneous ventricular activity. Thus it will only fire in backup situations when the ventricular rate is lower than its set point. The right ventricular wire is rarely if ever irritating itself and does not cause ventricular tachycardia. Since the patient has a single-chamber, nontriggered pacer, triggering after ventriculoatrial conduction is not possible. On the other hand, since the VVI only paces the ventricle, the normal physiologic augmentation of cardiac output by atrial contraction is lost. Moreover, atrial contraction will occur at the wrong time if the AV valve is closed, thereby leading to large *a* waves.

201. The answer is A-N, B-N, C-N, D-Y, E-Y. *(Wilson, ed 12. chap 184.)* Ventricular tachycardia (VT) generally accompanies some form of structural heart disease, most commonly chronic ischemic heart disease associated with a prior myocardial infarction. The ECG diagnosis of VT is suggested by a wide-complex tachycardia at a rate exceeding 100 beats per minute. It is important, however, to differentiate supraventricular tachycardia with aberration of intraventricular conduction from VT since the clinical implications and managements of these two entities are so different. If a tracing previously obtained during sinus rhythm demonstrates a bundle branch block pattern with the same morphologic features as those during the tachycardia, then supraventricular origin is favored. Characteristics of the 12-lead ECG during the arrhythmia that suggest a ventricular origin are (1) a QRS complex >0.14 s in the absence of antiarrhythmic therapy (although a QRS complex >0.20 s suggests a preexcitation syndrome); (2) AV dissociation or variable retrograde conduction; (3) a superior QRS axis; (4) a broad initial R wave in V_1; (5) a Q wave in V_6; and (6) concordance of the QRS pattern in all precordial leads. Intracardiac electrical recordings would be required to confirm this important distinction.

202. The answer is A-Y, B-Y, C-N, D-N, E-N. *(Wilson, ed 12. chap 190.)* The rate of occlusion of saphenous venous grafts is highest in the first postoperative year and declines subsequently. Internal mammary artery grafts to the left anterior descending artery have gained popularity, since the incidence of occlusion is lower than that with venous grafts. Angina is abolished or significantly reduced in the majority (85 percent) of patients after CABG. Impaired left ventricular (LV) function is not a contraindication to CABG; in fact, a reduction in mortality has been found in patients with three-vessel disease and moderate LV dysfunction. In the hands of an experienced surgical team, surgical mortality associated with CABG should be less than 1 percent.

203. The answer is A-Y, B-N, C-N, D-Y, E-Y. *(Wilson, ed 12. chap 183.)* The calcium channel blocker verapamil is a very effective agent in the treatment of atrial and AV nodal reentrant tachycardias, but can cause hemodynamic collapse if given to a patient with sustained VT or atrial fibrillation/flutter and preexcitation and can raise serum levels of digoxin. Therefore it should be used with extreme caution in any patient with a wide-complex tachycardia. Amiodarone is useful in the treatment of refractory atrial and ventricular tachyarrhythmias, but is associated with a host of side effects including prolonged QT interval, peripheral neuropathy, abnormalities of thyroid function, pulmonary fibrosis, and various ocular and cutaneous problems, including corneal deposits and skin pigmentation. Flecainide may result in AV block, polymorphic VT, or heart failure if given in the face of severe left ventricular dysfunction. Reversible agranulocytosis occurs rarely after institution of procainamide therapy, while thrombocytopenia may be associated with quinidine use. Quinidine can also cause elevation of serum digoxin levels. Disopyramide may cause blurred vision and narrow-angle glaucoma.

204. The answer is A-Y, B-N, C-N, D-Y, E-Y. *(Wilson, ed 12. chap 195.)* The Framingham heart study found that low plasma levels of high-density lipoprotein (HDL) are a potent risk factor for coronary artery disease. HDL levels are increased by exercise, intake of small amounts of alcohol, and administration of estrogens. Cigarette smoking and androgen therapy depress plasma HDL levels.

205. The answer is A-Y, B-N, C-Y, D-Y, E-N. *(Wilson, ed 12. chap 194.)* Hyperthyroidism is an important, reversible cause of cardiac disease. Some of the manifestations are hyperadrenergic in nature and may in part be related to increased numbers of beta receptors. Atrial arrhythmias are frequent. The diagnosis should be entertained particularly for persons whose cardiac disease is resistant to the usual treatments as well as for the elderly, in whom many of the typical manifestations of hyperthyroidism tend to be lacking. Low-voltage electrocardiograms and pericardial effusion are features of hypothyroidism.

206. The answer is A-N, B-Y, C-N, D-Y, E-N. *(Wilson, ed 12. chap 192.)* The symptoms of dyspnea in persons with asymmetrical septal hypertrophy are related as much to decreased left ventricular compliance as to the degree of obstruction. Use of calcium-channel blockers often relieves dyspnea by decreasing left ventricular stiffness. Sudden death in affected persons does not correlate with the degree of obstruction and is thought to be due to arrhythmias. On electrocardiography, Q waves commonly are seen and do not imply a coexistent infarction. Histologic abnormalities consist of disorganized arrangements of myocytes in the ventricular septum.

207. The answer is A-N, B-N, C-N, D-Y, E-Y. *(Wilson, ed 12. chap 188.)* In approximately two-thirds of patients with aortic regurgitation (AR), the disease is rheumatic in origin, although such an etiology is less common in those with isolated AR. Manifestations of the rapidly falling arterial pressure during late systole and diastole include Corrigan's "water-hammer" pulse, capillary pulsations visible at the root of nails (Quincke's pulse), a pistol-shot sound over the femoral arteries, and a to-and-fro murmur (Duroziez's sign) audible over a lightly compressed femoral artery. In addition to a midsystolic ejection murmur, a second associated murmur may be the Austin Flint murmur, a low-pitched, rumbling diastolic bruit. Such a murmur is produced by the anterior displacement of the anterior leaflet of the mitral valve by the aortic regurgitant stream (characteristically seen at echocardiography). Close followup by means of echocardiography is necessary to ensure that an operation is undertaken before irreversible left ventricular dysfunction occurs.

208. The answer is A-N, B-N, C-N, D-Y, E-N. *(Wilson, ed 12. chap 182. The CONSENSUS trial study group. N Engl J Med 316:1429, 1987.)* In advanced heart failure, left ventricular afterload is augmented because of increased levels of circulating catecholamines and activation of the renin-angiotensin system. Afterload reducing agents reduce aortic impedance, resulting in elevation of stroke volume and cardiac output, with reduction in the left ventricular filling pressure. As cardiac output increases, reflex sympathetic nerve activity and circulating catecholamine levels decrease, and the heart rate tends to slow. Hydralazine is a potent afterload reducing agent; nitrates primarily dilate the systemic veins and are, therefore, potent *preload* reducing agents. Captopril is a balanced vasodilator. At least one trial has shown a reduction in mortality (the Scandinavian CONSENSUS study) in patients with chronic CHF treated with enalapril compared with a control group.

209. The answer is A-N, B-Y, C-Y, D-N, E-N. *(Wilson, ed 12. chap 189.)* Creatine phosphokinase (CK) rises within 8 to 24 h of infarction and returns to normal in 2 or 3 days, while the lactic dehydrogenase (LDH) level rises at 2 to 3 days, but may remain elevated for 2 weeks. LDH isoenzyme 1 (LDH_1) predominates in the heart and is a relatively specific indicator of myocardial damage. Coronary reperfusion leads to a rapid washout (early sharp rise and quick fall) of serum CK levels. Hypothyroidism can actually account for misleadingly elevated CK levels.

210. The answer is A-N, B-Y, C-N, D-Y, E-Y. *(Wilson, ed 12. chap 189.)* With the advent of successful cardioversion and aggressive early treatment of active ischemia, the *routine* prophylactic use of lidocaine is no longer recommended. Suppression of ventricular ectopic beats is indicated in the following categories: (1) > 5 isolated ventricular ectopic beats per minute; (2) consecutive or multifocal ventricular ectopic beats; and (3) early diastolic ventricular ectopic beats (R-on-T phenomenon). In the case of sustained ventricular tachycardia and hemodynamic collapse, immediate cardioversion should be performed. If ventricular tachycardia is well tolerated, lidocaine should be employed. If lidocaine fails to abolish the arrhythmia, then bretylium can be given.

211. The answer is A-N, B-Y, C-Y, D-Y, E-Y. *(Wilson, ed 12. chap 191.)* Pulmonary hypertension due to chronic pulmonary vascular disease such as that produced by multiple pulmonary emboli produces characteristic findings on physical examination, including a loud pulmonary second heart sound, a prominent *a* wave in the jugular venous pulse, and the systolic murmur of tricuspid regurgitation (the abnormal jet of blood flow is easily detectable on Doppler echocardiography). Pulmonary function testing may reveal an enlarged dead space, but there are usually no abnormalities on spirometry. Usual findings on the ECG include P pulmonale (tall, peaked P waves) and right axis deviation. The hypertrophied right ventricle can be imaged on thallium 201 scintigraphy, whereas this chamber normally remains invisible because of the marked uptake of the left ventricle.

212. The answer is A-N, B-N, C-N, D-Y, E-N. *(Wilson, ed 12. chap 192.)* Chronic alcoholics may develop a clinical picture virtually identical to that of idiopathic dilated cardiomyopathy. Ceasing consumption of alcohol may well result in halting the progression of heart disease. With continued alcohol abuse, however, 75 percent of afflicted persons will die within 3 years. While beriberi heart disease leads to high output failure, alcoholic cardiomyopathy is associated with a low cardiac output. Atrial arrhythmias, particularly fibrillation, are the most common electrical disorder seen in what is termed "holiday heart syndrome."

213. The answer is A-N, B-Y, C-Y, D-Y, E-N. *(Wilson, ed 12. chap 193.)* The manifestations of pericardial tamponade include equalization of pressures in the pericardial space, right atrium, pulmonary artery wedge, right ventricle, and pulmonary artery during diastole. The systolic pressure in the left ventricle, unlike the diastolic, may be greater than the right-sided pressure. Right ventricular free-wall diastolic collapse is a characteristic echocardiographic feature of tamponade. The normal small decrease in left ventricular stroke volume during the negative intrathoracic pressure created by inspiration is magnified by the nondistensible sac comprising the diseased pericardium; this leads to pulsus paradoxus (a greater than 10 mmHg drop in systolic blood pressure with inspiration). In tamponade there is a prominent *x* descent with a small *y* descent on the jugular venous pressure contour.

214. The answer is A-N, B-Y, C-Y, D-N, E-Y. *(Wilson, ed 12. chap 194.)* The most common type of primary cardiac tumor is the benign myxoma, which most frequently arises in the left atrium. Auscultation may reveal a "tumor plop" in diastole as the tumor hits the ventricular wall. Although most myxomas are sporadic, some are familial with autosomal dominant inheritance. Features of the familial syndromes associated with cardiac myxomas include pigmented nevi, nodular disease of the adrenal cortex, mammary fibroadenomas, and testicular and pituitary tumors. Systemic symptoms that are typically confused with those of endocarditis, noncardiac malignancy, or collagen vascular disease may be associated with myxomas. Sarcoma is the most common primary malignant cardiac tumor.

215. The answer is A-Y, B-N, C-N, D-Y, E-N. *(Wilson, ed 12. chap 195. National Cholesterol Education Program, Arch Intern Med 148:36, 1988.)* An increasing risk of premature ischemic heart disease can be detected when the cholesterol level exceeds 5.2 mmol/L (200 mg/dL); men with levels above 6.21 mmol/L (240 mg/dL) have a threefold risk of death from myocardial infarction compared with men whose cholesterol is below 5.2 mmol/L (200 mg/dL). Pure hypertriglyceridemia does not appear to be an independent risk factor for atherosclerotic heart disease, but this condition can exacerbate the problem for those who have other risk factors such as uremia, smoking, and hypertension. Hyperlipidemia is best confirmed by measurement of total cholesterol, high-density lipoprotein cholesterol, and triglycerides in serum or plasma in a sample obtained after an overnight fast. Routine use of lipoprotein electrophoresis adds little information. Secondary causes of hyperlipidemia include uncontrolled diabetes mellitus, hypothyroidism, uremia, nephrotic syndrome, obstructive liver disease, dysproteinemias, and drugs (alcohol, estrogens, glucocorticoids, and antihypertensives). Such conditions must be considered and ruled out before an appropriate decision on treatment can be made. There is no compelling evidence that lowering blood sugar per se decreases the death rate from ischemic heart disease in those with diabetes.

216. The answer is A-N, B-Y, C-Y, D-Y, E-N. *(Wilson, ed 12. chap 196.)* The abrupt onset of severe hypertension or the onset of high blood pressure of any severity in a person under the age of 25 or after the age of 50 should lead to additional tests to exclude renovascular hypertension and pheochromocytoma. The presence of an abdominal bruit (though not a very sensitive screening test) should prompt a workup for renovascular hypertension. Any patient whose hypertension is not controlled by a two-drug regimen such as an angiotensin-converting enzyme inhibitor and a diuretic at adequate doses should undergo further workup. While evidence for left ventricular hypertrophy on physical examination or electrocardiography suggests long-standing hypertension, such a finding does not necessarily imply the presence of Cushing's syndrome, pheochromocytoma, or a renovascular disease.

217. The answer is A-Y, B-Y, C-N, D-N, E-N. *(Wilson, ed 12. chap 196.)* Though they are inexpensive and effective, thiazide diuretics have recently fallen out of favor as the drugs of first choice for the tretament of essential hypertension because of metabolic side effects, which include hypokalemia due to renal potassium loss, hyperuricemia due to renal uric acid retention, hypercalcemia, carbohydrate intolerance, and hyperlipidemia. Stimulation of alpha$_2$ receptors in the vasomotor centers of the brain (as accomplished by clonidine, aldomethyldopa, and guanethidine) reduces sympathetic outflow and causes a fall in blood pressure. Diazoxide, though structurally a thiazide, is not a diuretic (it actually causes sodium retention). Moreover, diazoxide can be given without monitoring, so it is a very good initial agent for malignant hypertension. Prazosin is a postsynaptic (alpha$_1$) receptor blocker and thus produces less reflex tachycardia than would a pure vasodilator, such as hydralazine. Angiotensin-converting enzyme inhibitors must be used with care in patients with any degree of renal insufficiency. Treatment with this class of drugs actually raises serum renin levels by relief of chronic feedback inhibition.

218. The answer is A-Y, B-Y, C-N, D-N, E-Y. *(Wilson, ed 12. chap 198.)* Pentoxifylline may have clinical utility in the treatment of claudication by increasing blood flow to the microcirculation through the mechanism of decreasing blood viscosity and enhancing red cell flexibility. Doppler measurements can be used to assess blood pressure in the ankle, which, in the absence of occlusive disease, is greater than that in the brachial artery. In addition to control of blood pressure and cholesterol level, patients with claudication should be advised to exercise regularly to progressively higher levels. Revascularization or angioplasty should be reserved for those patients who suffer from pain at rest or from progressive and disabling symptoms. Patency rates of femoral-popliteal saphenous vein bypass grafts approach 90 percent at 1 year and 70 to 80 percent at 5 years.

219–223. The answers are: 219-A, 220-B, 221-C, 222-D, 223-D. *(Wilson, ed 12, chap 179.)* Equalization of diastolic pressures in the four cardiac chambers occurs in pericardial tamponade and constrictive pericarditis. The dip-and-plateau pattern in the ventricles and steep *y* descent in the atria are features of constrictive pericarditis but not pericardial tamponade.

In persons who have restrictive cardiomyopathy, diastolic pressures may be nearly equal. Often, however, a separation of at least 5 mmHg exists or can be brought out by acute volume loading. The dip-and-plateau pattern in ventricular pressures is typical.

Acute mitral regurgitation is associated with tall regurgitant *v* waves, which reflect regurgitation of blood into a noncompliant left atrium during systole. They are often absent in more chronic mitral regurgitation—a dilated left atrium can accommodate large volumes of blood without a significant increase in pressure. A regurgitant *v* wave often slightly precedes the usual physiologic *v* wave, which reflects venous return to the atria while atrioventricular valves are closed. In ventricular septal rupture with left-to-right shunt, venous return to the left atrium increases and the *v* wave becomes exaggerated.

Slow *y* descent is due to delayed atrial emptying. This phenomenon occurs in mitral or tricuspid stenosis, atrial myxomas, and cor triatriatum.

224–227. The answers are: 224-C, 225-A, 226-B, 227-E. *(Wilson, ed 12. chaps 186, 209.)* Many hereditary conditions and exposures to infectious agents during pregnancy result in congenital heart disease. Marfan's syndrome is a disorder of connective tissue in which cardiac abnormalities produce the greatest mortality. Decreased strength of the aortic connective tissue results in dilatation with aortic regurgitation and aortic dissection. Prolapse of the aortic and mitral valves usually presents, the latter associated with mitral regurgitation.

Turner's syndrome is a chromosomal abnormality (45 XO) characterized by short stature and hypogonadism. Associated cardiac defects include coarctation of the aorta and bicuspid aortic valve.

Maternal rubella during pregnancy can result in deafness, microcephaly, and cataracts in the infant. The most common cardiovascular lesions are pulmonic stenosis, multiple pulmonary artery stenoses, and patent ductus arteriosus.

Cystic fibrosis is an autosomal recessive disease primarily affecting exocrine glands and results in chronic obstructive lung disease and pancreatic insufficiency. The prominent abnormalities of lung function may result in cor pulmonale.

228–231. The answers are: 228-E, 229-A, 230-C, 231-B. *(Wilson, ed 12. chaps 188, 191, 193.)* Right heart failure, or elevated right-heart filling pressure, can develop from many causes. Right heart failure most commonly occurs as a result of pulmonary artery hypertension. Pulmonary artery hypertension, in turn, arises either from increased pulmonary vascular resistance with lung disease, in which case the pulmonary capillary wedge pressure (left atrial pressure) is not elevated, or from left-sided failure or valvular disease, in which case left atrial pressure is increased. Massive right ventricular infarction can cause the right side of the heart to fail at low systolic pressures. With primary myocardial disease, both left and right atrial pressures are elevated; however, when diastolic pressures are *equal* in the left and right cardiac chambers, external compression, such as constrictive pericarditis, must be suspected as the cause.

Disorders of the Respiratory System

DIRECTIONS: Each question below contains five suggested responses. Select the **one best** response to each question.

232. The most useful and predictive tool in evaluating the condition of a patient with an acute asthmatic attack and in assessing response to therapy is

(A) chest radiography
(B) arterial blood gas measurement
(C) measurement of pulsus paradoxus
(D) observation of accessory muscle use
(E) measurement of peak expiratory flow or FEV_1

233. A 26-year-old garage mechanic has been ill for 3 days with fever, malaise, cough, and mild shortness of breath. On physical examination there is no evidence of pharyngitis or lymphadenopathy; only a few scattered pulmonary rhonchi, and no wheezes or rales, are heard on chest auscultation. Chest x-ray, however, shows changes of bronchopneumonia. Assuming the person has no history of drug allergy, oral antibiotic therapy should begin with

(A) chloramphenicol
(B) erythromycin
(C) tetracycline
(D) penicillin V potassium
(E) cephalexin

234. All the following mediators are produced by alveolar macrophages isolated from patients with idiopathic pulmonary fibrosis EXCEPT

(A) fibronectin
(B) platelet-derived growth factor
(C) alveolar macrophage–derived growth factor
(D) collagenase
(E) leukotriene B_4

235. A patient who is being evaluated for shortness of breath is found to have an arterial P_{O_2} of 59 mmHg while breathing room air at sea level and an arterial P_{O_2} of 61 mmHg while breathing 40% inspired O_2. In each case the arterial P_{CO_2} is normal. Which of the following conditions would be LEAST likely to account for these findings?

(A) Idiopathic pulmonary fibrosis
(B) Atelectasis
(C) *Klebsiella* pneumonia
(D) Cardiogenic pulmonary edema
(E) Osler-Rendu-Weber syndrome

236. A 63-year-old man has pneumococcal pneumonia with extensive air-space consolidation in the left upper and left lower lobes. He complains of extreme shortness of breath when positioned with his left side down. An arterial blood sample drawn in this position shows a P_{O_2} of 46 mmHg; 10 min earlier, an arterial blood sample drawn while his right side was dependent had revealed a P_{O_2} of 66 mmHg. The most likely explanation for the drop in P_{O_2} when the man was lying on his left side is

(A) increased blood flow to the dependent lung
(B) reduced ventilation to the dependent lung
(C) increased airway resistance in the dependent lung
(D) accumulation of interstitial edema in the dependent lung
(E) increased stiffness of the chest wall on the dependent side

237. A 21-year-old college student with no prior medical problems begins working as a laboratory technician. He subsequently presents because of several recent episodes of shortness of breath, cough, fever, chills, and malaise. Each episode has lasted several days. The patient is seen during the recovery phase of such an episode; findings at physical examination are normal. Chest x-ray reveals several ill-defined, diffuse, patchy infiltrates. The laboratory evaluation is positive only for an increased erythrocyte sedimentation rate. Pulmonary function studies display reduced lung volumes.

On further questioning it is learned that these episodes begin on days the patient is required to tend to experiments involving laboratory rats at the animal facility. What is the best treatment for this condition?

(A) Inhaled cromolyn sodium
(B) Prednisone
(C) Inhaled beclomethasone
(D) Discontinuation of visits to the animal facility
(E) No treatment

238. Asthmatic attacks may be precipitated in susceptible persons by a wide variety of stimuli. All the following have been demonstrated to produce airway obstruction in certain asthmatic subjects EXCEPT

(A) viral respiratory infections
(B) cold air
(C) sodium salicylate
(D) exercise
(E) airborne allergens

239. Although asthma is a heterogeneous disease, a given individual with asthma would be most likely to

(A) relate a personal or family history of allergic diseases
(B) conform to a characteristic personality type
(C) display a skin-test reaction to extracts of airborne allergens
(D) demonstrate nonspecific airway hyperirritability
(E) have supranormal serum immunoglobulin E

240. A diagnosis of allergic bronchopulmonary aspergillosis in a person who has asthma, recurrent pulmonary infiltrates, and eosinophilia would be supported by all the following findings EXCEPT

(A) delayed, tuberculin-type skin-test reaction to *Aspergillus fumigatus*
(B) sputum culture positive for *A. fumigatus*
(C) presence of serum precipitins to *A. fumigatus*
(D) marked elevation of serum immunoglobulin E level
(E) radiographic evidence of bronchiectasis

241. The dyskinetic ciliary syndromes, including Kartagener's syndrome, can produce all the following manifestations EXCEPT

(A) bronchiectasis
(B) pneumonia
(C) recurrent bronchitis
(D) interstitial pulmonary fibrosis
(E) infertility

242. Bronchospasm may be produced by exposure in the workplace to all the following EXCEPT

(A) cotton dust
(B) toluene diisocyanate
(C) fluorocarbons
(D) flax
(E) silica

243. Cavity formation is a common complication of pneumonia caused by

(A) anaerobic bacteria
(B) *Legionella pneumophila*
(C) *Streptococcus pneumoniae*
(D) *Mycoplasma pneumoniae*
(E) influenza virus

244. All the following characteristics distinguish small cell lung carcinoma from non-small cell lung carcinoma EXCEPT

(A) neuroendocrine properties (e.g., neuron-specific enolase staining, presence of dense core granules ultrastructurally) are more common in small cell tumors
(B) higher rate of response to chemotherapy in small cell tumors
(C) higher rate of response to radiation therapy in small cell tumors
(D) higher overall 5-year survival in small cell tumors
(E) more common loss of short arm of chromosome 3 in small cell tumors

Questions 245–246

A 60-year-old man with emphysema and bronchitis is brought to an emergency room by an ambulance crew that has been giving him oxygen by mask. Three days ago, he noted that his sputum had changed color and increased in amount. His wife called the ambulance when he became suddenly short of breath and confused. On arrival at the hospital he is somnolent. Mid-inspiratory crackles and diffuse expiratory wheezes are audible on examination of the chest, and he has marked peripheral edema and ascites. Hemoglobin is 180 g/L (18 g/dL). Arterial blood gases are pH 7.08, P_{O_2} 148 mmHg, and P_{CO_2} 106 mmHg.

245. The most appropriate immediate therapy for the man described above would be

(A) intravenous infusion of sodium bicarbonate
(B) endotracheal intubation and assisted ventilation
(C) administration of isoetharine by air-compressor nebulizer
(D) discontinuation of supplemental oxygen
(E) subcutaneous injection of epinephrine

246. For the man described above, manifestations of right ventricular heart failure would be treated with

(A) diazoxide
(B) digoxin
(C) hydralazine
(D) oxygen
(E) phlebotomy

247. A 34-year-old man complains of shortness of breath after minimal exertion. He has no systemic symptoms. He developed a nonproductive cough 10 months ago. A chest x-ray, which was reportedly normal, was done at that time. Examination now reveals a respiratory rate of 28 breaths per minute, and diffuse end-inspiratory crackles are heard over his lower lung fields. His chest x-ray is shown below. An arterial P_{O_2} measured while the patient is breathing room air is 55 mmHg, and arterial P_{CO_2} is 26 mmHg. Routine blood counts are normal. The next step in his evaluation should be

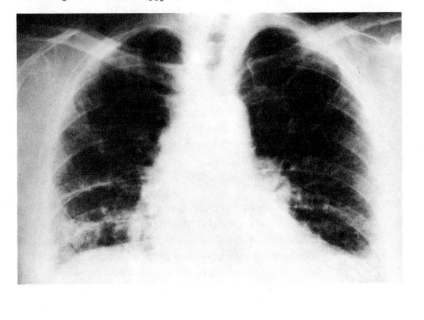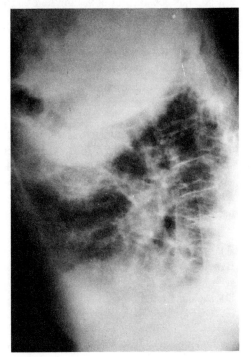

(A) angiotensin-converting enzyme level
(B) transbronchial biopsy
(C) bronchoalveolar lavage
(D) salivary gland biopsy
(E) serology for rheumatoid factor

248. A 23-year-old woman complains of dyspnea and substernal chest pain on exertion. Evaluation for this complaint 6 months ago included arterial blood-gas testing, which revealed pH 7.48, P_{O_2} 79 mmHg, and P_{CO_2} 31 mmHg. Electrocardiography then showed a right axis deviation. Chest x-ray now shows enlarged pulmonary arteries but no parenchymal infiltrates, and a lung perfusion scan reveals subsegmental defects that are thought to have a "low probability for pulmonary thromboembolism." Echocardiogram demonstrates right heart strain, but no evidence of primary cardiac disease. The most appropriate diagnostic test now would be

(A) open lung biopsy
(B) Holter monitoring
(C) right-heart catheterization
(D) transbronchial biopsy
(E) serum α_1–antitrypsin level

249. A 53-year-old man is noted to be tachypneic and confused 48 h after suffering multiple orthopedic and internal injuries in an automobile accident. Chest x-ray is interpreted as normal, but arterial blood-gas values are as follows: pH 7.49, P_{O_2} 52 mmHg, and P_{CO_2} 30 mmHg. The course of action most likely to confirm the diagnosis of this man's condition would be to

(A) order a ventilation-perfusion scan
(B) order pulmonary angiography
(C) order impedance plethysmography
(D) order blood testing for fibrin split products
(E) repeat the physical examination

250. A 42-year-old man who is a heavy cigarette smoker develops chills, malaise, and tenderness at the angle of the jaw a week after onset of a sore throat. On examination he is febrile and tachypneic, and a pleural friction rub is audible over the left chest. Chest x-ray reveals several nodular densities in both lung fields. The most likely diagnosis is

(A) osteoma of the tonsil
(B) retropharyngeal abscess
(C) peritonsillar cellulitis
(D) pharyngeal tuberculosis
(E) postanginal sepsis

251. A 52-year-old woman with long-standing rheumatoid arthritis is hospitalized for total knee replacement. On her admission chest x-ray, a 2-cm nodule is noted near the right hilus. She has smoked one pack of cigarettes daily for the last 32 years. The most appropriate management of this woman's pulmonary condition would be

(A) observation with chest x-rays every 4 months
(B) therapy for 2 months with oral corticosteroids
(C) an upper gastrointestinal series
(D) scalene node biopsy
(E) exploratory thoracotomy

252. The most sensitive noninvasive test for bilateral diaphragmatic paralysis is

(A) testing of vital capacity
(B) ''sniff test''
(C) chest x-ray
(D) fluoroscopy
(E) physical examination

253. All the following statements about obstructive sleep apnea syndrome are true EXCEPT

(A) men are affected more often than women
(B) systemic hypertension is a common finding
(C) alcohol can be a contributing factor
(D) estrogens are frequently useful
(E) personality changes may be the presenting complaint

254. A 54-year-old man has a nonproductive cough and exertional breathlessness. He also notes low-grade fever, malaise, and a 7 kg (15 lb) weight loss occurring over 6 weeks. His white blood cell count is 13,500/mm³. He has a history of mild asthma. A chest x-ray discloses peripheral lung infiltrates. The most likely diagnosis is

(A) idiopathic pulmonary fibrosis
(B) alveolar proteinosis
(C) polymyositis
(D) chronic eosinophilic pneumonia
(E) lymphangiomyomatosis

Questions 255–256

An 18-year-old man develops adult respiratory distress syndrome after a near drowning. Breathing room air, he has the following arterial blood-gas values: pH 7.50, P_{O_2} 48 mmHg, and P_{CO_2} 28 mmHg. Arterial blood gases obtained while he is breathing 80% oxygen by mask (measured in the nasopharynx) are pH 7.50, P_{O_2} 63 mmHg, and P_{CO_2} 29 mmHg.

255. The most important cause of hypoxemia in the man described above would be

(A) a block in alveolar-capillary diffusion
(B) right-to-left shunting
(C) ventilation-perfusion mismatch
(D) hypoventilation
(E) poor cardiac output

256. Owing to profound hypoxemia, tracheal intubation is performed on the man described above, and mechanical ventilation is begun. Inspired oxygen concentration is 80%. Initially, the man is agitated and fights the respirator. Arterial blood gases are obtained and show pH 7.21, P_{O_2} 70 mmHg, and P_{CO_2} 56 mmHg. The most appropriate management step at this time would be to

(A) add positive end-expiratory pressure (5 cmH₂O)
(B) sedate the man and control his ventilation
(C) infuse sodium bicarbonate intravenously
(D) raise the inspired oxygen concentration
(E) initiate extracorporeal membrane oxygenation

257. One week following a right total hip replacement a 65-year-old woman develops the sudden onset of shortness of breath. Workup reveals normotension, a prominent second heart sound, hypoxemia, sinus tachycardia with new right axis deviation on the electrocardiogram, and a normal chest x-ray. Oxygen is administered. Impedance plethysmography is consistent with a large proximal clot in the left leg.

Which of the following would be the most reasonable next step?

(A) Performance of a pulmonary angiogram
(B) Performance of perfusion scintigraphy
(C) Administration of tissue plasminogen activator
(D) Administration of heparin
(E) Administration of warfarin

DIRECTIONS: Each question below contains five suggested responses. For **each** of the five responses listed with every question, you are to respond either YES (Y) or NO (N). In a given item **all, some, or none of the alternatives may be correct**.

258. A 25-year-old woman comes to the hospital because of an acute exacerbation of her long-standing asthma. When examined, she is anxious and tachypneic. She is using accessory muscles of respiration to breathe, and diffuse wheezes are audible on expiration. Which of the following measures would be appropriate initial therapy for this woman?

(A) Administration of inhaled beclomethasone
(B) Administration of inhaled cromolyn sodium
(C) Administration of inhaled isoproterenol
(D) Intravenous infusion of aminophylline
(E) Intravenous administration of sedatives

259. The diagnosis of cystic fibrosis is best made by measurement of sweat chloride concentration. This measurement should be made in a boy who has chronic airway obstruction and which of the following?

(A) Intussusception
(B) Sinusitis
(C) Steatorrhea
(D) Dextrocardia
(E) Clubbing

260. Cystic fibrosis is correctly characterized by which of the following statements?

(A) It is unusual for an affected male to live past the age of 20 years
(B) It is inherited in a polygenic fashion
(C) Portal hypertension may occur in affected persons who lack pancreatic function
(D) Affected women are likely to have difficulty conceiving a child
(E) Meconium ileus occurs in approximately 5 percent of cases

Questions 261–262

A 35-year-old man seeks medical attention for breathlessness on exertion. He has never smoked cigarettes and has not been coughing. One sibling died at 40 years of age of respiratory failure. His three children are healthy. Physical examination reveals him to be tachypneic as he exhales through pursed lips. His chest is tympanitic to percussion, and breath sounds are poorly heard on auscultation. Chest x-ray shows flattened diaphragms with peripheral attenuation of bronchovascular markings most noticeable at the lung bases.

261. Expected results of the pulmonary function testing of the man described above would include

(A) increased lung elastic recoil
(B) increased total lung capacity
(C) reduced functional residual capacity
(D) reduced vital capacity
(E) increased diffusing capacity

262. Initial laboratory assessment of the man described above should include

(A) measurement of oxygen consumption during exercise
(B) measurement of sweat chloride concentration
(C) serum protein electrophoresis
(D) complete spirometry
(E) arterial blood-gas determination

263. In persons with chronic airway obstruction, prognosis can be improved by

(A) oxygen therapy
(B) exercise programs
(C) cessation of smoking
(D) phlebotomy
(E) use of oral expectorants

264. Correct statements concerning hemoptysis—expectoration of blood or blood-streaked sputum—include which of the following?

(A) The most common cause of hemoptysis is primary carcinoma of the lung
(B) Hemoptysis is rare in carcinoma that has metastasized to the lung
(C) Chronic, recurrent hemoptysis in a young, otherwise asymptomatic female suggests bronchiectasis
(D) Despite extensive evaluation including bronchoscopy, approximately 10 percent of patients with gross hemoptysis remain undiagnosed
(E) A patient with hemoptysis tends to keep the non-bleeding side in the superior position for drainage purposes

265. Correct statements concerning the pathogenesis of α_1–antitrypsin deficiency include which of the following?

(A) Emphysema results from an inability to inhibit alveolar destruction by neutrophils
(B) Clinical deficiency of α_1–antitrypsin usually results from one of several missense mutations that cause a truncated mRNA
(C) Most α_1–antitrypsin is synthesized by alveolar macrophages
(D) Mutations of the α_1-antitrypsin gene of the S type produce less severe emphysema than do mutations of the Z type
(E) Treatment with purified α_1–antitrypsin can raise serum levels to a level associated with lung protection

266. Hypoxemia occurring after pulmonary thromboembolism can result from

(A) lowered mixed venous P_{O_2} due to heart failure
(B) perfusion of atelectatic areas
(C) increased dead-space ventilation in the area of vascular occlusion
(D) perfusion of areas poorly ventilated because of airway constriction
(E) inadequate time for oxygen diffusion secondary to a reduction in the capillary bed

267. A middle-aged woman has a large central mass on chest x-ray. Sputum cytology is positive for squamous cell carcinoma. Which of the following conditions would be considered a contraindication for operation on this woman?

(A) Resting P_{CO_2} above 50 mmHg
(B) Syndrome of inappropriate antidiuretic hormone secretion
(C) Pleural effusion
(D) Recurrent laryngeal nerve paralysis
(E) Metastasis to lobar lymph nodes

268. Which of the following conditions would be likely to result in an increased residual volume on plethysmographic pulmonary function testing?

(A) Emphysema
(B) Sarcoidosis
(C) Cystic fibrosis
(D) Fracture of the cervical spine
(E) Kyphoscoliosis

269. In order to decrease the likelihood of drug toxicity, theophylline dosage should be reduced in a patient with asthma who is

(A) older than 70
(B) taking erythromycin for *Mycoplasma* pneumonia
(C) taking phenytoin for seizures
(D) a heavy abuser of marijuana
(E) taking allopurinol for gout

270. True statements about pleural effusions include which of the following?

(A) Although acid-fast bacilli rarely are seen on smears of fluid from postprimary tuberculous effusions, the fluid culture is positive in a majority of cases
(B) If eosinophils constitute more than 10 percent of cells in a pleural effusion, hypereosinophilic syndrome is a likely diagnosis
(C) The second most common malignancy-associated pleural effusion is due to lymphoma
(D) Low glucose concentration is a common finding in a rheumatoid pleural effusion
(E) Recurrent, malignancy-associated pleural effusions may be effectively treated via sclerosis with chloroquine

271. Health effects of exposure to asbestos fibers include

(A) pulmonary fibrosis
(B) pleural effusion
(C) oat cell carcinoma
(D) peritoneal mesothelioma
(E) pleural plaques

272. A 51-year-old man develops pancreatitis associated with the passage of a gallstone. His treatment includes meperidine and intravenous normal saline. Two days later, he becomes anxious, tachypneic, and short of breath. An emergency chest x-ray demonstrates diffuse, bilateral interstitial and alveolar infiltrates. A year ago, he suffered a myocardial infarction, but since then he has had no evidence of congestive heart failure. In this case, adult respiratory distress syndrome can be distinguished from cardiogenic pulmonary edema by

(A) measurement of lung water
(B) measurement of protein concentration in edema fluid
(C) measurement of pulmonary artery wedge pressure
(D) measurement of lung compliance
(E) calculation of the alveolar-arterial P_{O_2} difference

273. A 65-year-old man with chronic bronchitis presented to the emergency room 2 weeks ago with acute respiratory failure. He was intubated and treated with diuretics and antibiotics. However, after apparent improvement during a 1-week stay in the intensive care unit on mechanical ventilation, he has since failed three attempts at being weaned from the ventilator. Which of the following factors could account for the difficulty in removing this patient from the ventilator?

(A) Metabolic acidosis
(B) Benzodiazepines
(C) A P_{CO_2} too high prior to extubation
(D) Hypokalemia
(E) Hypothyroidism

274. True statements regarding idiopathic pulmonary fibrosis include

(A) the forced expiratory volume (FEV_1) is reduced
(B) therapy with corticosteroids and cyclophosphamide may be beneficial
(C) serial chest x-rays are helpful in following response to therapy
(D) the carbon monoxide diffusing capacity is a useful indicator of response to therapy
(E) lung transplantation should be considered

Disorders of the
Respiratory System

Answers

232. The answer is E. *(Wilson, ed 12. chap 204.)* Several investigators have shown that the most efficient means of assessing the severity of an asthmatic attack and of following the therapeutic response is the measurement of some parameter of respiratory function such as peak flow or forced expiratory volume in 1 s (FEV_1). The chest radiograph will frequently show only hyperinflation in attacks of varying degrees of severity. Arterial blood gases will reflect hypoxemia and hypocapnia in all but the most severe episodes, when they may reflect respiratory fatigue and severe obstruction as rising P_{CO_2} levels. Accessory muscle use and the presence of pulsus paradoxus reflect changes in intrathoracic pressure and the work of breathing, and they may actually disappear if the patient's breathing worsens to the point of becoming shallow. Thus, these signs may be misleading.

233. The answer is B. *(Wilson, ed 12. chap 154.)* Most authorities recommend using erythromycin in the treatment of persons who have community-acquired bronchopneumonia because the drug is effective therapy for pneumococcal as well as mycoplasmal infections, the leading causes. It also is an effective treatment for Legionnaires' disease. Tetracycline may not always be effective against pneumococci, and penicillin V potassium and cephalexin are not effective against mycoplasma. Chloramphenicol is too toxic for initial therapy of bronchopneumonia.

234. The answer is D. *(Wilson, ed 12. chaps 199, 211.)* An as-yet-unknown stimulus, possibly an immune complex formed locally, activates alveolar macrophages, which are believed to be the primary mediators of the pulmonary inflammation and fibrosis characteristic of idiopathic pulmonary fibrosis. The activated alveolar macrophages secrete leukotrienes, which act as chemoattractants for neutrophils and eosinophils. Among the many substances made by neutrophils, collagenase is responsible for disrupting existing structures prior to scar formation. Fibronectin, a dimeric glycoprotein that interacts with the intracellular matrix, is also released by macrophages. Fibroblasts are recruited and stimulated by the actions of at least two polypeptide mediators elaborated by macrophages. One factor responsible for recruiting fibroblasts, platelet-derived growth factor, is partially encoded for by the proto-oncogene c-*sis*. Alveolar macrophage–derived growth factor is believed to stimulate fibroblast proliferation, which is also required for scar formation.

235. The answer is A. *(Wilson, ed 12. chap 201.)* General mechanisms responsible for hypoxemia include alveolar hypoventilation, impaired diffusion, ventilation/perfusion inequality, and shunting (blood bypassing ventilated areas of the lung). In each of these cases, except for shunting, the arterial P_{O_2} increases significantly when the inspired P_{O_2} is raised. Examples of shunts (which could account for the lack of response to oxygen therapy described in the question) include congenital heart disease that produces direct right-to-left intracardiac flow (usually associated with pulmonary hypertension), intrapulmonary vascular shunting (i.e., congenital telangiectatic disorders such as Osler-Rendu-Weber syndrome), or most commonly perfused alveoli that are not ventilated because of atelectasis or fluid buildup (pneumonia or pulmonary edema). Since impaired diffusion is usually not severe enough to lead to disordered gas exchange except during exercise, most cases of normocapnic hypoxemia are due to ventilation-perfusion mismatch. Many processes that affect the lungs (alveolar disease, interstitial lung disease, pulmonary vascular disease, airway disease) do so unevenly, which leads to some areas with adequate perfusion and poor ventilation and some with good ventilation and poor perfusion.

236. The answer is A. *(Wilson, ed 12. chap 201.)* In a person standing erect, blood flow per unit volume increases from the apex of the lung to the base. Ventilation also increases from apex to base, but the gradient is less than that for blood flow, making the ventilation-perfusion ratio less at the bottom of the lung than at the top. Both ventilation and perfusion are affected by posture; as a general rule, the dependent regions are better perfused than ventilated and have the lowest ratio of ventilation to perfusion. Thus, a person with unilateral air-space disease may have an increase in venous admixture when the diseased lung is dependent. In that situation, blood flow increases to the diseased lung, perfusing atelectatic and poorly ventilated alveoli, and hypoxemia ensues.

237. The answer is D. *(Wilson, ed 12. chap 205.)* Given the temporal relationship of the symptoms to the work with rats, serologic evidence for inflammation, the nonspecific radiographic findings, and the restrictive pulmonary physiology suggested by spirographic examination, the most likely diagnosis is acute hypersensitivity pneumonitis with male rat urine probably the offending antigen. Without treatment, the patient could develop the subacute or chronic form of the disease with potentially serious physiologic impairment. While steroids can be helpful in severe or chronic cases, the best therapy is to remove the offending antigen or to remove the patient from an environment where exposure is inevitable. This approach is difficult when the patient's life-style or livelihood requires a radical change; in the case presented, however, simply restricting the student's laboratory efforts to those not involving direct animal care seems relatively nondisruptive.

238. The answer is C. *(Wilson, ed 12. chap 203.)* Respiratory infections, particularly those that are viral in origin, are common precipitants of acute asthmatic attacks. Bacterial infections are relatively less common precipitants; in fact, they may be implicated wrongly in acute asthma if purulent sputum due to sputum eosinophilia is mistakenly attributed to bacterial disease. Hyperventilation with cold air is now used as a broncho-provocation test in some pulmonary function laboratories to identify asthmatic subjects. Heat loss across the respiratory mucosa is believed to be the stimulus producing airway narrowing in asthmatic persons who breathe cold air and who have exercise-induced asthma. Although some persons with asthma develop bronchospasm after ingestion of acetylsalicylic acid or tartrazine dye, they tolerate sodium salicylate without symptoms. In allergic asthma subjects, inhalation challenge testing with appropriate antigens causes reproducible bronchospasm.

239. The answer is D. *(Wilson, ed 12. chap 204.)* The importance of immune mechanisms in the pathogenesis of asthma is suggested by the common association between the disease and the presence of allergic diseases, skin-test sensitivity, and increased serum IgE levels. In addition, many susceptible persons develop bronchospasm after inhalation challenge with airborne allergens. A large proportion of asthmatic subjects, however, have none of these markers of immunologic activity and are classified as having idiosyncratic asthma. When tested for bronchial hyperirritability with various nonantigenic bronchoprovocational agents (e.g., histamine or cold air), asthmatic subjects are found to be more sensitive than normal; the reason for this airway hyperirritability, which is a common feature of all asthmatic persons, is unknown. Although psychologic factors certainly influence the expression of asthma, no single personality type is considered "asthmatic."

240. The answer is A. *(Wilson, ed 12. chap 205. Greenberger, Chest 91:1655, 1987.)* Allergic bronchopulmonary aspergillosis is a hypersensitivity pneumonitis involving an allergic reaction to antigens from *Aspergillus* species, most commonly *A. fumigatus*. The diagnosis should be suspected in asthmatic persons who have recurrent pulmonary infiltrates associated with peripheral blood or sputum eosinophilia. Suggestive laboratory findings include serum immunoglobulin E levels elevated many times normal and the presence of aspergilli in the sputum. Antigenic skin testing is positive both in immediate (type I, wheal and flare) reaction and reaction evident after 4 to 6 h (type III, erythema and induration). Delayed, tuberculin-type (type IV, cell-mediated) reactions, however, do not occur. Serum precipitins to aspergilli are found in a majority of affected persons. The inflammatory response leads to dilatation of central airways and often is evident radiographically as mucoid impaction.

241. The answer is D. *(Wilson, ed 12. chap 208.)* Cilia, responsible for the motility and mucous clearance functions of many cell types, are composed of a double tubular structure. Abnormalities in one or another of the anatomic components of cilia can lead to a lack of coordinated ciliary action. Kartagener's syndrome, the best known of the dyskinetic ciliary syndromes, is caused by an absence of the inner or outer dynein arms normally present in functional cilia. Impaired ciliary motion is most prominently reflected in the lack of sperm motility and in the impaired epithelial function of the fallopian tubes and respiratory tract. Infertility results from impaired motility of sperm and epithelial function of fallopian tubes, while chronic sinopulmonary infections result from impaired function of the respiratory tract. Recurrent bronchitis and pneumonia due to impaired removal of airway secretions can lead to diffuse bronchiectasis with abnormally dilated airways and copious sputum production, but not to interstitial pulmonary fibrosis.

242. The answer is E. *(Wilson, ed 12. chap 206.)* Occupational respiratory illness resulting from inhalation of cotton dust or flax is first evident as a drop in airflow, with chest tightness and wheezing occurring on the first day of the work week. If exposure continues, symptoms may persist through the week. Persons exposed for 10 years or more may have irreversible airflow obstruction. Toluene diisocyanate exposure during production of polyurethane may produce persistent asthma in susceptible persons. Fluorocarbons, transmitted by a worker's hands to his or her cigarettes, are volatilized as the cigarette burns and may cause polymer fume fever, characterized by fever, malaise, and wheezing. Intense exposure to silica may produce acute silicosis with extensive pulmonary fibrosis that often terminates in respiratory failure in less than 2 years. Long-term exposure to lower levels of silica will cause nodular pulmonary fibrosis with hilar adenopathy. The fibrosis is usually greatest in the upper lobes. However, silica does not cause bronchospasm.

243. The answer is A. *(Wilson, ed 12. chap 207.)* Anaerobic organisms often cause pneumonia that features a gradually developing, almost indolent course characterized by weight loss and fever. However, single or multiple cavities are common complications usually occurring in lung segments that were dependent at the time of the initial aspiration. In contrast, cavitation is uncommon in pneumococcal pneumonia, rare in *Mycoplasma* pneumonia and in pneumonia due to *Legionella pneumophila*. Viral infections usually do not produce cavitation.

244. The answer is D. *(Wilson, ed 12. chap 215. Seifter, Semin Oncol 15:278, 1988.)* The distinction between small cell (also called oat cell) and non-small cell (adenocarcinoma, large cell, squamous cell) is made on morphologic, biochemical, and biologic grounds. While these differences bear heavily on the understanding of the neoplastic process, they also have important clinical implications because major treatment decisions rest on the differentiation of small cell and non-small cell lung tumors. Most small cell tumors present at a stage beyond the limits of reasonable resectability; however, they are much more responsive to radiation therapy and sensitive to chemotherapy than are the non-small variants. Complete regression of a non-small cell lung tumor would be rare with either modality, but such regression occurs about half the time with small cell tumors. Some 10 to 20 percent of patients with small cell disease limited to one hemithorax are long-term survivors; however, because most patients present with incurable, extensive disease, the overall 5-year survival for both non-small cell and small cell variants is under 10 percent. Small cell tumors are believed to originate from neuroendocrine cells because of the frequent presence of neuron-specific enolase, chromogranin, and secretory granules, as well as neuropeptides such as vasopressin and ACTH. Perhaps also indicative of the distinctive pathogenesis of small cell tumors is the frequent finding of retinoblastoma gene abnormalities and deletions in the long arm of chromosome 3.

245. The answer is B. *(Wilson, ed 12. chap 210.)* Certain persons with severe obstructive lung disease appear to respond to uncontrolled oxygen therapy by dangerously reducing their minute ventilation. Because they are relatively insensitive to changes in arterial P_{CO_2}, hypoxemia is the major ventilatory stimulus in these persons. When hypoxemia is suddenly treated with supplemental oxygen therapy given in an uncontrolled fashion, ventilation drops, arterial P_{CO_2} rises, acidosis results, and coma may develop. However, abrupt removal of supplemental oxygen may precipitate life-threatening hypoxemia. Because acidosis must nevertheless be rapidly reversed by increasing ventilation, endotracheal intubation should be performed, followed by mechanical ventilation of sufficient amount to return arterial pH to physiologic range. Inhaled bronchodilators cannot be given to comatose, unintubated persons. Epinephrine is relatively ineffective in persons with acute or chronic respiratory failure and is dangerous in elderly, acidemic patients.

246. The answer is D. *(Wilson, ed 12. chap 210.)* Right ventricular failure in persons with chronic pulmonary disease is usually evident as edema and ascites—that is, signs of increased extravascular water. Evidence also suggests that increased right ventricular filling pressures contribute to increases in lung water. Treatment should be aimed at reducing the afterload of the right ventricle. This goal can be accomplished most physiologically by increasing alveolar oxygen tension with supplemental oxygen therapy. Although hydralazine and diazoxide are vasodilators with important effects on the pulmonary circulation, they would not be needed in the case described and may, in fact, worsen gas exchange. Although the usefulness of digoxin therapy in cor pulmonale is debated, the drug generally is reserved for treating persons who have coexisting left ventricular disease. Phlebotomy, although it may improve oxygen delivery in persons with right ventricular failure and elevated hemoglobin concentrations (>200 g/L [20 g/dL]), would not be a reliable remedy for the ascites and edema in the patient presented.

247. The answer is B. *(Wilson, ed 12. chap 211. Crystal, N Engl J Med 310:154, 235, 1985.)* The chest x-rays presented show diffuse, severe interstitial infiltrates without hilar adenopathy. Although sarcoidosis may produce this radiographic picture, it is also compatible with idiopathic interstitial pneumonitis, hypersensitivity pneumonitis, collagen vascular disease, inhalation of inorganic dusts, and many other processes. The degree of respiratory system dysfunction demonstrated by this patient necessitates rapid evaluation and a definitive histologic diagnosis so that appropriate therapy can be initiated. Angiotensin-converting enzyme levels, although elevated in many patients with sarcoidosis, are not sufficiently sensitive or specific to replace tissue biopsy in the workup of persons with interstitial infiltrates. Although biopsy of extrapulmonary tissue may demonstrate noncaseating granulomas in patients with sarcoidosis, such biopsies may be negative in patients with active disease. A pathologic diagnosis is absolutely required in patients presenting with interstitial lung disease of uncertain etiology. Fiberoptic bronchoscopy should be performed to rule out infection or malignancy; an accompanying transbronchial biopsy may yield a diagnosis about 25 percent of the time. Bronchoalveolar lavage to assess the degree of inflammation may be helpful in monitoring disease activity, but its precise role in interstitial lung disease remains to be defined. Despite its relatively low yield, the relatively low risk makes an attempt at transbronchial biopsy reasonable prior to definitively obtaining tissue at open lung biopsy.

248. The answer is C. *(Wilson, ed 12. chap 212. Rich, Prog Cardiovasc Dis 31:205, 1988.)* Primary pulmonary hypertension is an uncommon disease that usually affects young women. Early in the illness affected persons often are diagnosed as psychoneurotic because of the vague nature of presenting complaints—for example, dyspnea, chest pain, and evidence of hyperventilation without hypoxemia on arterial blood-gas testing. However, progression of the disease leads to syncope in approximately one-half of cases and signs of right heart failure on physical examination. Chest x-ray typically shows enlarged central pulmonary arteries with or without attenuation of peripheral markings. The diagnosis of primary pulmonary hypertension is made by documentation of elevated pressures by right heart catheterization and by exclusion of other pathologic processes. Lung disease of sufficient severity to cause pulmonary hypertension would be evident by history and on examination. Major differential diagnoses include thromboemboli and heart disease; outside the United States, schistosomiasis and filariasis are common causes of pulmonary hypertension, and a careful travel history should be taken.

249. The answer is E. *(Wilson, ed 12. chap 213. Moylan, Annu Rev Med 28:85, 1977.)* The clinical triad of dyspnea, confusion, and petechiae in a person who has had recent long-bone fractures establishes the diagnosis of fat embolism syndrome. This disorder, which usually occurs within 48 h of injury, may lead to respiratory failure and death. Petechiae most often are found across the neck, in the axillae, and in the conjunctivae; however, their appearance is often evanescent. No laboratory test is specific for fat embolism.

250. The answer is E. *(Wilson, ed 12. chaps 91, 108, 214.)* Postanginal sepsis is a complication of acute bacterial pharyngitis in which a tonsillar abscess leads to infection of the ipsilateral carotid sheath and suppurative thrombophlebitis of the jugular vein. Anaerobic organisms are most commonly cultured from the blood and metastatic foci of infection. At the time of dissemination of infection the pharynx may not be painful, so the origin of the infection may be unsuspected.

251. The answer is E. *(Wilson, ed 12. chap 215.)* A solitary lung nodule in a middle-aged person who is a cigarette smoker requires surgical resection. Although a rheumatoid nodule would be in the differential diagnosis of the lesion described in the case, such nodules are usually subpleural and are more common in men than in women. The central location and small size of the lesion described make it relatively inaccessible to nonsurgical biopsy techniques. Because 95 percent of malignant solitary nodules originate in the lung, an undirected search for a primary source is likely to be fruitless. Mediastinoscopy has largely replaced scalene node biopsy in most centers, but because the incidence of mediastinal metastases in malignant solitary nodules is less than 10 percent, surgical exploration would be indicated for the woman described in the question.

252. The answer is E. *(Wilson, ed 12. chap 216.)* When the diaphragm is completely paralyzed, it behaves as a floppy membrane. With inspiration, the intercostal and other accessory muscles of respiration contract, causing intrathoracic pressure to become more negative. A floppy diaphragm would then be drawn upward into the chest, and the anterior abdominal wall would move inward. This ''paradoxical'' motion of the abdominal wall, which is best seen while an affected person is supine, is the most sensitive sign of bilateral diaphragmatic paralysis. Other disorders, such as severe obstructive lung disease, may also produce paradoxical motion of the anterior abdominal wall; however, the paradoxical motion usually improves when a person with this disorder is supine.

253. The answer is D. *(Wilson, ed 12. chap 217. Thawley, Med Clin North Am 69 (6), 1985.)* Obstructive sleep apnea syndrome is a complex entity that involves intermittent upper-airway obstruction during sleep. Most of the manifestations, such as hypertension, cor pulmonale, chronic fatigue, personality changes, and disordered sleep behavior, resolve when obstruction is bypassed by a tracheostomy or endotracheal tube. Although the syndrome is more common in men, the prevalence increases in women after menopause. Alcohol and sedatives can exacerbate ventilatory obstruction by decreasing upper-airway muscle tone. Treatment of severe obstructive sleep apnea includes tricyclics to improve upper-airway muscle tone, uvulopalatopharyngoplasty to create a more spacious airway, continuous nasal positive airway pressure to prevent muscular collapse, and tracheostomy to completely bypass the obstruction. Estrogens, once thought beneficial in improving respiratory drive, are not now considered a mainstay of treatment.

254. The answer is D. *(Wilson, ed 12. chaps 205, 211.)* Chronic eosinophilic pneumonia is an interstitial lung disorder of unknown cause that produces a systemic illness characterized by fever, weight loss, and malaise. Although lung biopsy shows an eosinophilic infiltrate involving both the interstitium and the alveolar space, there may not be an associated eosinophilia in the peripheral blood. The diagnosis should be suggested by the ''photonegative pulmonary edema'' pattern, with central sparing and nonsegmental, patchy infiltrates in the lung periphery. This disorder often responds dramatically to corticosteroid therapy. Idiopathic pulmonary fibrosis and polymyositis produce diffuse reticular, nodular, or reticulonodular infiltrates on chest x-ray. Alveolar proteinosis is a rare disorder that most often produces a diffuse air-space filling pattern radiating from hilar regions on chest x-ray, often with air bronchograms. Alveolar proteinosis does not cause fever unless complicated by infection such as nocardiosis. Lymphangiomyomatosis is also rare. It occurs exclusively in women of childbearing age. The chest x-ray shows reticulonodular infiltration but the lungs often appear hyperinflated. Lymphangiomyomatosis is complicated by pleural effusion and pneumothorax, but not fever.

255. The answer is B. *(Wilson, ed 12. chap 218.)* With mild respiratory distress syndrome, or early in the clinical picture, ventilation-perfusion abnormalities are primarily responsible for hypoxemia; therefore, modest increases in the inspired oxygen tension would produce significant increases in arterial oxygenation. As the disease becomes fully developed, however, diffuse alveolar collapse occurs, and right-to-left shunts are created. Under these circumstances, hypoxemia would be insensitive to small changes in inspired oxygen concentration.

256. The answer is B. *(Wilson, ed 12. chaps 218, 219.)* Some persons who become agitated or anxious while on a mechanical ventilator receive inadequate ventilation because they are breathing out of phase with the machine. The man described in the question has adequate oxygenation—a P_{O_2} of 70 mmHg means his hemoglobin is more than 90 percent saturated. However, he is hypoventilating and has developed an acute respiratory acidosis. Positive end-expiratory pressure (PEEP) improves oxygenation by raising the lung volume and reducing shunting but it does not have a large effect on carbon dioxide clearance. Therefore, the appropriate first step in management would be to administer a sedative and control the man's ventilation, in order to reduce arterial P_{CO_2} and raise pH.

257. The answer is D. *(Wilson, ed 12. chap 213.)* Patients at high risk for thromboembolic disease include those who have had recent anesthesia, recent childbirth, heart failure, leg fracture, prolonged bed rest, obesity, estrogen use, or cancer. The clinical scenario presented is highly consistent with a pulmonary embolism arising from venous thrombosis of a proximal lower extremity in a postoperative patient. While the electrocardiogram is usually normal except for sinus tachycardia, the finding of new right heart strain is compatible with a significant pulmonary embolus. The positive impedance plethysmogram for an above-the-knee venous thrombosis obviates the need for additional diagnostic testing. The patient must receive antithrombotic therapy (heparin) in an attempt to inhibit clot growth, promote resolution, and prevent recurrence. Warfarin requires several days to achieve anticoagulation and is therefore not appropriate for the acute setting. While thrombolytic therapy can clearly hasten the resolution of thrombi and may be appropriate for large, deep venous thromboses and pulmonary embolisms large enough to cause hypotension, its role in altering the natural history of this disorder remains to be defined. Furthermore, recent surgery is a contraindication to the use of thrombolytic agents, which, even in the case of more specific newer agents such as tissue plasminogen activator, carry significant hemorrhagic risk.

258. The answer is A-N, B-N, C-Y, D-Y, E-N. *(Wilson, ed 12. chap 204.)* Immediate drug therapy for a severe asthmatic attack consists primarily of intravenous administration of aminophylline and administration by inhalation or subcutaneous injection of a beta-adrenergic agent. Isoproterenol is a potent beta agonist highly effective when given by inhalation during an acute attack. Both the steroid beclomethasone and the mast-cell inhibitor cromolyn sodium are often effective when given by inhalation to asthmatic patients during periods of relative remission; however, both preparations actually can worsen airway function when administered during an acute attack. Because of the danger of respiratory depression, sedatives should not be used during acute exacerbations of asthma. Oral or intravenous steroids are useful in treating acute episodes of asthma but are not effective until several hours after initial administration.

259. The answer is A-Y, B-Y, C-Y, D-N, E-Y. *(Wilson, ed 12. chap 209.)* Although the majority of patients with cystic fibrosis receive their diagnosis in childhood, a significant number of patients will not be identified until their late teens, twenties, or even thirties. Accurate diagnosis requires that the sweat chloride test be given to all patients with clinical features of cystic fibrosis. Airway obstruction resulting from bronchiectasis is associated with sinusitis and infertility in males with both cystic fibrosis and the immotile cilia syndrome, but only males with immotile cilia have Kartagener's syndrome (bronchiectasis, sinusitis, and dextrocardia). Patients with cystic fibrosis may have any of several gastrointestinal manifestations including intussusception, fecal impaction, volvulus, portal hypertension, and steatorrhea. Steatorrhea is a manifestation of pancreatic insufficiency. Nearly all patients with cystic fibrosis show clubbing.

260. The answer is A-N, B-N, C-Y, D-Y, E-Y. *(Wilson, ed 12. chap 209. Riordan, Science 245:1066, 1989.)* Since 1948, the life expectancy of persons who have cystic fibrosis has improved from 2 years to more than 19 years. This rise can be attributed to two factors. First, owing to increased physician awareness and more aggressive screening programs, a population of older persons with slowly developing disease has now been identified. Second, meticulous treatment regimens, including regular pulmonary toilet and nutritional support with pancreatic enzymes, are improving survival. The lungs of affected persons are normal at birth, but poor clearance of secretions leads to chronic airway infections and destruction. Only 20 percent of persons with cystic fibrosis have persistent pancreatic function; the others are subject to malabsorption and may also develop portal hypertension. Nearly all men with cystic fibrosis (97 percent) are infertile because of structural defects in the reproductive system. Women with cystic fibrosis are likely to have difficulty conceiving a child, but a number of pregnancies have occurred and been carried to term. Meconium ileus occurs in 5 percent of cases and is a common mode of presentation. Cystic fibrosis, which is an autosomal recessive disorder, is associated with mutations in a gene on chromosome 7.

261. The answer is A-N, B-Y, C-N, D-Y, E-N. *(Wilson, ed 12. chap 210.)* The man described in the question presents physical signs (pursed lip breathing, chest hyperexpansion) and radiographic evidence (flattened diaphragms, attenuated markings) suggestive of obstructive lung disease with loss of lung tissue. Reduced expiratory air-flow rates are produced by narrowing of airways (e.g., in asthma), by loss of airways (e.g., in bronchiolitis obliterans), or by loss of elastic tissue (e.g., in emphysema). Pathophysiologically, these conditions cause increased resistance as airways are narrowed or collapse, as well as decreased driving pressure, representing loss of elastic recoil. Air-trapping and reduced lung recoil lead to an increase in both total lung capacity (TLC) and functional residual capacity (FRC), which is the volume at which the tendency of the lung to recoil inward is just balanced by the tendency of the chest to recoil outward. Although TLC is increased, vital capacity, the maximum amount of gas that can be exhaled from the lungs with a single breath, is reduced owing to the great increase in residual volume produced by gas trapping. Not only is vital capacity reduced, but it takes longer to empty the lungs; thus, forced expiratory volume in 1 s (FEV_1) is reduced as a percentage of vital capacity. When alveolar capillaries are destroyed by emphysema, the diffusing capacity, which reflects in part the surface area of alveolar membrane available for gas exchange, is reduced.

262. The answer is A-N, B-N, C-Y, D-Y, E-Y. *(Wilson, ed 12. chap 210.)* To establish baseline information in persons who have emphysema, spirometry should be performed, and for those persons with significant complaints or physical findings, arterial blood gases also should be checked. Although cigarette smoking accounts for the vast majority of cases of emphysema, a small percentage of persons who develop this illness have had no exposure to tobacco products. A subset of this nonsmoking, emphysematous population is deficient in α_1-antitrypsin, which is a protease inhibitor normally found in the serum. It is currently believed that release of proteolytic enzymes from inflammatory cells accounts for the lung destruction that typifies emphysema, and α_1-

antitrypsin deficiency, a familial disorder diagnosed by serum protein electrophoresis, permits this destruction to occur unimpeded. Exercise testing is not necessary as an initial screening test for emphysema but should be considered before oxygen therapy is prescribed. A male who has emphysematous respiratory failure, gives no history of respiratory infections, and who has children would not have cystic fibrosis (affected men are sterile); therefore, a sweat chloride test would not be a useful procedure.

263. The answer is A-Y, B-N, C-Y, D-N, E-N. *(Wilson, ed 12. chap 210.)* All persons suffer a gradual decline in expiratory flow rates with age, but smoking can cause some persons to lose function three or more times faster than in nonsmokers. Although lost function cannot be restored, cessation of smoking can reduce the rate at which function is lost, thereby improving the prognosis for persons who have chronic airway obstruction. In a subset of persons with air-flow obstruction—those whose resting P_{O_2} is less than 60 mmHg on room air—oxygen therapy has been shown to improve prognosis (this effect is not attributable to cessation of smoking). These two interventions, oxygen therapy and abstinence from smoking, can thus prolong life expectancy in selected persons. Exercise programs, phlebotomy, and use of oral expectorants may improve exercise performance and provide symptomatic relief, but none has a positive impact on survival in chronic airway obstruction.

264. The answer is A-N, B-Y, C-N, D-Y, E-Y. *(Wilson, ed 12. chap 35. Adelman, Ann Intern Med 102:829, 1985.)* Most patients with hemoptysis should be subject to in-depth evaluation until a cause is identified. Even after extensive workup, 5 to 15 percent of patients with gross hemoptysis remain undiagnosed. If patients with blood-tinged sputum as well as gross hemoptysis are included, the most common causes are bronchitis and bronchiectasis. If the definition is restricted to gross hemoptysis, then primary lung carcinoma is a more prominent etiology. Patients with cancer that metastasizes to the lung do not usually have hemoptysis. Historical clues can be helpful when pursuing the etiology. For example, a young, generally asymptomatic woman with repeated episodes of gross hemoptysis probably has a bronchial adenoma, whereas foul-smelling sputum suggests a lung abscess. In order to avert gravitational drainage and aspiration into the uninvolved lung, patients with hemoptysis tend to lie with the affected lung in the dependent position.

265. The answer is A-Y, B-N, C-N, D-Y, E-Y. *(Wilson, ed 12. chaps 199, 211. Crystal, Chest 95:196, 1989.)* Reduced serum levels of the antiprotease α_1-antitrypsin, which is primarily synthesized in the liver, are associated with an inability to control the alveolar-damaging effects of neutrophil elastase and clinical emphysema. α_1-Antitrypsin is encoded by a 7 exon gene spanning 12.2 kilobases on chromosome 14. Common disease-producing mutations of the normal M gene are the Z type, in which a single amino-acid substitution results in a hyperaggregative, improperly processed protein, and the S type, which results in a product with a shortened half-life and is also due to a single amino-acid change. Since the S type produces less clinical antiprotease ''deficiency,'' the pulmonary disease produced in SS homozygotes is much less than that seen in patients whose genotype is ZZ. Intravenous administration of normal human purified α_1-antitrypsin can increase serum levels to a point at which sufficient antiprotease activity is provided to protect alveoli from elastase-induced damage.

266. The answer is A-Y, B-Y, C-N, D-Y, E-N. *(Wilson, ed 12. chap 213.)* Hypoxemia occurs commonly after massive pulmonary thromboembolism, although normal arterial oxygen tension does not exclude the diagnosis. The most important mechanism producing hypoxemia in this setting is an increase in venous admixture due to continued perfusion of poorly ventilated areas. Ventilation may be decreased by atelectasis or by airway constriction in response to the release of bronchoactive mediators. A fall in cardiac output producing a low mixed venous P_{O_2} can increase the effect of venous admixture. Increased dead-space ventilation would not be a cause of hypoxemia.

267. The answer is A-Y, B-N, C-N, D-Y, E-N. *(Wilson, ed 12. chap 215.)* Although persons with pulmonary lesions often require sophisticated pulmonary function testing to determine their suitability for surgery, hypercapnia at rest usually is considered a contraindication to resection. Obviously, metabolic and other causes of hypoventilation must be excluded. The presence of systemic syndromes, including syndrome of inappropriate antidiuretic hormone secretion (SIADH), does not rule out surgery; in fact, these syndromes often remit following surgical resection of the pulmonary lesion. Pleural effusion in the absence of cytologic or histologic evidence of pleural metastasis also is not a contraindication to surgery. Paralysis of either the recurrent laryngeal nerve or the phrenic nerve indicates that the affected person has nonoperable disease. Although metastatic invasion of mediastinal lymph nodes usually is considered an indication not to operate, metastatic spread to lobar lymph nodes that could be included in the surgical block resection does not rule out surgery.

268. The answer is A-Y, B-N, C-Y, D-Y, E-N. *(Wilson, ed 12. chap 201.)* The volume remaining in the lungs at the conclusion of a complete forced expiration is termed the *residual volume* and can be determined either by the body plethysmography or helium dilution methods. At the residual volume there is a balance between the intrinsic outward recoil of the chest wall and the force maintained by the respiratory muscles to decrease lung volumes further. Therefore, increases in the residual volume can result from the functionally weak musculature of the chest wall that might be observed in neuromuscular disorders that affect the ability to expire forcefully (Guillain-Barré syndrome, muscular dystrophies, cervical spine injury). Furthermore, diseased airways will collapse at low lung volumes, preventing further emptying and also producing an abnormally high residual volume. Thus, any condition in which airway obstruction plays a major role (chronic bronchitis, emphysema, asthma, cystic fibrosis) may be associated with increased residual volume. On the other hand, pulmonary parenchymal disease (e.g., sarcoidosis) produces normal expiration and reduced lung volumes. If inspiratory dysfunction is the primary chest wall problem (as in kyphoscoliosis and obesity), then residual volume will be relatively unaffected or slightly decreased.

269. The answer is A-Y, B-Y, C-N, D-N, E-Y. *(Wilson, ed 12. chap 204.)* Although inhaled sympathomimetics are now considered the first-choice treatment for acute asthmatic attacks, the methylxanthines such as theophylline are effective bronchodilators and continue to be extensively used in this disorder. The therapeutic plasma concentration is 10 to 20 μg/mL, but the dose required to achieve these levels varies widely depending on the clinical situation. Theophylline dosage should be reduced in any condition in which the clearance of this drug is significantly impaired, such as in the very young, the elderly, and in those with liver or cardiac dysfunction. Many drugs interfere with the metabolism of theophylline. Commonly used agents including allopurinol, propranolol, cimetidine, and erythromycin all interfere with theophylline clearance and thereby lead to increased levels of this methylxanthine. Drugs that activate hepatic microsomal enzymes—such as cigarettes, marijuana, phenobarbital, and phenytoin—may lower theophylline levels.

270. The answer is A-N, B-N, C-N, D-Y, E-N. *(Wilson, ed 12. chap 216.)* Pleural fluid culture is positive in less than 25 percent of cases of postprimary tuberculous pleural infection. For this reason, a closed pleural biopsy should be performed in suspected cases of tuberculous pleuritis. Eosinophils are a nonspecific finding in pleural effusion and often occur in large numbers after thoracentesis. Eosinophils also may be found in effusions associated with viral or bacterial pneumonias, pancreatitis, and carcinomatous involvement of the pleura. Glucose concentration less than 0.83 mmol/L (15 mg/dL) is characteristic of rheumatoid pleural effusion. This low glucose concentration is due to a defect in glucose transport across the pleural surface and is not sensitive to changes in serum glucose levels. Pleural effusions in patients with malignant disease are most often due to pleural metastasis or to lymphatic or bronchial obstruction caused by tumor. Malignant pleural effusions are typically exudative and hemorrhagic. If repeated thoracenteses and systemic antineoplastic therapy fail to alleviate symptoms associated with a large effusion, sclerosis with tetracycline after chest tube drainage is usually effective. After lung cancer, breast cancer is the most common cause of malignant pleural effusion; lymphoma, which is the third most common cause, may be associated with chylothorax, the accumulation of triglyceride-laden particles due to thoracic duct obstruction.

271. The answer is A-Y, B-Y, C-N, D-Y, E-Y. *(Wilson, ed 12. chap 206.)* Inhalation of asbestos fibers for 10 years or more may lead to interstitial fibrosis that typically begins in the lower lobes, later spreading to mid and upper lung fields. This fibrosis is associated with a restrictive pattern on pulmonary function testing. The chest x-ray shows linear densities, thickening or calcification of the pleura (pleural plaques), and, in severe cases, honeycombing. Exposure to asbestos may also cause exudative pleural effusions. These effusions are often blood-stained and may be painful. The diagnosis may be elusive if a careful occupational exposure is not obtained. These effusions are benign, but affected persons may later sustain malignant mesotheliomas of the pleura or peritoneum. Unlike pulmonary fibrosis, pleural effusions and mesotheliomas may develop after brief exposures to asbestos, often of 1 to 2 years. Mesotheliomas are not associated with cigarette smoking, but the combination of exposure to asbestos and cigarette smoking has a multiplicative effect on the risk of development of lung cancer. Exposure to asbestos increases the risk for both adenocarcinoma and squamous cell (but not oat cell) carcinoma of the lung, which suggests that lung cancer screening may be useful in selected individuals.

272. The answer is A-N, B-Y, C-Y, D-N, E-N. *(Wilson, ed 12. chap 218. Raffin, Hosp Pract 22:65, 1987.)* The adult respiratory distress syndrome (ARDS) is a clinical triad of hypoxemia, diffuse lung infiltrates, and reduced lung compliance not attributable to congestive cardiac failure. This syndrome's many causes suggest its complex pathogenesis. However, the pathologic outcome is the same: an increase in lung water due to an increase in alveolar capillary permeability. This noncardiogenic pulmonary edema is identical to congestive cardiac pulmonary edema in its effect on the mechanical properties of the lung and on gas exchange. Just as in cardiac pulmonary edema, the increase in lung water associated with ARDS produces interstitial edema and alveolar collapse, so the affected lung becomes stiff and the alveolar-arterial oxygen tension difference widens. Unlike cardiac edema, however, the increase in lung water in ARDS occurs as a result of an increase in alveolar capillary permeability and is not due to an increase in hydrostatic forces. Edema fluid in ARDS, therefore, often contains macromolecules (such as serum proteins), and measurement of pulmonary artery wedge pressure is normal or low. In clinical practice, determination of pulmonary artery wedge pressure is the most helpful discriminant between ARDS and cardiac failure.

273. The answer is A-N, B-Y, C-N, D-Y, E-Y. *(Wilson, ed 12. chap 210.)* There are many reasons why patients fail removal from assisted ventilation. Sedatives, commonly prescribed earlier in the hospital stay for agitation or sleep, may not yet have been discontinued or metabolized and could contribute to impairment of respiratory drive. Persistent secretions that could be removed by suctioning might also contribute to the problem. A very important issue is maintenance of a continued drive to breathe. The central respiratory centers are sensitive to blood pH and will promote ventilation when sufficient acidosis (greater than that normally noted in the bronchitic patient with chronic CO_2 retention) ensues. Thus, creation of metabolic alkalosis with diuretic therapy or running the assisted minute ventilation too high (i.e., lower P_{CO_2} and higher pH than normal for the patient) could account for failed extubation. Neuromuscular weakness caused by diuretic-induced hypokalemia, malnutrition, and occult hypothyroidism are potential factors leading to difficulty in independent ventilation and trouble in weaning.

274. The answer is A-N, B-Y, C-N, D-Y, E-Y. *(Wilson, ed 12. chap 211. Toronto Lung Transplant Group, JAMA 259:2258, 1988.)* A nonproductive cough, dyspnea, hypoxemia with normo- or hypocapnia at rest, bibasilar reticular infiltrates on chest x-ray, and restrictive pulmonary function tests (normal or increased FEV_1, reduced lung volumes) should suggest the diagnosis of idiopathic pulmonary fibrosis. This diagnosis can only be confirmed after the host of other entities causing interstitial lung disease are excluded by appropriate clinical and pathologic examination. Inasmuch as activated alveolar macrophages (possibly owing to an immune complex) are believed to be pathogenetically responsible for this disease, it is not surprising that immunosuppressive therapy with corticosteroids with or without cyclophosphamide has been beneficial. While chest x-ray correlates poorly with disease activity, the carbon monoxide diffusing capacity, usually reduced in idiopathic pulmonary fibrosis, is a useful test in assessing therapeutic response. Given the initial success with the procedure, lung transplantation (heart-lung or single-lung) should be considered in severe or unresponsive cases.

Disorders of the Kidney and Urinary Tract

DIRECTIONS: Each question below contains five suggested responses. Choose the **one best** response to each question.

275. Laboratory evaluation of a 19-year-old man being worked up for polyuria and polydipsia yields the following results:

> Serum electrolytes (mmol/L): Na^+ 144; K^+ 4.0; Cl^- 107; HCO_3^- 25
> BUN: 6.4 mmol/L (18 mg/dL)
> Blood glucose: 5.7 mmol/L (102 mg/dL)
> Urine electrolytes (mmol/L): Na^+ 28; K^+ 32
> Urine osmolality: 195 mosmol/kg water

After 12 h of fluid deprivation, body weight has fallen by 5 percent. Laboratory testing now reveals the following:

> Serum electrolytes (mmol/L): Na^+ 150; K^+ 4.1; Cl^- 109; HCO_3^- 25
> BUN: 7.1 mmol/L (20 mg/dL)
> Blood glucose: 5.4 mmol/L (98 mg/dL)
> Urine electrolytes (mmol/L): Na^+ 24; K^+ 35
> Urine osmolality: 200 mosmol/kg water

One hour after the subcutaneous administration of 5 units of pitressin, urine values are as follows:

> Urine electrolytes (mmol/L): Na^+ 30; K^+ 30
> Urine osmolality: 199 mosmol/kg water

The likely diagnosis in this case is

(A) nephrogenic diabetes insipidus
(B) osmotic diuresis
(C) salt-losing nephropathy
(D) psychogenic polydipsia
(E) none of the above

276. A 70-year-old woman who has adult-onset diabetes is brought to an emergency room in an unresponsive state. Her family states that several days ago she got a "cold" and then became increasingly weak and finally disoriented. She has not been taking insulin or any other medication. Admission vital signs are temperature 38.3°C (101°F), pulse 100 beats per minute, respiratory rate 36 breaths per minute, and blood pressure 110/70 mmHg. Her weight is 70 kg (154 pounds). Laboratory values include the following:

> Serum electrolytes (mmol/L): Na^+ 142; K^+ 3.2; Cl^- 102; HCO_3^- 26
> Blood glucose: 67 mmol/L (1200 mg/dL)
> BUN: 12.4 mmol/L (35 mg/dL)
> Serum creatinine: 141 μmol/L (1.6 mg/dL)

A reasonable estimate of this woman's total body water and sodium deficits would be

(A) 5 L water, 50 mmol sodium
(B) 5 L water, 150 mmol sodium
(C) 5 L water, 350 mmol sodium
(D) 10 L water, 150 mmol sodium
(E) 10 L water, 350 mmol sodium

277. A 70-year-old man with diabetes mellitus and hypertension has the following serum chemistries:

> Electrolytes (mmol/L): Na^+ 138; K^+ 5.0; Cl^- 106; HCO_3^- 20
> Glucose: 11 mmol/L (200 mg/dL)
> Creatinine: 176 μmol/L (2.0 mg/dL)

All the following may contribute to worsening hyperkalemia EXCEPT

(A) propranolol
(B) indomethacin
(C) captopril
(D) digitalis
(E) carbenicillin

278. A 35-year-old man with a history of alcoholism and hepatic cirrhosis is hospitalized because of massive ascites and severe pitting edema of the lower extremities and sacrum. Admission laboratory values are as follows:

Serum electrolytes (mmol/L): Na^+ 135; K^+ 3.0; Cl^- 95; HCO_3^- 28
Serum chemistries: BUN 5.4 mmol/L (15 mg/dL); creatinine 176 μmol/L (2.0 mg/dL)

During the first hospital day the man makes 400 mL of urine with a sodium concentration of 6 mmol/L and an osmolality of 638 mosmol/kg. Which of the following measures is likely to be most beneficial in the treatment of the sodium-retaining state described?

(A) Oral furosemide, 120 mg twice daily
(B) Intravenous furosemide, 120 mg twice daily
(C) Intravenous mannitol, 25 g twice daily
(D) Abdominal paracentesis to drain 2 L of fluid daily
(E) Bed rest and a low-sodium diet

279. The following laboratory serum values are obtained:

Electrolytes (mmol/L): Na^+ 122; K^+ 4.2; Cl^- 88; HCO_3^- 24
BUN: 2.8 mmol/L (8 mg/dL)
Creatinine: 71 μmol/L (0.8 mg/dL)
Osmolality: 245 mosm/kg

These findings are most consistent with

(A) multiple myeloma
(B) acute bacterial meningitis
(C) congestive heart failure
(D) Addison's disease
(E) diabetes mellitus

280. Which of the following case histories would most likely be associated with the urine sediment depicted?

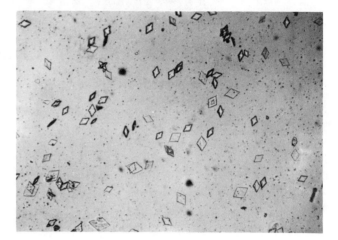

(A) A 23-year-old man with newly diagnosed lymphoblastic lymphoma who is found to have a rising creatinine level 2 days after the administration of combination chemotherapy
(B) A 23-year-old woman 1 year after surgery performed because of morbid obesity
(C) A 45-year-old woman with a history of multiple urinary tract infections with urea-splitting organisms
(D) A 40-year-old man with edema, hypoalbuminemia, and proteinuria
(E) An 18-year-old man with flank pain, hematuria, and a positive family history for renal stones occurring in youth

281. A 72-year-old man becomes oliguric following surgery for repair of an abdominal aortic aneurysm. He is alert, oriented, and able to take fluids and medications by mouth. Laboratory testing done on the fourth postoperative day reveals the following:

> Serum electrolytes (mmol/L): Na^+ 139; K^+ 5.1; Cl^- 104; HCO_3^- 17
>
> Serum chemistries: BUN 32 mmol/L (90 mg/dL); creatinine 740 μmol/L (8.4 mg/dL); calcium 2.0 mmol/L (8.0 mg/dL); phosphorus 3.4 mmol/L (10.4 mg/dL); uric acid 1070 μmol/L (18.0 mg/dL); glucose 7.8 mmol/L (140 mg/dL)
>
> Urine volume: approximately 400 mL/d (Foley catheter in place)
>
> Urine electrolytes (mmol/L): Na^+ 50; K^+ 30; Cl^- 40

All the following orders would be appropriate in the management of this man EXCEPT

(A) discontinue drainage by Foley catheter
(B) give oral aluminum hydroxide gel (Amphogel), 60 mL four times daily
(C) give oral allopurinol, 300 mg once daily
(D) limit total fluid intake to 800 mL per day
(E) ensure daily intake of at least 100 g of carbohydrate

282. In patients with chronic renal failure, all the following are important contributors to bone disease EXCEPT

(A) impaired renal production of 1,25-dihydroxyvitamin D_3
(B) hyperphosphatemia
(C) aluminum-containing antacids
(D) loss of vitamin D and calcium via dialysis
(E) metabolic acidosis

283. A 45-year-old woman who has had slowly progressive renal failure begins to complain of increasing numbness and prickling sensations in her legs. Examination reveals loss of pinprick and vibration sensation below the knees, absent ankle jerks, and impaired pinprick sensation in her hands. Serum creatinine concentration, checked during her most recent clinic visit, is 790 μmol/L (8.9 mg/dL). The woman's physician should now recommend

(A) a therapeutic trial of phenytoin
(B) a therapeutic trial of pyridoxine (vitamin B_6)
(C) a therapeutic trial of cyanocobalamin (vitamin B_{12})
(D) initiation of maintenance hemodialysis
(E) neurologic referral for nerve conduction studies

284. The condition of a 50-year-old obese woman with a 5-year history of mild hypertension controlled with a thiazide diuretic is being evaluated because proteinuria was noted on her routine yearly medical visit. Physical examination disclosed a height of 167.6 cm (66 in); weight 91 kg (202 lb); blood pressure 130/80 mmHg; and trace pedal edema. Laboratory values are as follows:

Serum creatinine: 106 μmol/L (1.2 mg/dL)
BUN: 6.4 mmol/L (18 mg/dL)
Creatinine clearance: 87 mL/min
Urinalysis: pH 5.0; specific gravity 1.018; protein 3+; no glucose; occasional coarse granular cast
Urine protein excretion: 5.9 g/d

A renal biopsy was performed and the results are as shown below. Sixty percent of the glomeruli appeared as shown (by light microscopy); the remainder were unremarkable.

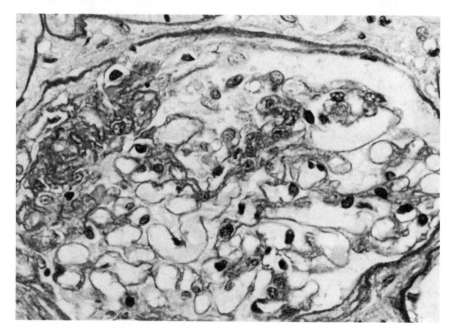

The most likely diagnosis is

(A)   hypertensive nephrosclerosis
(B)   focal and segmental sclerosis
(C)   minimal-change (nil) disease
(D)   membranous glomerulopathy
(E)   crescentic glomerulonephritis

285. In a person who has carcinoma of the lung and the depicted urinalysis, renal biopsy would most likely show

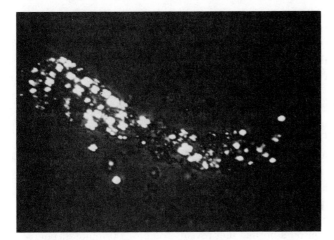

(A) minimal change disease
(B) diffuse proliferative glomerulonephritis
(C) membranoproliferative glomerulonephritis
(D) membranous glomerulopathy
(E) focal glomerulosclerosis

286. A 19-year-old U.S. Marine, who has had a feeling of malaise for a few hours, begins passing coffee-colored urine. During the next 2 days pedal edema develops. Urinalysis reveals 4+ hematuria, 3+ proteinuria, and a sediment containing many red-cell and white-cell casts. Serum testing shows that the BUN level is 14 mmol/L (40 mg/dL) and creatinine concentration is 350 μmol/L (4.0 mg/dL). Renal biopsy reveals diffuse endocapillary proliferative lesions with infiltration of glomeruli by polymorphonuclear leukocytes. All the following conditions could produce this clinical picture EXCEPT

(A) infectious mononucleosis
(B) streptococcal infection
(C) heroin abuse
(D) acute viral hepatitis
(E) falciparum malaria

287. All the following represent potential complications of chronic hemodialysis EXCEPT

(A) autonomic neuropathy
(B) cerebral vascular accidents
(C) osteomalacia
(D) gastrointestinal bleeding
(E) dementia

288. A 40-year-old woman who has never had significant respiratory disease is hospitalized for evaluation of hemoptysis. Urinalysis reveals 2+ proteinuria and microscopic hematuria. BUN concentration is 7.1 mmol/L (20 mg/dL), and serum creatinine concentration is 177 μmol/L (2.0 mg/dL). Serologic findings include normal complement levels, increased immunoglobulin A levels, and a negative assay for fluorescent antinuclear antibodies. Renal biopsy reveals granulomatous necrotizing vasculitis with scattered immunoglobulin and complement deposits. The most likely diagnosis in this case is

(A) mesangial lupus glomerulonephritis
(B) Henoch-Schönlein purpura
(C) microscopic polyarteritis
(D) Wegener's granulomatosis
(E) Goodpasture's syndrome

289. All the following patients are at risk of developing destruction of renal papillae with concomitant tubulointerstitial damage EXCEPT

(A) a middle-aged man who has consumed "moonshine" alcohol distilled in automobile radiators
(B) an older man with repetitive episodes of acute urinary retention due to prostatic hypertrophy
(C) a young adult woman with sickle cell anemia
(D) an older woman who uses analgesics for chronic headaches
(E) a middle-aged woman with a history of multiple urinary tract infections associated with pyuria, flank pain, fever, and poor response to short courses of oral antibiotics

290. A marked decline in renal function due to acute interstitial nephritis has been reported in association with all the following drugs EXCEPT

(A) methicillin
(B) cephalothin
(C) heparin
(D) ampicillin
(E) furosemide

291. A patient being examined for acute renal failure has a urine sodium concentration of 15 mmol/L and a urine osmolality of 510 mosmol/kg. These findings might be consistent with all the following conditions EXCEPT

(A) acute poststreptococcal glomerulonephritis
(B) acute partial urinary obstruction
(C) cholesterol embolization of the kidneys
(D) rhabdomyolysis
(E) cirrhosis of the liver with ascites

292. A 30-year-old woman with diabetic nephropathy received a cadaveric renal allograft. On the third postoperative day her serum creatinine concentration was 160 μmol/L (1.8 mg/dL). She is being treated with cyclosporine and prednisone. On the sixth postoperative day she experiences a decrease in urine output from 1500 mL/d to 1000 mL/d; the serum creatinine concentration increases to 194 μmol/L (2.2 mg/dL). Her blood pressure remains stable at 170/90 mmHg and her temperature is 37.2°C (99.0°F). The best initial step in management would be to

(A) decrease the dose of cyclosporine
(B) obtain ultrasonography of the renal allograft
(C) obtain a biopsy of the renal allograft
(D) administer pulsed steroid therapy
(E) administer an intravenous bolus of furosemide

293. A 55-year-old man undergoes intravenous pyelography (IVP) as part of a workup for hypertension. A solitary radiolucent mass, 3 cm in size, is noted in the left kidney; the study otherwise is normal. The man complains of no symptoms referable to the urinary tract, and examination of urine sediment is within normal limits. Which of the following studies should be performed next?

(A) Repeat intravenous pyelography in 6 months
(B) Early-morning urine collections for cytology (three samples)
(C) Selective renal arteriography
(D) Renal ultrasonography and, if warranted, needle aspiration of the mass
(E) CT scanning (with contrast enhancement) of the left kidney

294. Risk factors for carcinoma of the bladder include all the following EXCEPT

(A) exposure to cigarette smoke
(B) use of cyclophosphamide
(C) exposure to dyes
(D) positive family history
(E) schistosomal infestation

295. A 10-year-old girl complaining of profound weakness, occasional difficulty walking, and polyuria is brought to her pediatrician. Her mother is sure her daughter has not been vomiting frequently. The girl takes no medicines. She is normotensive and no focal neurologic abnormalities are found. Serum chemistries include sodium 142 mmol/L; potassium 2.5 mmol/L; bicarbonate 32 mmol/L; chloride 100 mmol/L. A 24-h urine collection on a normal diet reveals sodium 200 mmol/d, potassium 50 mmol/d, and chloride 30 mmol/d. A stool phenolphthalein test and urine screen for diuretics are negative. Plasma renin levels are found to be elevated. Which of the following conditions is most consistent with the above data?

(A) Conn's syndrome
(B) Chronic ingestion of licorice
(C) Bartter's syndrome
(D) Wilms's tumor
(E) Proximal renal tubular acidosis

DIRECTIONS: Each question below contains five suggested responses. For **each** of the five responses listed with **each** item, you are to respond either YES (Y) or NO (N). In a given item **all, some, or none of the alternatives may be correct.**

296. A 43-year-old construction worker is noted to be anuric following a crush injury to the lower extremities. Serum electrolytes (mmol/L) obtained 8 h following admission are Na^+ 138, K^+ 8.8, Cl^- 100, and HCO_3^- 19. Electrocardiography reveals peaked T waves, prolongation of the PR interval, and widening of the QRS complex. Which of the following measures would rapidly lower serum potassium concentration in the man described?

(A) Intravenous infusion of 10 mL of a 10% calcium gluconate solution
(B) Intravenous infusion of 10 mL of a 10% magnesium sulfate solution
(C) Intravenous infusion of 50 mL of a 50% glucose solution with 10 units of regular insulin
(D) Intravenous infusion of 2 ampules of sodium bicarbonate
(E) Administration by nasogastric tube of 60 mL of a potassium-binding resin

297. Rhabdomyolysis or acute myoglobinuric renal failure can develop as a result of

(A) strenuous muscular exercise
(B) barbiturate overdose
(C) ethanol ingestion
(D) hypokalemia
(E) volume depletion

298. A 38-year-old man who has diverticulitis develops azotemia after 7 days of inpatient therapy with gentamicin. His BUN and serum creatinine concentrations, normal on admission, now are 21 mmol/L (60 mg/dL) and 450 μmol/L (5.1 mg/dL), respectively. His urine output never has been less than 2 L per day. Which of the following statements about this case are true?

(A) About 25 percent of persons with acute renal failure are not oliguric
(B) Oliguric and nonoliguric renal failure carry similar prognoses
(C) Nonoliguric renal failure is characteristic of gentamicin toxicity
(D) The maximum BUN achieved by this man would be less than that expected if he developed oliguria
(E) Urine sodium concentration would probably be less than 10 mmol/L and urine osmolality greater than 400 mosmol/kg

299. Patients in whom the mechanism leading to their urinary incontinence puts them at risk for hydronephrosis include those with

(A) Alzheimer's dementia
(B) Guillain-Barré syndrome
(C) normal pressure hydrocephalus
(D) diabetes mellitus
(E) hypothyroidism

300. A previously healthy 55-year-old man presents with confusion that began 2 days ago. Serum values (in mmol/L) include Na^+ 120, K^+ 4.0, Cl^- 90, and HCO_3^- 23. The patient is not edematous. Which of the following conditions could explain the preceding information?

(A) Subdural hematoma
(B) Occult alcoholism with hepatic cirrhosis
(C) Lung cancer
(D) Addison's disease
(E) Hypothyroidism

301. Serum complement levels typically are low during the acute or active phase of which of the following diseases?

(A) Diffuse proliferative glomerulonephritis associated with systemic lupus erythematosus
(B) Membranous glomerulopathy
(C) Poststreptococcal glomerulonephritis
(D) Membranoproliferative glomerulonephritis
(E) Immunoglobulin A nephropathy

302. Metabolic abnormalities associated with the nephrotic syndrome include

(A) increased serum lipid levels
(B) increased serum thyroxine levels
(C) reduced serum calcium levels
(D) reduced serum zinc levels
(E) increased serum antithrombin III (heparin cofactor) levels

303. True statements about acute poststreptococcal glomerulonephritis (PSGN) include which of the following?

(A) The latent period appears to be longer when PSGN is associated with cutaneous rather than with pharyngeal infections
(B) Serologic evidence of a streptococcal infection may not be forthcoming if antimicrobial therapy is begun early
(C) Antimicrobial therapy for streptococcal infection is without value once the presence of renal disease is established
(D) Long-term antistreptococcal prophylaxis is indicated following documented cases of PSGN
(E) Lasting and progressive deterioration in renal function is more common in adults than in children with PSGN

304. A 23-year-old woman develops gross hematuria following an upper respiratory tract infection. Urinalysis shows 4+ hematuria and 2+ proteinuria with a sediment containing red-cell casts. Gross hematuria resolves during the next several days. Renal biopsy shows diffuse mesangial deposition of immunoglobulin A (IgA). True statements about this woman's disease include

(A) elevation of circulating IgA levels would be unusual
(B) IgA deposits are often found in dermal capillaries
(C) further episodes of gross hematuria typically would be associated with flulike infections or with exercise
(D) the nephrotic syndrome occasionally develops
(E) the disease leads to dialysis or transplantation in 10 percent of cases

305. A 27-year-old woman whose diabetes was diagnosed when she was 9 years old has had 1+ to 2+ proteinuria without abnormality of the urine sediment for the last 3 years. During the last year her serum creatinine concentration has doubled, so that now it is 210 μmol/L (2.4 mg/dL). Blood pressure has risen from 95/70 to 125/95 mmHg. Presuming the diagnosis of diabetic nephropathy is established, which of the following statements concerning the woman's condition would be true?

(A) Ophthalmologic examination would likely reveal retinal microvascular disease
(B) Rigorous control of hypertension would likely slow the progression of renal failure
(C) Rigorous control of blood sugar levels would likely slow the progression of renal failure
(D) Insulin requirement would likely decline with worsening renal failure
(E) Dialysis or transplantation would likely be required within 5 years

306. The inheritance of a tendency to develop adult polycystic kidney disease is correctly described by which of the following statements?

(A) A mutation on the short arm of chromosome 16 has been linked to the disease
(B) A polymorphic locus near the alpha-globin gene cluster has been linked to the disease
(C) Most cases are due to new mutations
(D) Adult polycystic kidney disease displays autosomal recessive inheritance
(E) A person found to be homozygous at the polymorphic locus linked to the disease cannot be analyzed for predisposition to the disease

307. Which of the following patients could be appropriately matched with the urine sediment depicted?

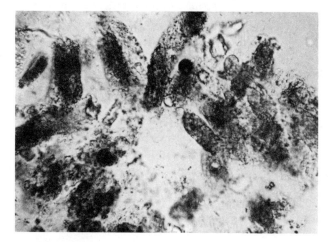

(A) A 75-year-old man 1 day after complicated surgery for the repair of an abdominal aortic aneurysm
(B) A 75-year-old man with a porcine aortic valve prosthesis, malaise, fever, and positive blood cultures
(C) A 50-year-old man with a history of chronic alcoholism who presents with stupor and a history of having been found on the street with multiple bruises
(D) A 75-year-old man with known benign prostatic hypertrophy and inability to void who presents with an enlarged bladder and a creatinine level of 220 μmol/L (2.5 mg/dL)
(E) A 35-year-old woman with idiopathic dilated cardiomyopathy and an ejection fraction of 15 percent who is awaiting cardiac transplantation

308. A 45-year-old black woman on chronic hemo-dialysis for renal failure due to uncontrolled hypertension has a hematocrit of 22 percent with a mean red cell volume (MCV) of 89. Correct statements about her condition include which of the following?

(A) A trial of erythropoietin is unlikely to improve her hematocrit because erythropoiesis is relatively unresponsive to this hormone in the face of chronic uremia

(B) The patient may be experiencing chronic blood loss because of the use of heparin with dialysis or the abnormal hemostasis associated with chronic renal failure

(C) Folic acid deficiency is possible, even though the anemia is normocytic

(D) Multiple blood transfusions could lead to direct heart damage

(E) If the patient requires surgery, vasopressin or cryoprecipitate could be used to ameliorate the bleeding tendency

309. A 48-year-old woman is hospitalized for elective knee surgery. Routine preoperative laboratory evaluation reveals the following:

Serum electrolytes (mmol/L): Na^+ 142; K^+ 4.3; Cl^- 110; HCO_3^- 20
Blood glucose: 5.2 mmol/L (95 mg/dL)
Serum creatinine: 160 μmol/L (1.8 mg/dL)
BUN: 7.1 mmol/L (20 mg/dL)
Urinalysis: pH 6.0; specific gravity 1.005; protein 1+; glucose 2+; 3 to 5 white blood cells per high-power field

This woman says she voids several times during the night but is unaware of any problem with her kidneys. Disorders associated with the findings in this case would include

(A) multiple myeloma
(B) diabetic nephropathy
(C) Sjögren's syndrome
(D) penicillamine-induced nephropathy
(E) analgesic abuse

310. True statements concerning renal artery stenosis as a cause of hypertension include which of the following?

(A) It is more likely to occur in persons less than 30 years of age or more than 50 years of age than in other persons

(B) It is often associated with a tendency towards hyperkalemia

(C) Captopril is a useful agent in the control of the blood pressure

(D) Administration of captopril may precipitate acute renal failure

(E) Intravenous pyelography is the most sensitive and specific screening procedure

311. Renal involvement in persons with scleroderma can be described correctly by which of the following statements?

(A) Serious renal insufficiency develops in a small minority of persons with scleroderma

(B) Accelerated hypertension is the most common presentation of renal disease in scleroderma

(C) Proliferative glomerulonephritis is the typical morphologic finding

(D) Aggressive antihypertensive therapy has been shown to preserve renal function

(E) Renal transplantation is generally contraindicated because of the risk of recurrent disease in the allograft

312. A 45-year-old woman presents with her third episode of nephrolithiasis. Laboratory studies disclose the following:

> Serum electrolytes (mmol/L): Na^+ 134; K^+ 2.5; Cl^- 106; HCO_3^- 18
>
> Serum chemistries: creatinine 97 μmol/L (1.1 mg/dL); calcium 2.4 mmol/L (9.5 mg/dL); albumin 40 g/L (4.0 g/dL)
>
> Arterial blood gas values: P_{CO_2} 4 kPa (30 mmHg); P_{O_2} 14 kPa (108 mmHg); pH 7.30
>
> Urine pH: 7.2

A plain film of the abdomen is shown below. Correct statements about this clinical picture include which of the following?

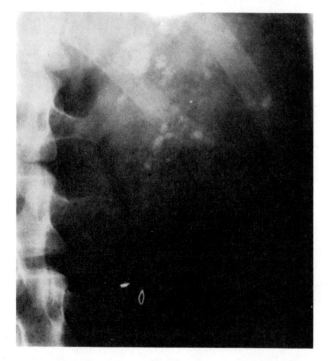

(A) The findings are consistent with the presence of multiple myeloma
(B) The findings are consistent with the presence of medullary sponge kidney
(C) There is evidence for type I distal renal tubular acidosis (RTA)
(D) Family members should be screened for electrolyte disorders
(E) Intravenous pyelography would provide further useful information

313. Correct statements regarding renal allografting include which of the following?

(A) A potential living donor that does not share the same blood type as the recipient cannot be considered even if the tissue types are HLA-identical
(B) The degree of HLA mismatch with cadaveric donor kidneys is a determinant of long-term graft survival
(C) Progressive renal failure in a transplant recipient, termed *chronic rejection,* is associated with renal vascular damage
(D) Allopurinol must be coadministered with azathioprine to prevent urate nephropathy associated with drug-induced cell turnover
(E) Cyclosporine A inhibits IL-2 production by helper T cells

314. A previously healthy 45-year-old man who developed weight gain, fatigue, and vomiting within the past week presents to his physician. He had been seen 3 months earlier for a routine check-up, at which time a physical examination, complete blood count, and serum chemistries were all normal. Relevant physical findings now include a blood pressure of 155/110 mmHg and periorbital edema. Serum studies reveal a BUN of 30 mmol/L (85 mg/dL) and a creatinine of 796 μmol/L (9 mg/dL). Urinalysis reveals 2+ proteinuria and the sediment findings depicted below. True statements about this man's condition include

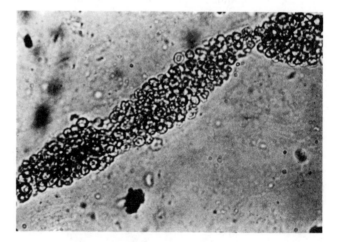

(A) renal biopsy is indicated
(B) poststreptococcal glomerulonephritis is an important diagnostic consideration
(C) extracapillary proliferation is probable
(D) spontaneous resolution of the renal disease is likely
(E) a trial of high-dose glucocorticoids is indicated

315. A 42-year-old man with a history of hypertension presents to the emergency room with his third episode of severe right flank pain over the past 5 years. Correct statements include which of the following?

(A) It is likely that a scout film of the abdomen will be positive

(B) If the pain is due to a renal stone and does not remit, direct removal will be necessary

(C) The patient should be asked about a history of bowel surgery

(D) After resolution of the acute episode, urine calcium, creatinine, uric acid, citrate, and oxalate should be measured

(E) If the patient is found to have calcium stones, thiazide diuretics should be avoided

DIRECTIONS: The group of questions below consists of lettered headings followed by a set of numbered items. For each numbered item select the **one** lettered heading with which it is **most** closely associated. Each lettered heading may be used **once, more than once, or not at all.**

Questions 316–318

For each case history that follows, select the set of laboratory values with which it is most likely to be associated.

	Na$^+$	K$^+$	Cl$^-$	HCO$_3$$^-$	Serum Creatinine	pH	
	(Serum, mmol/L)				(μmol/L [mg/dL])	(Arterial blood)	(Urine)
(A)	143	4.8	100	10	265 (3.0)	7.25	5.0
(B)	135	4.5	107	21	265 (3.0)	7.37	5.0
(C)	140	2.5	114	14	265 (3.0)	7.30	6.2
(D)	139	5.1	104	21	265 (3.0)	7.37	5.0
(E)	139	6.3	108	19	265 (3.0)	7.35	5.0

316. A 28-year-old man, comatose, is believed to have been drinking ethylene glycol

317. A 48-year-old woman has been given amphotericin B for treatment of disseminated coccidioidomycosis

318. A 19-year-old man is recovering from acute poststreptococcal glomerulonephritis

Disorders of the Kidney and Urinary Tract

Answers

275. The answer is A. *(Wilson, ed 12. chap 49.)* Failure to concentrate urine despite substantial hypertonic dehydration suggests a diagnosis of diabetes insipidus. A nephrogenic origin would be postulated if there is no response in urine concentration to exogenous vasopressin. The only useful mode of therapy is a low-salt diet and use of a thiazide diuretic agent. The resultant volume contraction presumably enhances proximal reabsorption and thereby reduces urine flow.

276. The answer is E. *(Wilson, ed 12. chap 50.)* The woman described has nonketotic hyperosmolar coma. The calculated effective extracellular fluid (ECF) osmolality is approximately 350 mosmol/kg ([2 × sodium concentration in mmol/L] + [glucose concentration in mmol/L]). This calculated ECF osmolality is about 25 percent above normal, meaning that about one-fifth of the woman's intracellular water has been lost. In addition, owing to the osmotic diuretic effect of glucose, there have presumably been significant losses of sodium and extracellular water. Loss of extracellular volume is reflected in the elevated BUN/creatinine ratio. A rough estimate of the magnitude of the changes accompanying the development of the hyperosmolar state in the case described would be as follows:

	Prior to illness	In emergency room
Weight (kg)	81	70
Intracellular vol (L)	35	28
Extracellular vol (L)	16	13.5
ECF Na$^+$ (total mmol)	2500	2100

277. The answer is E. *(Wilson, ed 12. chap 50.)* This man's electrolyte pattern is consistent with the "syndrome of hyporeninemic hypoaldosteronism," or type IV renal tubular acidosis. Inhibition of the renin-angiotensin system by nonsteroidal anti-inflammatory agents, converting enzyme inhibitors, and beta-adrenergic blockade can contribute to hyperkalemia. Beta blockade can also interfere with intracellular potassium uptake. Potassium can leak out of cells owing to the digitalis-induced poisoning of the Na, K-ATPase. Use of carbenicillin can lead to hypokalemia since this drug acts as an unresorbed anion, thereby promoting the potassium loss associated with distal tubular secretion.

278. The answer is E. *(Wilson, ed 12. chaps 50, 223.)* In a cirrhotic patient, massive extracellular volume expansion and low urine sodium excretion are evidence of inappropriate sodium retention. If serum creatinine concentration is elevated in addition, the possibility of incipient renal failure—the so-called hepatorenal syndrome—should be entertained. Attempts at rapid volume reduction in this setting can precipitate renal failure and thus are contraindicated. Current treatment recommendations call for rest, observation, a possible trial of plasma expansion, and then gentle diuresis if renal function remains stable.

279. The answer is B. *(Wilson, ed 12. chap 50.)* The differential diagnosis of hyponatremia depends on exclusion of artifactual causes followed by an assessment of volume status. Artifactual hyponatremia can occur in the setting of hyperlipidemia (where a portion of any volume of plasma taken for analysis will be sodium-free lipid) or extreme hyperproteinemia (plasma proteins occupy more than the normal 7 percent of plasma volume) as in multiple myeloma. In these cases plasma osmolality should not be depressed. Actually, modern sodium-selective electrodes eliminate artifactual hyponatremia by measuring the sodium concentration in plasma volume only, not total plasma volume.

In diabetes with very high blood sugars, plasma osmolality may actually be increased in the face of significant hyponatremia. Plasma sodium can become diluted by the movement of water outside cells in the presence of any osmotically active solute. For every elevation of 5.5 mmol/L (100 mg/dL) of plasma glucose, plasma sodium will decrease by 1.6 mmol/L.

In congestive heart failure or any edema-forming state in which the "effective" arterial blood volume is depressed, hyponatremia may ensue. This situation is generally accompanied by alkalosis and hypokalemia because mineralocorticoid secretion is high. On the other hand, acidosis and hyperkalemia would be associated with the hyponatremia of Addison's disease (adrenal insufficiency) with insufficient aldosterone present to cause the distal tubular reabsorption of sodium bicarbonate and the concomitant extrusion of potassium chloride.

The inappropriate secretion of vasopressin, or ADH (SIADH), may occur in multiple settings including head trauma, drug use (vincristine, narcotics), pain, or bacterial meningitis. Vasopressin has little effect on the renal excretion of potassium and hydrogen ions. Patients with SIADH must be euvolemic. Thus, hyponatremia in this setting is usually not accompanied by changes in concentrations of BUN or creatinine (if anything, they are low-normal), potassium, or bicarbonate.

280. The answer is A. *(Wilson, ed 12. chaps 223, 232.)* Cystine crystals appear as flat hexagonal plates and are found in association with cystine stones, which are caused by a hereditary deficiency in tubular cystine transport. Struvite stones result from chronic urinary tract infection with *Proteus* species. These bacteria degrade urea to carbon dioxide and ammonia, which alkalinizes the urine, thereby favoring the formation of the insoluble triple salt $MgNH_4PO_4$. Struvite crystals can appear in the urine as rectangular prisms. Patients with proteinuria due to albuminuria exhibit a sediment characteristic of the nephrotic syndrome with oval fat bodies. Patients with intestinal malabsorption with concomitant steatorrhea, such as in the case of a jejunoileal bypass done for obesity, may hyperabsorb oxalate and form calcium oxalate renal stones. Calcium oxalate crystals appear bipyramidal or as biconcave ovals. The sediment depicted here displays flat square plates, which represent one of the several forms uric acid crystals may manifest. Hyperuricemia may accompany rapid cell turnover (as occurs in the rapid lysis of lymphomas with large tumor burdens after chemotherapy). In such settings aggressive hydration, the use of allopurinol, and urinary alkalinization may be effective prophylaxis against uric acid nephropathy.

281. The answer is C. *(Wilson, ed 12. chap 223.)* The management of oliguric acute renal failure is largely conservative, although some clinicians believe that early dialysis and hyperalimentation lessen morbidity and speed recovery. Fluid intake should match output plus estimated insensible losses; food intake should be encouraged to lessen tissue catabolism. Continuous drainage by Foley catheter should not be routinely employed because it increases the risk of infection; however, if supervening bladder outlet obstruction is suspected, recatheterization should be considered. Reduction of high serum phosphate levels usually is recommended to reduce the risk of soft-tissue calcification. Reduction of high uric acid levels, however, is unnecessary, both because symptomatic gout is very unusual in persons with oliguric renal failure and because there is no evidence that kidneys are damaged by hyperuricemia that develops after an acute reduction in the glomerular filtration rate.

282. The answer is D. *(Wilson, ed 12. chap 224. Sherrard, Semin Nephrol 12:56, 1986.)* Impaired renal production of 1,25-dihydroxy-vitamin D_3 leads to decreased calcium absorption from the gut. Impaired renal phosphate excretion contributes to increased calcium entry into bone. The resultant decreased serum calcium concentration leads to secondary hyperparathyroidism. Chronic metabolic acidosis leads to dissolution of bone buffers and decalcification. Aluminum administered in long-term therapy, although useful in controlling hyperphosphatemia and, thereby, controlling hypocalcemia, can be taken up by bone and contribute to altered bone matrix. There is *no* significant loss of vitamin D or calcium associated with presently employed dialysis techniques.

283. The answer is D. *(Wilson, ed 12. chap 224.)* Development of advancing peripheral neuropathy is an indication for dialysis. Delaying dialysis could allow development of irreversible motor deficits, such as foot drop. Prompt institution of dialysis, on the other hand, usually prevents progression of uremic peripheral neuropathy and may ameliorate early sensory defects. No pharmacologic agent would be of significant benefit in the clinical situation described.

284. The answer is B. *(Wilson, ed 12. chap 227.)* The characteristic pattern of focal and segmental glomerular scarring is shown. The history and laboratory features are also consistent with this lesion, i.e., some associated hypertension, diminution in creatinine clearance, and a relatively inactive urine sediment. The "nephropathy of obesity" may be associated with this lesion secondary to hyperfiltration. Hypertensive nephrosclerosis exhibits more prominent vascular changes and patchy ischemic, totally sclerosed glomeruli. In addition, nephrosclerosis seldom is associated with nephrotic-range proteinuria. Minimal-change disease is usually associated with symptomatic edema and normal-appearing glomeruli as demonstrated by light microscopy. This patient's presentation is consistent with that of membranous nephropathy but the biopsy is not. With membranous glomerular nephritis all glomeruli are uniformly involved with subepithelial dense deposits. There are no features of crescentic glomerulonephritis present.

285. The answer is D. *(Wilson, ed 12. chap 227.)* Persons who have solid tumors and develop nephrotic syndrome usually have membranous glomerulopathy. Diagnosis of the nephrotic syndrome may precede the recognition of the primary tumor. In several cases, tumor antigens have been discovered in the glomerular deposits; the nephrotic syndrome may remit following effective tumor therapy.

286. The answer is C. *(Wilson, ed 12. chap 227.)* The presentation and renal pathology described in the question are typical of acute glomerulonephritis. This syndrome, both when originally described and currently, occurs most often in association with streptococcal infection. Antibodies generated in response to *Streptococcus* are assumed to compose part of the immune deposits seen in damaged glomeruli. More recently, acute glomerulonephritis has been noted in association with a number of other infectious illnesses, which presumably also give rise to immune complexes capable of damaging glomerular capillaries. Heroin abuse is associated with focal and segmental glomerulosclerosis (focal sclerosis), not acute glomerulonephritis; proteinuria and a decline in renal function usually are the first signs.

287. The answer is A. *(Wilson, ed 12. chap 225.)* Almost 100,000 Americans require chronic dialysis, with about 85 percent receiving hemodialysis. Long-term complications of hemodialysis include dialysis dementia and osteomalacia, which is believed to be secondary to the aluminum to which the patient is exposed either in the dialysate or in oral preparations designed to lower serum phosphate. Immunological derangements lead to an increased incidence of hepatitis B antigenemia, which in some cases can lead to liver failure or portal hypertension with resultant variceal bleeding. Morover, the heparin required to maintain access patency also predisposes to bleeding. The high incidence of heart attack and stroke in dialysis patients is probably due to the prevalence of risk factors in the uremic patient, such as hypertension and hyperlipidemia. Peripheral neuropathy, present in many with chronic failure, is a consequence of uremia and represents an indication for the institution of dialytic therapy.

288. The answer is D. *(Wilson, ed 12. chap 228.)* A variety of diseases involve both pulmonary and renal (and, often, also dermal) microvasculature and may present with either prominent pulmonary or renal manifestations. When a firm diagnosis cannot be made serologically or by biopsy of skin or upper respiratory-tract lesions, renal biopsy may be necessary. In the case described in the question, the serologic findings, though not specific, are typical of Wegener's granulomatosis, a diagnosis established by the renal biopsy report. Granulomas are an uncommon microscopic finding in polyarteritis as well as in lupus nephritis and in Henoch-Schönlein purpura, though a spectrum of pathological abnormalities may be seen in the latter two conditions. The renal biopsy in Goodpasture's syndrome usually reveals linear immunoglobulin deposits.

289. The answer is A. *(Wilson, ed 12. chap 229.)* Patients with damage to renal papillae may be unable to excrete maximally concentrated urine owing to chronic tubular damage. Moreover, the necrosed papillae can lead to the gradual development of renal failure. Although renal papillary necrosis has been classically associated with long-term abuse of analgesics (phenacetin or acetaminophen), such a finding can also be present in those with sickle cell anemia, diabetic nephropathy, or obstructive uropathy (as in the man with prostate disease) or after many episodes of pyelonephritis due to urinary tract infections. Aspirin can potentiate the deleterious effects of chronic analgesic abuse by inhibiting the production of renal vasodilatory prostaglandins. Ingestion of lead, such as that caused by leaching out from an unusual distilling apparatus, can lead to a nephropathy manifested by tubular atrophy and fibrosis of small renal arteries.

290. The answer is C. *(Wilson, ed 12. chap 229. Adler, Am J Kidney Dis 5:75, 1985.)* Methicillin therapy is the most frequently reported cause of acute renal failure resulting from interstitial inflammation. This condition usually is associated with prominent eosinophilia and other features of an immune hypersensitivity disorder, although eosinophilia and other common signs such as fever and skin rash need not be present. Cases of interstitial nephritis also have been reported in connection with the use of many other drugs, including some antibiotics (e.g., cephalothin, ampicillin, and penicillin), certain nonsteroidal anti-inflammatory agents, and furosemide. Thus, medication effects must be included in the differential diagnosis of an unexplained decline in renal function. Heparin therapy has not yet been implicated in the development of interstitial nephritis.

291. The answer is D. *(Wilson, ed 12. chap 49.)* Cholesterol embolization of the kidneys and cirrhosis fit clearly into the "prerenal" azotemia category, with a low urine sodium concentration and high urine osmolality. Cholesterol emboli cause "plugging" of renal arterioles and cirrhosis causes hypoalbuminemia, hypovolemia, and possibly a humorally mediated reduction of renal perfusion. However, it is important to recall that other disorders associated with abrupt decline in renal function but with intact tubular integrity, such as acute partial urinary obstruction and acute glomerulonephritis, can also give urinary solute values similar to those in prerenal states if evaluated early in the process. When rhabdomyolosis causes renal damage, it typically produces the picture of acute tubular necrosis, with a urine osmolality less than 400 mosmol/kg and a urinary sodium exceeding 20 mmol/L.

292. The answer is B. *(Wilson, ed 12. chap 225.)* In the first week after renal transplantation, the differential diagnosis of graft dysfunction includes early rejection, hypovolemia, cyclosporine intoxication, acute tubular necrosis, urinary obstruction, and renal artery thrombosis. Cyclosporine can mask many of the classic signs of rejection, such as fever and graft tenderness; renal biopsy is often needed to make the diagnosis. However, renal ultrasonography should precede any manipulation to rule out mechanical outflow obstruction, as it should in any patient with acute deterioration of renal function.

293. The answer is D. *(Wilson, ed 12. chap 234.)* The most important differential diagnosis in the case presented is between a renal cell carcinoma and a benign cystic lesion. Urinalysis may be normal in the presence of renal cell carcinoma, and urinary cytology is unfortunately of little value in the diagnosis of this lesion. Ultrasonography will reveal whether or not the lesion is cystic. If the lesion appears cystic on both IVP and ultrasonographic examination and the patient does not have hematuria, the cyst can be considered benign with a diagnostic accuracy of 97 percent. If greater assurance is required or if there are changes on follow-up radiologic studies, then needle aspiration should be carried out. If the ultrasound appearance is not consistent with a simple cyst, then contrast-enhanced CT scanning, the optimal test for diagnosis and staging of renal cell carcinoma, should be performed.

294. The answer is D. *(Wilson, ed 12. chap 234.)* Older men are the most frequent victims of carcinoma of the bladder. Transitional cell carcinoma, the most common histologic subtype of cancer of the bladder in this country, is associated with a more favorable prognosis than is adenocarcinoma or squamous carcinoma. Squamous carcinomas are more frequent in Egypt, where the prevalence of *Schistosoma haematobium* is high. The prognosis in cancer of the bladder is highly linked to the stage of the disease at presentation: muscular or perivascular fat invasion offers a much bleaker outlook (45 percent 5-year survival) than does disease confined to the mucosa. Risk factors for cancer of the bladder include exposure to the aromatic amines (cigarette smoke and products of the dye, rubber, and chemical industries), but not positive family history, as in the case of renal carcinoma. Chronic bladder irritation, such as that produced by the metabolites of cyclophosphamide as well as by recurrent stones or infections, also leads to a higher incidence of carcinoma of the bladder.

295. The answer is C. *(Wilson, ed 12. chaps 50, 231. Narins, Am J Med 72:496, 1982.)* The evaluation of patients with hypokalemia should first include consideration of redistribution of body potassium into cells as occurs in alkalosis, insulin excess, vitamin B_{12} therapy, and periodic paralysis. In the last condition serum bicarbonate is normal. If urinary excretion of potassium is elevated (>20 mmol/d), then the blood pressure should be measured. If the patient is hypertensive and plasma renin is elevated, renovascular hypertension or a renin-secreting tumor (including Wilms's) must be considered and appropriate imaging studies carried out. If plasma renin levels are low, mineralocorticoid effect may be high, either due to endogenous hormone (glucocorticoid overproduction or aldosterone overproduction as in Conn's syndrome) or exogenous agents (licorice or steroids). In the normotensive patient a high serum bicarbonate excludes renal tubular acidosis. A high urine chloride excretion makes gastrointestinal losses less likely and implies primary renal potassium loss as might be seen in diuretic abuse (ruled out by the urine screen) or Bartter's syndrome. In Bartter's syndrome, hyperplasia of the granular cells of the juxtaglomerular apparatus leads to high renin levels and secondary aldosterone elevations. Such hyperplasia appears to be secondary to chronic volume depletion caused by a hereditary (autosomal recessive) defect interfering with salt reabsorption in the thick ascending loop of Henle. Chronic potassium depletion, which frequently initially presents in childhood, leads to polyuria and weakness.

296. **The answer is A-N, B-N, C-Y, D-Y, E-N.** *(Wilson, ed 12. chaps 50, 223.)* Intravenous calcium infusion, although the correct treatment for the cardiac disturbances caused by hyperkalemia, does not lower serum potassium concentration. Sodium bicarbonate infusion, on the other hand, lowers serum potassium levels rapidly by causing potassium to move into cells. Intravenous infusion of glucose and insulin achieves the same result though slightly less rapidly. Potassium-binding resins effectively remove potassium from the body but are slow, particularly when instilled into the stomach. Persons who are in acute renal failure and have a large potassium load due to severe muscle damage may require emergency dialysis.

297. **The answer is A-Y, B-Y, C-Y, D-Y, E-Y.** *(Wilson, ed 12. chap 223. Koffler, Ann Intern Med 85:23, 1976.)* Muscle cells may be sufficiently taxed during strenuous exercise (e.g., distance running) to result in cell breakdown and myoglobin release. Muscle breakdown associated with sedative overdose is generally attributed to ischemia caused by muscle compression in immobile, comatose patients. Not only can ethanol ingestion promote muscle breakdown in a similar manner, but also ethanol itself has a direct toxic effect on muscle. Hypokalemia and hypophosphatemia decrease muscle-cell energy production and thus increase the risk of rhabdomyolysis in any setting. Volume depletion can contribute to decrease muscle perfusion and, more importantly, increase the susceptibility of the kidneys to damage from myoglobin and other muscle breakdown products.

298. **The answer is A-Y, B-N, C-Y, D-Y, E-N.** *(Wilson, ed 12. chap 223. Anderson, N Engl J Med 296:1134, 1977.)* Nonoliguric acute renal failure (urine volume greater than 800 mL/day) occurs in 25 to 50 percent of cases of acute renal failure and is most commonly associated with the use of nephrotoxic drugs, such as gentamicin. It generally is associated with less severe elevations of blood urea nitrogen and serum creatinine levels than is oliguric renal failure; urine composition, however, is similar to that in the more common oliguric type. Prognosis of nonoliguric renal failure is better than that of oliguric renal failure.

299. **The answer is A-N, B-Y, C-N, D-Y, E-Y.** *(Wilson, ed 12. chap 49. de Groat, Ann Intern Med 92:312, 1980.)* The force for bladder emptying is provided by the detrusor muscle, which is innervated by parasympathetic outflow from the sacral plexus. The involuntary control that prevents automatic bladder emptying emanates from sympathetic innervation of the bladder outlet. A sacral spinal reflex arc mediates automatic detrusor contraction when the intravesical pressure exceeds 20 cmH$_2$O (a volume of 400 mL) unless inhibited by cortical centers via the reticulospinal tracts. Diseases leading to damage of inhibitory neural pathways in the brain or spinal cord, such as multiple strokes, Alzheimer's disease, brain tumors, and normal pressure hydrocephalus, create detrusor instability. In this situation the bladder will empty automatically before it is filled owing to unchecked operation of the spinal reflex arc. On the other hand, conditions leading to chronic overflow incontinence caused by obstruction at the bladder neck or a hypotonic bladder caused by autonomic neuropathy could result in hydronephrosis and impaired renal function. The most common example of outflow obstruction is benign prostatic hypertrophy. Examples of conditions in which autonomic peripheral neuropathy could lead to overflow incontinence include diabetes mellitus, hypothyroidism, uremia, collagen vascular diseases, Guillain-Barré syndrome, and exposure to certain toxins (including alcohol). Cholinergic agents, such as bethanechol, can sometimes aid bladder emptying in those with overflow incontinence.

300. **The answer is A-Y, B-N, C-Y, D-Y, E-Y.** *(Wilson, ed 12. chap 50.)* Hepatic cirrhosis associated with hyponatremia almost always would be associated with edema, thereby defining a state of inappropriate water and sodium retention. The differential diagnosis of hypovolemic hyponatremia includes disorders associated with volume depletion in extrarenal or renal (renal failure, diuretic excess, osmotic loads, Addison's disease) losses. In almost all such cases, plasma bicarbonate and potassium tend to be elevated. The differential diagnosis of euvolemic hyponatremia includes syndromes in which vasopressin is secreted inappropriately either by the pituitary (head trauma, meningeal infection, brain disease, drugs, pulmonary disease) or directly by certain tumors (e.g., oat cell carcinoma of the lung). The endocrine disorders Addison's disease and hypothyroidism should also be included in the etiology of euvolemic hyponatremia.

301. **The answer is A-Y, B-N, C-Y, D-Y, E-N.** *(Wilson, ed 12. chaps 227, 228.)* Serum complement levels usually are normal in persons who have membranous and immunoglobulin A nephropathies. The complement level is depressed during the acute phase of acute poststreptococcal glomerulonephritis but returns to normal about 8 weeks after onset of the disease. Serum complement concentration tends to fall during exacerbation of lupus nephritis. Most patients with membranoproliferative glomerulonephritis have reduced serum levels of complement component C3.

302. The answer is A-Y, B-N, C-Y, D-Y, E-N. *(Wilson, ed 12. chap 227.)* Persons who have nephrotic syndrome may lose a variety of serum proteins other than albumin. Loss of thyroxine-binding globulin leads to reduced serum thyroxine levels, and loss of cholecalciferol-binding protein may combine with a decrease in albumin-bound calcium to reduce serum calcium levels. Loss of antithrombin III has been implicated in hypercoagulability, which affects some persons who have nephrotic syndrome. Hyperlipidemia is associated commonly with nephrotic syndrome; the cause remains uncertain, though it may be the loss of certain plasma proteins involved in the regulation of lipid metabolism. Loss of metal-binding proteins may lead to zinc or copper deficiency.

303. The answer is A-Y, B-Y, C-N, D-N, E-Y. *(Wilson, ed 12. chap 227.)* Studies during epidemics of streptococcal disease have shown the latent period between symptomatic pharyngitis and the appearance of poststreptococcal glomerulonephritis (PSGN) to be between 6 and 10 days. The latent period following cutaneous infection is more difficult to establish but appears to be longer. Persons who receive early antimicrobial therapy for streptococcal infection may develop glomerulonephritis but not mount the immune response to streptococcal enzymes (e.g., streptolysin O) on which laboratory testing for antecedent streptococcal infection is based. Antimicrobial therapy is recommended for persons who have acute glomerulonephritis and continuing streptococcal infection. Long-term prophylaxis, however, is unwarranted, because affected persons are not markedly predisposed to recurrent episodes of PSGN. For unknown reasons, PSGN leads to permanent, progressive renal insufficiency more often in adults than in children.

304. The answer is A-N, B-Y, C-Y, D-Y, E-N. *(Wilson, ed 12. chap 227.)* When first described, Berger's disease was thought to be a relatively benign glomerulopathy characterized by episodes of gross hematuria most often associated with viral illness or exercise. More recently, however, it has become apparent that as many as half the persons affected by this disorder progress to end-stage renal failure. The nephrotic syndrome is associated occasionally with immunoglobulin A (IgA) nephropathy; elevated circulating IgA levels and dermal IgA deposition are common. The latter phenomenon has led to the suggestion that a common immunopathologic mechanism may underlie Berger's disease and Henoch-Schönlein purpura.

305. The answer is A-Y, B-Y, C-N, D-Y, E-Y. *(Wilson, ed 12. chap 228.)* Diabetic nephropathy invariably progresses to end-stage renal failure. Although no available therapy can prevent progression of diabetic nephropathy, careful blood pressure control has been shown to slow the loss of renal function. However, rigorous blood sugar control has unfortunately not been shown to retard progression of renal disease once it has become clinically apparent. As renal failure becomes more severe, insulin requirements may decrease, owing in part to reduced insulin catabolism by the kidneys. The course from onset of proteinuria to end-stage renal failure averages about 7 years. Retinal microvascular disease is usually present by the time urinalysis first shows proteinuria.

306. The answer is A-Y, B-Y, C-N, D-N, E-N. *(Wilson, ed 12. chap 220. Reeders, Nature 317:542, 1985.)* Many instances of adult polycystic kidney disease, which displays autosomal dominant inheritance but which is sometimes due to new mutations, have been mapped to a single genetic locus on the short arm of chromosome 16. This particular locus is close to the gene coding for the alpha-globin chain. A highly polymorphic (genetic variability among individuals; less than 1 percent of the population is homozygous) locus is associated with the alpha-globin gene cluster. Thus, in an individual family with members manifesting the disease, a given polymorphic allele can be shown to be coinherited with the disease. Since such a polymorphism is inherited as a germ line sequence, DNA from any tissue in the body can be extracted, cut with the proper restriction enzyme, electrophoresed, and probed with a radioactive sequence at the polymorphic region. The presence of a fragment of the size previously established to be associated with the disease suggests a predisposition to the disease. If a person lacks the relevant fragment, even if he or she is homozygous at the polymorphism, the likelihood of disease is very low because of the proximity of this locus to the disease-specific gene.

307. The answer is A-Y, B-N, C-Y, D-N, E-Y. *(Wilson, ed 12. chap 223.)* The granular casts seen in the photograph are the hallmark of acute tubular necrosis (ATN). The most common cause of ATN is prerenal failure. Such an occurrence is not infrequent in major intravascular volume loss of a real or effective nature (burns, trauma, surgery with major blood loss or aortic compromise, severe pancreatitis, pregnancy-related catastrophe, or severe heart failure). A second important cause of ATN is that brought on by agents directly toxic to the tubules. These agents include endogenous pigments such as hemoglobin (released in hemolytic crises) or myoglobin (released in rhabdomyolysis due to any cause, including heat stroke, multiple trauma, severe exercise, or hypokalemia/hypophosphatemia). Certain antibiotics (such as gentamicin), radiographic contrast, organic solvents, and heavy metals represent examples of direct tubular toxins. The renal disease caused by endocarditis would produce red blood cell casts on urinalysis. Obstructive uropathy, as exemplified by the man with prostatism, would tend to produce few abnormalities in the urine sediment.

308. The answer is A-N, B-Y, C-Y, D-Y, E-Y. *(Wilson, ed 12. chap 224. Eschback, N Engl J Med 316:73, 1987.)* Debilitating normochromic, normocytic anemia experienced by most patients with chronic renal failure (CRF) is a significant clinical problem. Fortunately, much recent evidence supports the use of recombinant human erythropoietin as a safe and effective therapy, even though bone marrow responsiveness may be somewhat decreased owing to the presence of uremic toxins. Former reliance on multiple blood transfusions was fraught with several dangers, including contracting HIV, HTLV-1, or hepatitis as well as hemochromatosis (chronic iron overload), which can damage many organs, including the heart and gonads. Folic acid deficiency is not uncommon in these patients even though their MCV is not elevated. Clotting problems in uremia are multifactorial; however, impaired platelet function can be improved safely with the administration of cryoprecipitate or desmopressin.

309. The answer is A-Y, B-N, C-Y, D-N, E-Y. *(Wilson, ed 12. chap 229.)* Glycosuria (with a normal blood glucose concentration) and hyperchloremic acidosis ("normal anion gap acidosis") are evidence of renal tubular dysfunction. Frequent nocturia, presumably resulting from impaired ability to concentrate urine, also suggests renal insufficiency caused by a tubulointerstitial disease. Multiple myeloma may present in this manner, and similar renal abnormalities may be associated with analgesic abuse and Sjögren's syndrome. The findings presented in the case are not characteristic of primary glomerular diseases, such as diabetic nephropathy, or the membranous glomerulopathy induced by penicillamine.

310. The answer is A-Y, B-N, C-Y, D-Y, E-N. *(Wilson, ed 12. chap 230. Hollenberg, Am J Kidney Dis 11 [suppl 1]:52, 1987.)* Clinical features of hypertension developing secondary to renal artery stenosis include an age of onset of under 30 years (usually fibromuscular dysplasia as a cause) or over the age of 50 years (usually of atherosclerotic etiology), poor response to medical therapy, and abdominal bruit. Routine laboratory evaluation usually discloses evidence of secondary hyperaldosteronism with hypokalemia. Captopril is particularly effective in treating renovascular hypertension, but it may cause renal failure in patients with bilateral renal artery stenosis or stenosis of the artery to a solitary kidney. Intravenous pyelography is a relatively insensitive screening procedure with only about one-fourth of patients with renovascular hypertension demonstrating the classic "triad" of late appearance of contrast in a small kidney and late hyperconcentration of contrast material in the renal pelvis. If clinical suspicion of renovascular hypertension is high, the best initial study might be digital subtraction angiography.

311. The answer is A-N, B-Y, C-N, D-Y, E-N. *(Wilson, ed 12. chap 230.)* Renal impairment, though rarely the presenting feature of scleroderma, eventually affects about half the persons with the disease. Renal involvement often is heralded by accelerated hypertension ("malignant hypertension"). Characteristic renal lesions in such cases include arterial and arteriolar narrowing and degeneration, not proliferative glomerulonephritis. Recent studies have shown that aggressive vasodilator therapy may preserve renal function. Transplantation has been performed successfully in persons with scleroderma; maintaining vascular access for hemodialysis, however, is often difficult.

312. The answer is A-N, B-Y, C-Y, D-Y, E-Y. *(Wilson, ed 12. chaps 229, 231.)* This patient with recurrent renal calculi and nephrocalcinosis has a normal serum calcium concentration. The serum electrolyte pattern is typical of distal (type 1) renal tubular acidosis with evidence of renal potassium wasting, hyperchloremic metabolic acidosis, and an alkaline urine. The nephrocalcinosis and distal RTA could be consistent with hypervitaminosis D, medullary sponge kidney, hyperparathyroidism, sarcoidosis, or multiple myeloma. However, in all of these conditions except medullary sponge kidney, an increased serum calcium concentration is responsible for the nephrocalcinosis. Intravenous pyelography would better define the defect seen in medullary sponge kidney; it shows a typical "paintbrush" pattern in the renal papillae with tiny papillary cysts containing the calcium deposits. Although medullary sponge kidney is usually not inherited, type 1 distal RTA is often hereditary and relatives should be screened.

313. The answer is A-N, B-Y, C-Y, D-N, E-Y. *(Wilson, ed 12. chap 225.)* Living volunteer donors should be healthy, have normal renal arteries, and have the same blood group as the recipient. The one exception to the last rule is in the case of a type O donor who could donate to a recipient with any blood group, since no endothelial antigens in the ABH system would be present to engender rejection. The donor and recipient should be as closely HLA-matched as possible and the mixed lymphocyte response should be absent. In the case of cadaveric donor kidneys, there is a direct relationship between the degree of HLA incompatibility and graft loss. For example, there is a projected 10-year graft survival rate of 27 percent if there are five HLA mismatches, but a 52 percent rate if there is only one mismatched loci. Chronic rejection is frequently due to nephrosclerosis, often initially characterized by proliferation of the intima (with eventual fibrosis) in the renal vasculature. Prophylaxis against rejection includes the use of cyclosporine A, which inhibits production of the immunostimulatory molecule IL-2 by helper-inducer T lymphocytes and the mercaptopurine analogue azathioprine. Azathioprine is metabolized by the purine degradative pathway to uric acid via the action of xanthine oxidase. Thus, coadministration of the xanthine oxidase inhibitor allopurinol could interfere with drug catabolism and lead to a dangerously toxic effect of a given dose of azathioprine.

314. The answer is A-Y, B-Y, C-Y, D-N, E-Y. *(Wilson, ed 12. chap 227.)* The syndrome described is typical of rapidly progressive glomerulonephritis with rapid onset of acute renal failure in the setting of glomerular disease (manifested by red blood cell casts and proteinuria). The patient's vomiting is consistent with the development of azotemia over a short time period. Renal biopsy is highly recommended early in the course of such a disease for the purpose of defining the nature and severity of the glomerular lesion both for prognostic and therapeutic purposes. The hallmark pathologic lesion associated with this clinical scenario is that of crescentic glomerulonephritis, the manifestation of extracapillary endothelial proliferation. Such a finding on renal biopsy carries an ominous prognosis, especially if crescents are present in more than 70 percent of glomeruli or if the GFR is <5 mL/min. Spontaneous resolution rarely occurs except in those cases associated with an infectious cause, such as endocarditis or streptococcal disease. Though controlled trials are lacking, it appears that high-dose methylprednisolone given parenterally ("pulse steroids") can stave off the need for hemodialysis in some patients.

315. The answer is A-Y, B-N, C-Y, D-Y, E-N. *(Wilson, ed 12. chap 232.)* The clinical scenario is certainly consistent with distention/irritation of the renal collecting system due to stone passage. Since about 75 percent of all renal stones are caused by either calcium oxalate or calcium phosphate, it is likely that the scout film of the abdomen will be positive. While surgical removal (either directly or by retrograde passage of a basket) was the primary approach in the treatment of a renal stone that led to intractable pain, obstruction, bleeding, or infection, lithotripsy (stone dissolution by sound waves) is becoming the preferred alternative. Ultrasound can be applied directly via a cystoscopically placed transducer, via percutaneous flank incision, or by extracorporeal means. The composition of the kidney stone should be directly assessed, if possible. Outpatient evaluation should consist of measurements of serum electrolytes, creatinine, uric acid, serum and urine calcium, and urine oxalate and citrate. In this fashion one will screen for idiopathic hypercalciuria (the most common reason for nephrolithiasis), primary hyperparathyroidism, hyperuricosuria, distal renal tubular acidosis, and hyperoxaluria (associated with fat malabsorption, including that due to ileal resection or bypass). If the patient is found to have idiopathic hypercalciuria, thiazide diuretics are a reasonable therapeutic approach because they lower calcium excretion.

316–318. The answers are: 316-A, 317-C, 318-D. *(Wilson, ed 12. chap 51.)* All the sets of laboratory values presented in the question indicate renal insufficiency with metabolic acidosis. Calculation of unmeasured anions (anion gap) is helpful in determining the etiology of the acidosis. Ethylene glycol ingestion, for example, not only causes acute renal failure but leads to rapid accumulation of metabolic acids. Acidosis is disproportionate to the degree of renal insufficiency and is characterized by a high anion gap (choice A). Amphotericin B also causes renal insufficiency with disproportionate metabolic acidosis. Acidosis, however, is due to a distal tubular acidification defect (distal, or type I, renal tubular acidosis) and is characterized by hyperchloremia, a normal anion gap, and inability to lower the urine pH (choice C). Urinary potassium loss also may be excessive. With moderate renal insufficiency caused by glomerulonephritis, metabolic acidosis is usually mild and the anion gap is only slightly, if at all, elevated (choice D).

The set of laboratory data in choice E illustrates moderate renal insufficiency with disproportionate hyperkalemia and hyperchloremic acidosis, so-called type IV renal tubular acidosis. A number of causes of renal insufficiency, most notably diabetic nephropathy but usually not acute glomerulonephritis, can produce these findings. The laboratory values in choice B illustrate an apparent reduction of the anion gap, which has been reported most frequently in association with multiple myeloma. The apparent reduction in unmeasured anions is due to the presence of abnormal circulating paraprotein that bears a positive charge.

Disorders of the Alimentary Tract and Hepatobiliary System

DIRECTIONS: Each question below contains five suggested responses. Choose the **one best** response to each question.

319. A 56-year-old woman has had profuse, watery diarrhea for 3 months. Laboratory studies of fecal water show the following:

  Sodium: 39 mmol/L
  Potassium: 96 mmol/L
  Chloride: 15 mmol/L
  Bicarbonate: 40 mmol/L
  Osmolality: 270 mosmol/kgH$_2$O (serum osmolality: 280 mosmol/kgH$_2$O)

The most likely diagnosis is

(A) villous adenoma
(B) lactose intolerance
(C) laxative abuse
(D) pancreatic insufficiency
(E) nontropical sprue

320. All the following can inhibit secretion of gastric acid EXCEPT

(A) reduction of the intragastric pH below 3.0
(B) somatostatin
(C) secretin
(D) histamine
(E) presence of fat in the duodenum

321. All the following statements regarding the association of *Helicobacter* (formerly *Campylobacter*) *pylori* and gastritis are true EXCEPT

(A) growth of *H. pylori* in the stomach is believed to be a cause of chronic gastritis, whereas growth in the duodenum is not clearly implicated in the pathogenesis of duodenal ulcer
(B) *H. pylori* is a gram-negative bacillus that invades the gastric mucosa, thereby producing mucosal inflammation
(C) *H. pylori* can be identified by its ability to cleave urea
(D) eradication of the bacteria results in histologic improvement of gastric mucosa
(E) the antibiotics ampicillin or metronidazole can eradicate *H. pylori*

322. A 57-year-old man seeks emergency-room attention for weakness and melena, which he has had for 3 days. He says he has not had significant abdominal pain and had no prior gastrointestinal bleeding. On examination he is disheveled and unshaven, appears older than his stated age, and has a 20 mmHg orthostatic drop in blood pressure. Findings include bilateral temporal wasting, anicteric and pale conjunctivae, cheilosis, spider angiomas on his upper torso, muscle wasting, hepatosplenomegaly, and hyperactive bowel sounds without abdominal tenderness to palpation. Stool is melenic. Nasogastric aspiration reveals coffee-grounds material, which quickly clears with lavage. Hematocrit is 30 percent and mean corpuscular volume is 105 fL. Saline gastric lavage is initiated. The appropriate next step in the management of this man's illness would be to

(A) perform gastroscopy
(B) pass a Sengstaken-Blakemore tube and begin an intravenous infusion of pitressin
(C) order an upper gastrointestinal series
(D) order immediate visceral angiography
(E) insert a large-bore intravenous line and type and cross-match the man's blood

323. A 45-year-old man says that for the past year he occasionally has regurgitated food particles eaten several days earlier. His wife complains that his breath has been foul-smelling. He has had occasional dysphagia for solid foods. The most likely diagnosis is

(A) gastric outlet obstruction
(B) scleroderma
(C) achalasia
(D) Zenker's diverticulum
(E) diabetic gastroparesis

324. During the last year, a 55-year-old man has experienced vague postprandial epigastric fullness. For the last several months, he has been anorectic and has lost 4.5 kg (10 lb). Physical examination is unrevealing except for faintly guaiac-positive stool. Hematocrit is 26 percent. A representative x-ray from his upper gastrointestinal series is reproduced below. The man's physician should now

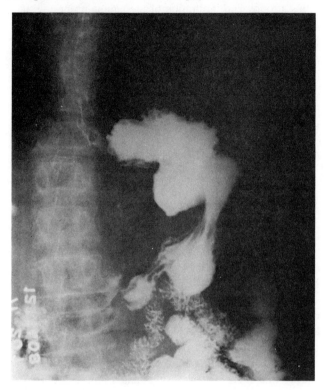

(A) prescribe cimetidine
(B) prescribe metoclopramide
(C) perform a double-contrast upper gastrointestinal series
(D) perform gastroscopy
(E) recommend total gastrectomy

325. The differential diagnosis of chylous ascites includes all the following EXCEPT

(A) lymphoma
(B) nephrotic syndrome
(C) tuberculosis
(D) trauma
(E) congestive heart failure

326. A 42-year-old woman presents with a complaint of watery diarrhea that has occurred intermittently over the past 4 years. After the passage of three or four loose stools in the morning, she feels well for the rest of the day and never has nocturnal diarrhea. Physical examination reveals an anxious woman with a tender left lower abdominal quadrant and no fecal material in the rectum; the results are otherwise normal. Sigmoidoscopic examination discloses excess mucus, but the mucosa appears normal. Barium enema is normal except for sigmoid spasticity, and examination of a stool specimen reveals well-formed feces that are negative for blood, pathogenic bacteria, and parasites. Results of thyroid studies are normal. A trial of milk restriction results in no change in symptoms.

At this point the physician should

(A) consider a trial of diphenoxylate or paregoric to control symptomatic diarrhea
(B) tell the patient that her symptoms are largely emotional in origin
(C) consider a trial of psyllium to increase stool bulk
(D) obtain stool electrolytes and osmolality
(E) perform a jejunal aspirate and analyze the fluid for parasites

327. When operation is performed for suspected appendicitis and that diagnosis proves incorrect, the most common condition discovered is

(A) mesenteric lymphadenitis
(B) pelvic inflammatory disease
(C) acute gastroenteritis
(D) ruptured ovarian cyst
(E) no organic disease

328. All the following statements about achalasia are true EXCEPT

(A) the underlying abnormality appears to be defective innervation of the esophageal body and lower esophageal sphincter
(B) dysphagia, chest pain, and regurgitation are the predominant symptoms
(C) chest x-rays often reveal a large gastric air bubble
(D) manometry reveals a normal or elevated pressure of the lower esophageal sphincter
(E) nifedipine is effective in controlling symptoms in many patients

329. Conditions associated with an increased risk of squamous cell cancer of the esophagus include all the following EXCEPT

(A) achalasia
(B) smoking
(C) Barrett's esophagus
(D) tylosis
(E) head and neck cancer

330. Four months ago, a 36-year-old man with a peptic ulcer underwent a Billroth II anastomosis, antrectomy, vagotomy, and gastrojejunostomy. He now returns for evaluation of a stomal (anastomotic) ulcer. Fasting serum gastrin level is 350 ng/L; 5 min after intravenous infusion of secretin the serum gastrin level is 100 ng/L. The man should be advised that the most appropriate treatment for his condition is

(A) total vagotomy
(B) total gastrectomy
(C) resection of the distal antrum attached to the duodenal stump
(D) laparotomy to search for a gastrin-producing tumor
(E) medical therapy with liquid antacids

331. All the following statements regarding eosinophilic enteritis are true EXCEPT

(A) peripheral blood eosinophilia is present
(B) it may affect the stomach, small intestine, and colon
(C) the majority of patients have a history of food allergies or asthma
(D) treatment with corticosteroids is often effective
(E) it may be difficult to distinguish from regional enteritis

332. Which of the following diagnostic studies for malabsorption is usually normal in persons who have bacterial overgrowth syndrome?

(A) Fecal fat quantitation (24 h)
(B) Stage II Schilling test (intrinsic factor given with vitamin B_{12})
(C) D-Xylose absorption test
(D) Lactulose breath test
(E) Quantitative cultures of jejunal aspirates

333. A 26-year-old man who has juvenile-onset diabetes complains of postprandial epigastric discomfort and bloating. An upper gastrointestinal series fails to reveal an ulcer, but the fluoroscopist notes delayed gastric emptying. Which of the following therapies would be best at this stage of the man's illness?

(A) Antacids
(B) Cimetidine
(C) Metoclopramide
(D) Propantheline
(E) Gastrojejunostomy

334. For the last 6 months, a 50-year-old man has had diarrhea and migratory arthralgias and has lost 9.1 kg (20 lb). An upper gastrointestinal barium study shows a malabsorption pattern in the small bowel. Stool fat content is 35 g per 24 h. Following oral administration of 25 g of D-xylose, a 5-h urine collection contains 0.8 g of D-xylose. A peroral small-bowel biopsy reveals subtotal villus atrophy and infiltration of the lamina propria with macrophages that stain positively with periodic acid Schiff (PAS) stain. The man's physician should now

(A) start him on a gluten-free diet
(B) prescribe prednisone, 60 mg/d and tapered over 2 months
(C) prescribe prednisone, 60 mg/d indefinitely
(D) prescribe trimethoprim-sulfamethoxazole for at least 1 year
(E) recommend an exploratory laparotomy with splenectomy and biopsy of retroperitoneal nodes

335. A 70-year-old Irish consular official seeks local medical attention for diarrhea and weight loss, which have been present for 2 years. He says he has always been in good health "even though I'm the runt of the litter" (he is the smallest of eight siblings). Laboratory studies include normal complete blood cell count and serum electrolyte concentrations. Serum D-xylose concentration is 0.76 mmol/L (15 mg/dL) 2 h after an oral challenge, and 24-h fecal fat determination is 12 g with the man on a 100-g fat diet. A representative biopsy specimen of his small bowel is shown below. All the following are true statements about the man's illness EXCEPT

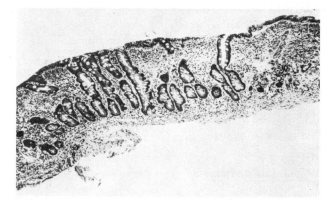

(A) this condition is associated with specific HLA genotypes
(B) abdominal pain, arthralgia, low-grade fever, and lymphadenopathy are frequently present
(C) corticosteroid therapy can reverse jejunal pathology and lessen clinical symptoms
(D) adherence to a strict gluten-free diet usually results in normalization of malabsorption tests and reversal of jejunal pathology
(E) a majority of affected persons complain of bloating after ingesting milk

336. A 62-year-old physician was well until 3 weeks ago when she developed a urinary tract infection. She was treated with ampicillin for 10 days, taking her last dose 7 days ago. Four days ago, she developed abdominal pain, fever, and bloody diarrhea. On examination, she appears acutely ill; her temperature is 38.3°C (101°F) and her abdomen is diffusely tender. Sigmoidoscopy demonstrates a hyperemic mucosa studded with plaquelike lesions. The most likely diagnosis is

(A)   *Shigella* superinfection
(B)   pseudomembranous colitis
(C)   amebic colitis
(D)   ischemic colitis
(E)   toxic megacolon

337. A 28-year-old man has had diarrhea and crampy right lower quadrant abdominal pain for the last 4 weeks. During the last 10 days, he also has had episodic low-grade fever, abdominal distention, and anorexia without vomiting but leading to a weight loss of 3.2 kg (7 lb). On examination, he is mildly uncomfortable. Vital signs are temperature, 37.8°C (100.1°F); pulse, 100 beats per minute; and blood pressure, 110/60 mmHg. His sclerae are anicteric, and there is no palpable lymphadenopathy. A tender, indistinct fullness is palpable in the right lower quadrant of the abdomen, but otherwise the abdomen is soft and without rebound tenderness or palpable hepatosplenomegaly. Rectal examination reveals no masses or focal tenderness, but the stool is guaiac-positive. Laboratory values include a hematocrit of 30 percent and a white blood cell count of 11,300/mm³ with a shift to the left. Flat-plate and upright x-rays of the abdomen show some air-filled loops of small bowel but no air-fluid levels. Sigmoidoscopy is unremarkable. On barium enema examination, barium fails to reflux into the terminal ileum, but the colon is otherwise normal. A representative film from a small-bowel barium examination is shown below.

Which of the following disorders is most consistent with the clinical picture described?

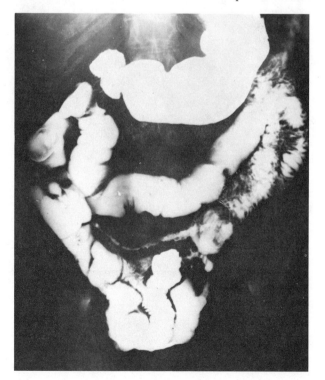

(A)   Perforated appendix with appendiceal abscess
(B)   Whipple's disease
(C)   Regional enteritis
(D)   Adenocarcinoma of the small intestine
(E)   Lymphoma of the small intestine

338. A 20-year-old man was found to have ulcerative proctitis 2 years ago. Mild rectal bleeding was well controlled on daily steroid enemas, which were discontinued a year ago. For the last 3 months, he has had increasingly frequent bloody diarrhea (now 6 to 10 times a day), lower abdominal cramps, low-grade fever, anorexia, and a 5-kg (11-lb) weight loss. Physical examination of this thin, pale young man, who appears acutely ill, reveals these vital signs: temperature, 37.8°C (100°F); pulse, 110 beats per minute; and blood pressure, 120/70 mmHg. The lower abdomen is mildly and diffusely tender, but there is no rebound tenderness and bowel sounds are active. Stool is grossly bloody. Sigmoidoscopy, limited to 10 cm because of discomfort, shows marked mucosal erythema and friability; diffuse ulceration is present, and an exudate contains pus and blood.

Three hours after a barium enema, which shows ulcerations throughout the colon, the man's abdominal pain markedly worsens. Vital signs now are temperature, 39.6°C (103.2°F); pulse, 130 beats per minute; and blood pressure, 90/60 mmHg. On examination the abdomen is distended and diffusely tender with rebound; bowel sounds are infrequent. An abdominal flat-plate x-ray is pictured below.

The most likely diagnosis for the disorder described above is

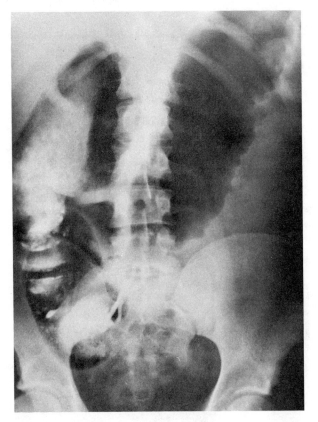

(A) acute colonic perforation
(B) inferior mesenteric artery occlusion
(C) nonthrombotic mesenteric ischemia
(D) volvulus
(E) toxic megacolon

339. All the following are risk factors for development of cancer of the colon EXCEPT

(A) Crohn's colitis
(B) adenomatous polyps
(C) uterosigmoidostomy
(D) ulcerative colitis
(E) juvenile polyposis

340. All the following statements regarding primary biliary cirrhosis (PBC) are true EXCEPT

(A) a positive antimitochondrial antibody test is present in more than 90 percent of patients
(B) increased serum cryoprotein concentrations are frequently present
(C) the majority of patients are women
(D) administration of D-penicillamine appears to be an effective treatment
(E) rheumatoid arthritis, CRST syndrome, and scleroderma occur with increased frequency in patients with PBC

341. The most common organism isolated from the ascitic fluid of patients with spontaneous bacterial peritonitis is

(A) *Streptococcus pneumoniae*
(B) *Staphylococcus aureus*
(C) *Escherichia coli*
(D) *Bacteroides fragilis*
(E) *Klebsiella* sp.

342. A 27-year-old man has had ulcerative colitis for 11 years. His symptoms have been reasonably well controlled on antispasmodic medications and sulfasalazine (Azulfidine). During the last 2 months, however, he has experienced fatigability and a weight loss of 6.8 kg (15 lb). A recent barium enema x-ray is reproduced below. The most appropriate next step in the management of this man's illness would be to

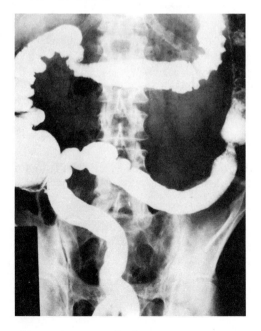

(A) order an air-contrast barium enema
(B) perform colonoscopy
(C) obtain a serum carcinoembryonic antigen level
(D) begin high-dose, intravenous steroid therapy
(E) begin azathioprine therapy

343. A 37-year-old man with chronic alcoholism is admitted to the hospital with acute pancreatitis. On the third hospital day, sudden, complete blindness develops in the left eye. The most likely explanation is

(A) alcohol withdrawal symptoms
(B) transient ischemic attack (transient monocular blindness)
(C) occlusion of the retinal vein
(D) acute glaucoma
(E) Purtscher's retinopathy

344. Mechanical obstruction of the colon is most commonly caused by

(A) adhesions
(B) carcinoma
(C) volvulus
(D) hernia
(E) sigmoid diverticulitis

345. In which of the following causes of fatty liver is microvesicular fat seen in liver biopsy specimens?

(A) Jejunoileal bypass for morbid obesity
(B) Acute fatty liver of pregnancy
(C) Massive tetracycline therapy
(D) Prolonged intravenous hyperalimentation
(E) Carbon tetrachloride poisoning

346. Magnetic resonance imaging (MRI) of the liver can be particularly helpful in all the following conditions EXCEPT

(A) hereditary hemochromatosis
(B) Wilson's disease
(C) thalassemia intermedia
(D) halothane hepatitis
(E) chronic exposure to vinyl chloride

347. Of the following agents that can account for drug-induced hepatitis, which one produces liver injury in a predictable and dose-dependent fashion?

(A) Halothane
(B) Chlorpromazine
(C) Methyldopa
(D) Acetaminophen
(E) Erythromycin

348. In a patient with hepatic cirrhosis, hepatic encephalopathy can be precipitated by all the following factors EXCEPT

(A) gastrointestinal bleeding
(B) metabolic acidosis
(C) renal insufficiency
(D) vomiting
(E) viral hepatitis

349. One month ago, a 21-year-old woman was begun on daily isoniazid therapy because of a positive tuberculin skin test. She now feels well and her physical examination is unremarkable. Routine laboratory data include the following: serum alanine aminotransferase (ALT), 2.5 μkat/L (150 Karmen units/mL); total bilirubin, 17 μmol/L (1.0 mg/dL); and alkaline phosphatase, 25 units. The most appropriate action by the woman's physician would be to order

(A) another antituberculous drug
(B) corticosteroids
(C) a liver biopsy
(D) an ultrasound of the gallbladder
(E) continuation of isoniazid therapy

350. A 45-year-old man with Laennec's cirrhosis and a history of hepatic encephalopathy comes to the local emergency room because of alcoholic intoxication. Physical examination is remarkable for palmar erythema, spider angiomas, and bilateral gynecomastia. Liver span is 8 cm and the edge cannot be felt; a spleen tip, however, is palpable. Stool is guaiac-negative. He has no asterixis. Laboratory studies include the following:

Hematocrit: 38 percent
Mean corpuscular volume: 104 fL
White blood cell count: 4000/mm³
Platelet count: 97,000/mm³
Prothrombin time: 17.5 s
Total serum bilirubin: 14 μmol/L (0.8 mg/dL)
Serum aspartate aminotransferase (AST): 0.5 μkat/L (45 U/L)
Serum alkaline phosphatase: 34 units

The man is given intravenous hydration and vitamin and mineral supplements, including folic acid (1 mg), thiamine (100 mg), magnesium (2 g), and vitamin K (10 mg). After spending the night in the hospital's detoxification unit, he awakens sober and alert. Repeat prothrombin time is 12 s.

The most likely explanation for the elevation in the man's initial prothrombin time is

(A) alcoholic hepatitis
(B) folate deficiency
(C) intestinal malabsorption
(D) disseminated intravascular coagulation
(E) laboratory error

351. A 67-year-old woman, who has previously been healthy, undergoes emergency surgery for a ruptured abdominal aortic aneurysm. Intraoperatively she requires 8 units of packed red blood cells to maintain her blood pressure and hematocrit. Following surgery she is hemodynamically stable. On the third postoperative day she appears jaundiced, but abdominal examination is unremarkable and she is afebrile. Total serum bilirubin concentration at this time is 141 μmol/L (8.3 mg/dL) (direct, 107 μmol/L [6.3 mg/dL]). Serum alkaline phosphatase level is 110 units, and serum AST level is 0.85 μkat/L (51 Karmen units/mL). The most likely explanation for the woman's jaundice is

(A) a stone in the common bile duct
(B) halothane hepatitis
(C) posttransfusion hepatitis
(D) acute hepatic infarct
(E) benign intrahepatic cholestasis

352. A 35-year-old former hemodialysis nurse is seen because of a 6-month history of fatigue and amenorrhea. On examination she has a scleral icterus, a mildly tender liver, and a tibial rash consistent with erythema nodosum. ALT and AST levels are both in the range of 1.5 μkat/L (100 U/L) and bilirubin is 51.3 μmol/L (3 mg/dL), while alkaline phosphatase and serum albumin levels are normal. Hepatitis serology detects HBsAg and IgG anti-HBcAg. Liver biopsy discloses a mononuclear cell portal infiltrate and hepatocyte destruction at the periphery of lobules.

Which of the following therapeutic strategies is best?

(A) Administration of low-dose cyclophosphamide, 50 mg/d for 2 months
(B) Administration of prednisone, 20 to 40 mg/d for 2 months and then taper-based on response
(C) Administration of prednisone, 10 mg every other day for 3 months
(D) Administration of acyclovir, 400 mg every 6 h for 2 weeks
(E) Referral to medical center participating in a trial of alpha interferon

353. A 50-year-old man with a history of organomegaly and an elevated hematocrit without apparent secondary cause was well until the sudden onset of right upper quadrant pain. On examination the patient is afebrile and has clear lungs, normal cardiac function, an abdominal fluid wave, splenomegaly, and a markedly enlarged liver with a palpable, very tender edge. Liver function tests are normal except for mild elevation of hepatic transaminases.

Which of the following is the most appropriate procedure for purposes of establishing a diagnosis?

(A) CT scan of the liver
(B) Abdominal ultrasound
(C) Radionuclide liver-spleen scan
(D) Hepatic venography
(E) Paracentesis

354. Chronic active hepatitis is distinguished most reliably from chronic persistent hepatitis by the presence of

(A) extrahepatic manifestations
(B) hepatitis B surface antigen in the serum
(C) antibody to hepatitis B core antigen in the serum
(D) a significant titer of anti-smooth-muscle antibody
(E) characteristic liver histology

355. Cholecystectomy is advisable in all the following patients EXCEPT

(A) a patient with the calcified outline of the gallbladder visible on plain abdominal x-ray
(B) a patient hospitalized for treatment of biliary colic four times in the last 2 months
(C) a patient with a history of a recent episode of acute cholecystitis who responded favorably to a 7-day course of intravenous antibiotics
(D) a diabetic patient without abdominal symptoms in whom gallstones were incidentally noted on ultrasound done to assess renal size
(E) a patient with a history of pancreatitis caused by gallstone

356. All the following conditions may lead to an elevation of the serum amylase EXCEPT

(A) diabetic ketoacidosis
(B) intestinal obstruction
(C) hypertriglyceridemia
(D) lung cancer
(E) pregnancy

357. All the following statements regarding abdominal angiography in the evaluation and treatment of gastrointestinal hemorrhage are true EXCEPT

(A) blood loss at a rate of 0.5 to 1.0 mL/min is required to demonstrate a bleeding site
(B) intraarterial administration of vasoconstrictors often is effective in controlling bleeding from mucosal bleeding sites
(C) vasopressin injected into the superior mesenteric artery is more effective than peripheral intravenous vasopressin in controlling hemorrhage from esophageal varices
(D) hemostatic agents may be delivered through the catheter to control hemorrhage from a duodenal ulcer
(E) angiography can successfully identify actively bleeding lesions in regions of the gastrointestinal tract not accessible to endoscopy

358. A 52-year-old woman is hospitalized for medical management of severe alcoholic hepatitis. On the ninth hospital day she develops a temperature of 38.3°C (101°F) and generalized abdominal discomfort. Abdominal examination reveals significant and diffuse abdominal tenderness without guarding; hepatosplenomegaly is present but is unchanged from the admission examination. Rectal and pelvic examinations reveal no area of localized tenderness; stool guaiac testing is positive. Hematocrit is 27 percent, white blood cell count is 12,000/mm^3, and liver function tests are unchanged from admission—total serum bilirubin, 214 μmol/L (12.5 mg/dL); serum AST, 2.5 μkat/L (150 Karmen units/mL); and serum alkaline phosphatase, 180 units.

The procedure most likely to yield diagnosis information in this case would be

(A) serum amylase determination
(B) blood culture
(C) supine and upright x-rays of the abdomen
(D) abdominal sonography
(E) paracentesis

359. A 38-year-old woman is hospitalized for an upper gastrointestinal hemorrhage. Following an uneventful recovery, an upper gastrointestinal series (part of which is reproduced below) is obtained. The abnormality demonstrated in the x-ray suggests which of the following diagnoses?

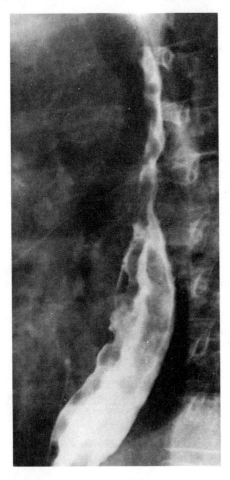

(A) Erosive gastritis
(B) Laennec's cirrhosis
(C) Hiatal hernia
(D) Gastric ulcer
(E) Reflux esophagitis

360. All the following conditions are known to predispose to the formation of cholesterol gallstones EXCEPT

(A) obesity
(B) hypercholesterolemia
(C) clofibrate therapy
(D) oral contraceptive therapy
(E) surgical resection of the ileum

361. A 58-year-old man with biopsy-proven Laennec's cirrhosis is hospitalized because of massive ascites and pedal edema. There is no evidence of respiratory compromise or hepatic encephalopathy. Initial laboratory values are as follows:

Serum electrolytes (mmol/L): Na^+ 130; K^+ 3.6; Cl^- 85; HCO_3^- 30
Serum creatinine: 88 μmol/L (1.0 mg/dL)
Blood urea nitrogen: 6.4 μmol/L (18 mg/dL)

Bed rest and sodium and water restriction produce no significant weight change after 5 days.
Which of the following therapeutic measures would be most appropriate at this time?

(A) Intravenous furosemide, 80 mg now
(B) Oral spironolactone, 100 mg/d
(C) Oral acetazolamide, 250 mg/d
(D) Placement of a peritoneovenous (LeVeen) shunt
(E) Therapeutic paracentesis

362. A 65-year-old man with long-standing, stable, biopsy-proven postnecrotic cirrhosis develops abdominal pain of the right upper quadrant and abdominal swelling. He is afebrile. Palmar erythema, spider telangiectasias, and mild jaundice are noted on physical examination. His abdomen is distended, shifting dullness is present, a tender, firm liver edge is felt 3 fingerbreadths below the right costal margin, and a spleen tip is palpable. A faint bruit is heard over the liver. Laboratory values include the following:

Hematocrit: 34 percent
White blood cell count: 4300/mm³
Platelet count: 104,000/mm³
Serum albumin: 26 g/L (2.6 g/dL)
Serum globulins: 46 g/L (4.6 g/dL)
Alkaline phosphatase: 400 units

Paracentesis reveals blood-tinged fluid.
The serum marker most specifically associated with this man's condition is

(A) antinuclear antibody
(B) α-fetoprotein
(C) antimitochondrial antibody
(D) 5'-nucleotidase
(E) chorionic gonadotropin

363. Administration of which of the following drugs or classes of drugs has been shown to prolong survival in persons with acute pancreatitis?

(A) Cimetidine
(B) Aprotinin (Trasylol)
(C) Antibiotics
(D) Anticholinergics
(E) None of the above

364. A 64-year-old man with insulin-dependent adult-onset diabetes mellitus seeks emergency medical treatment after 2 days of increasingly severe abdominal pain of the right upper quadrant, which has spread over the entire abdomen and is associated with nausea, vomiting, fever, and chills. On examination, he is alert and oriented but appears to be quite acutely distressed. Vital signs are temperature, 39.4°C (103°F); pulse, 140 beats per minute; and blood pressure, 100/60 mmHg. His sclerae are mildly icteric. His abdomen is diffusely tender with marked guarding in the right upper quadrant; there is no palpable hepatosplenomegaly, and there are no audible bowel sounds. Rectal examination reveals no focal tenderness; stool is guaiac-negative. Laboratory values are as follows:

Hematocrit: 34 percent
White blood cell count: 22,500/mm^3 with a marked left shift
Plasma glucose: 17.8 mmol/L (325 mg/dL)
Blood urea nitrogen: 10.5 μmol/L (30 mg/dL)
Serum AST: 2.1 μkat/L (125 Karmen units/mL)
Serum alkaline phosphatase: 210 units
Serum amylase: 3.3 μkat/L (200 U/dL)

His abdominal flat-plate x-ray is shown below. During the first 4 h of hospitalization, the man's condition is stabilized somewhat with the administration of intravenous fluids and insulin. A nasogastric tube is inserted, blood cultures are drawn, and he is begun on broad-spectrum antibiotics.

The most appropriate management at this point would be to order

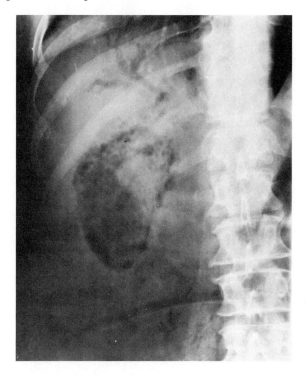

(A) conservative medical measures only for the next 48 to 72 h
(B) an abdominal ultrasound examination
(C) an upper gastrointestinal examination with Gastrografin dye
(D) endoscopic retrograde cholangiopancreatography
(E) preparations for an emergency laparotomy

365. Complications of chronic pancreatitis include all the following EXCEPT

(A)   gastric varices
(B)   erythema nodosum
(C)   vitamin B_{12} malabsorption
(D)   pleural effusion
(E)   jaundice

366. All the following factors portend a poor survival rate during an attack of acute pancreatitis EXCEPT

(A)   hyperbilirubinemia
(B)   hypoalbuminemia
(C)   hypocalcemia
(D)   hypoxemia
(E)   discolored peritoneal fluid

367. All the following may be manifestations of a gastrointestinal carcinoid tumor EXCEPT

(A)   bowel obstruction
(B)   steatorrhea
(C)   peripheral edema
(D)   wheezing
(E)   cutaneous flushing

368. A 52-year-old woman has hepatomegaly. Percutaneous liver biopsy reveals "adenocarcinoma," but the woman refuses further evaluation or treatment. A year later she presents with weight loss (13.6 kg, 30 lb) and a skin rash that has waxed and waned. Examination shows angular stomatitis and a firm, enlarged liver. An erythematous, bullous, necrotic skin rash (Color Plate A) is present on the face, perineum, and legs. Sonography reveals an enlarged pancreas. Hematologic testing shows the woman to be anemic.

The diagnostic test of choice would be

(A)   serum amylase determination
(B)   plasma glucagon determination
(C)   plasma vasoactive intestinal polypeptide (VIP) determination
(D)   plasma gastrin determination
(E)   pancreatic arteriography

DIRECTIONS: Each question below contains five suggested responses. For **each** of the **five** responses listed with every question, you are to respond either YES (Y) or NO (N). In a given item **all, some, or none of the alternatives may be correct.**

369. True statements regarding delta hepatitis virus (HDV) include

(A) HDV is a defective RNA virus
(B) HDV can infect only persons infected with HBV
(C) the HDV genome is partially homologous with HBV DNA
(D) HDV infection has been isolated only in limited areas of the world
(E) simultaneous infection with HDV and HBV results in an increased risk of development of chronic hepatitis

370. Causes of upper gastrointestinal bleeding that usually are missed by routine upper gastrointestinal x-rays but can be diagnosed by endoscopy include

(A) Mallory-Weiss tears
(B) duodenal ulcers
(C) gastric ulcers
(D) erosive gastritis
(E) Osler-Rendu-Weber syndrome

371. True statements about the management of variceal hemorrhage include which of the following?

(A) Owing to the risk of perforation, endoscopy sclerotherapy should be reserved for patients who rebleed after surgery
(B) Peripheral-vein infusion of vasopressin is as effective as superior mesenteric artery infusion in controlling variceal hemorrhage
(C) The presence of preoperative jaundice and ascites increases the risk of immediate postoperative mortality in persons undergoing surgical shunting procedures for variceal hemorrhage
(D) Elective portacaval shunt surgery prevents recurrent variceal hemorrhage but does not improve life expectancy
(E) The selective, distal splenorenal shunt appears to be associated with a lower incidence than the portacaval shunt of postoperative hepatic encephalopathy

372. Chronic reflux esophagitis can lead to the development of

(A) gastrointestinal bleeding
(B) an esophageal peptic stricture
(C) a lower esophageal ring
(D) Barrett's esophagus (esophagus lined by columnar epithelium)
(E) adenocarcinoma

373. True statements regarding the prophylaxis of viral hepatitis include which of the following?

(A) Although immune globulin (IG) is effective in preventing clinically apparent type A hepatitis, not all IG preparations have adequate anti-HAV titers to be protective
(B) If given soon enough after exposure to hepatitis B, hepatitis immune globulin (HBIG) is effective in preventing infection
(C) HBIG and hepatitis B vaccine can be effectively administered simultaneously
(D) Hepatitis B vaccine is effective in preventing delta hepatitis infection in persons who are not HBsAg carriers
(E) IG prophylaxis after needle-stick, sexual, or perinatal exposure to non-A, non-B hepatitis is effective in preventing infection

374. A ''bald'' tongue (i.e., one devoid of papillae) may be observed in which of the following clinical scenarios?

(A) A 45-year-old man with recent onset of glucose intolerance and change in shoe size
(B) An 18-year-old man with abnormal facies, developmental delay, and myeloblasts noted on peripheral blood smear
(C) A 55-year-old woman with painful joints, eye irritation, and dental caries
(D) A 30-year-old man from Africa with recent mental deterioration, gummatous infiltration of the palate, and a positive rapid plasma reagin (RPR) test
(E) A 25-year-old man with macrocytic anemia and a history of major abdominal surgery

375. Which of the following antiemetics will act on the chemoreceptor trigger zone in the brain?

(A) Tetrahydrocannabinol
(B) Metoclopramide
(C) Prochlorperazine
(D) Scopolamine
(E) Promethazine

376. Gastrointestinal manifestations of scleroderma (progressive systemic sclerosis) include

(A) reflux esophagitis
(B) pancreatitis
(C) steatorrhea
(D) gallstones
(E) pneumatosis intestinalis

377. A gastric ulcer can safely be called benign if it

(A) heals significantly after a 6-week course of antacid therapy
(B) has a benign appearance on upper gastrointestinal air contrast barium study
(C) is located on the lesser gastric curvature
(D) is less than 2 cm in diameter
(E) shows no evidence of malignancy after six biopsies and brush cytology examinations

378. Primary intestinal lymphoma can be characterized by which of the following statements?

(A) It may develop as a late complication of nontropical sprue
(B) Hepatosplenomegaly and peripheral adenopathy are frequently present
(C) Steatorrhea and malabsorption may be the presenting symptoms
(D) The diagnosis is best made by endoscopic biopsies
(E) Perforation and bleeding are unusual

379. A patient with scleral icterus and a positive reaction for bilirubin by urine dipstick testing could have which of the following disorders or conditions?

(A) Autoimmune hemolytic anemia
(B) Dubin-Johnson syndrome
(C) Crigler-Najjar type II disorder
(D) Thalassemia intermedia
(E) Use of oral contraceptives

380. Correct statements concerning the diagnosis of the Zollinger-Ellison syndrome (gastrinoma) include which of the following?

(A) It should be considered in the differential diagnosis of chronic diarrhea
(B) It should be considered in the presence of large mucosal folds observed at radiographic examination of the upper gastrointestinal tract
(C) Endoscopic retrograde pancreaticoduodenography is helpful in identifying gastrinomas missed on selective arteriography or CT
(D) A patient with recurrent duodenal ulcer whose fasting gastrin is 50 ng/L (repeat 100 ng/L) should undergo a secretin test
(E) If gastrin levels are measured at 15-min intervals before and after the feeding of a standard meal in a patient with gastrinoma, the hormone level rises by 200 ng/L

381. True statements about gastric cancer include which of the following?

(A) Most gastric cancers begin as benign polyps or benign ulcers
(B) The risk of gastric cancer is increased following a Billroth II partial gastrectomy
(C) The incidence of gastric cancer is higher in persons with blood group O than in other persons
(D) Gastric lymphoma accounts for 5 to 10 percent of malignancies in the stomach
(E) If achlorhydria persists despite pentagastrin stimulation in a person with a gastric ulcer, then it is likely that the ulcer is malignant

382. True statements concerning the short bowel syndrome include which of the following?

(A) Following massive small-bowel resection, a transient syndrome of gastric hypersecretion may develop
(B) If more than 100 cm of ileum have been resected, dietary fat intake should be reduced to 40 g/d
(C) Ileal malabsorption of bile salts results in enhanced fluid and electrolyte absorption in the colon
(D) Antiperistaltic agents would aid fluid and electrolyte absorption
(E) Loss of ileal tissue is better tolerated than loss of an equal length of jejunal tissue

383. Extraintestinal complications associated with regional enteritis but *not* associated with ulcerative colitis include

(A) pericholangitis
(B) bilirubin gallstones
(C) hypocalcemia
(D) uveitis
(E) oxalate kidney stones

384. The medical therapy of Crohn's disease can be described by which of the following statements?

(A) Metronidazole may be useful if the perineal area is involved
(B) Azathioprine is ineffective as a single agent
(C) Corticosteroids are more effective in the treatment of Crohn's disease of the small intestine than in the treatment of Crohn's disease of the colon
(D) In persons in whom a remission in disease activity has been achieved, sulfasalazine decreases the frequency of relapse
(E) Sulfasalazine is contraindicated in the treatment of pregnant women who have Crohn's disease

385. A 40-year-old man has a history of ulcerative colitis. Features of his illness that would contribute to an increased risk of developing colon cancer include

(A) disease duration of more than 10 years
(B) history of toxic megacolon
(C) presence of pancolitis (total colonic involvement)
(D) presence of pseudopolyps on colonoscopy
(E) high steroid requirements

386. True statements about carcinoembryonic antigen (CEA) include which of the following?

(A) Most persons with colon cancer have elevated serum CEA levels
(B) A normal serum CEA level excludes a diagnosis of gastrointestinal malignancy
(C) A decline in serum CEA level suggests a favorable response to therapy
(D) Serum CEA level is elevated in some persons who have benign biliary disease
(E) Serum CEA level is elevated in some persons who have inflammatory bowel disease

387. Subacute ischemic colitis can be described by which of the following statements?

(A) The usual presenting symptom is severe abdominal pain
(B) Rectal bleeding may be the presenting symptom
(C) Involvement of the rectum is uncommon
(D) Symptoms and signs of nonocclusive ischemic colitis resolve in 2 to 4 weeks
(E) Angiography is the definitive diagnostic procedure

388. True statements describing Meckel's diverticulum include which of the following?

(A) It is the most frequent congenital anomaly of the digestive tract
(B) Mechanical obstruction due to intussusception may occur
(C) In young adults, inflammatory complications may produce a clinical syndrome indistinguishable from acute appendicitis
(D) Conventional gastrointestinal barium x-rays can demonstrate the diverticulum in more than 85 percent of cases
(E) Technetium scans are valuable in the diagnosis of those diverticula associated with gastrointestinal bleeding

389. True statements regarding acute bleeding from colonic diverticula include which of the following?

(A) Diverticulitis usually is present
(B) The source of hemorrhage is more likely to be on the right side than on the left side of the colon
(C) Bleeding usually abates spontaneously
(D) Angiographic detection of bleeding usually is unsuccessful
(E) It is the most common cause of acute lower gastrointestinal bleeding in elderly persons

390. An 18-year-old man develops watery diarrhea shortly after returning from a vacation in Africa. Physical examination reveals a temperature of 37.8°C (100°F) and generalized abdominal tenderness. A stool sample stained with methylene blue reveals abundant mixed bacterial organisms and polymorphonuclear leukocytes. Which of the following diagnoses would be compatible with the findings described?

(A) Amebic colitis
(B) Cholera
(C) Bacillary dysentery
(D) Ulcerative colitis
(E) Giardiasis

391. Percutaneous needle liver biopsy would be indicated in a diagnostic workup for

(A) unexplained hepatosplenomegaly
(B) persistently abnormal liver function tests
(C) suspected hepatic angioma
(D) suspected miliary tuberculosis
(E) suspected obstruction of the common bile duct

392. Which of the following conditions would likely be associated with the set of serum values presented below?

Total bilirubin: 26.5 μmol/L (1.5 mg/dL)
AST: 1.0 μkat/L (60 U/L)
Alkaline phosphatase: 450 units

(A) Primary biliary cirrhosis
(B) Stricture of the common bile duct
(C) Acute viral hepatitis
(D) Acetaminophen overdose
(E) Chlorpromazine therapy

393. Adenomatous polyps of the colon are correctly characterized by which of the following statements?

(A) Most adenomatous polyps are clinically silent
(B) The majority of adenomatous polyps occur in the rectosigmoid colon
(C) The size of an adenomatous polyp correlates with the risk of malignancy
(D) Villous adenomas are more likely than tubular polyps to be malignant
(E) Colonoscopic polypectomy is adequate therapy of an adenoma that has evidence of carcinoma in situ

394. Acute viral hepatitis can be described by which of the following statements?

(A) There is a direct correlation between peak rise in AST and ALT and the degree of hepatocellular damage
(B) A serum bilirubin concentration greater than 340 μmol/L (20 mg/dL), in the absence of hemolysis, is a poor prognostic sign
(C) A serum sickness–like syndrome may precede the onset of clinical jaundice caused by hepatitis B virus infection
(D) The presenting symptoms and signs are useful in predicting the specific etiologic agent responsible
(E) Steroid therapy has been shown to shorten the clinical course of the illness

395. True statements regarding non-A, non-B hepatitis include which of the following?

(A) It accounts for approximately 90 percent of all cases of posttransfusion hepatitis
(B) Its mean incubation period is longer than that of hepatitis A but shorter than that of hepatitis B
(C) It can be spread by both percutaneous and nonpercutaneous exposure
(D) It is associated with chronic carrier states in asymptomatic persons
(E) The presence of the causative agent can be detected serologically in some cases

396. An 18-year-old man is evaluated because of weight loss and diarrhea. On examination he was found to have pedal edema and decreased breath sounds at the right lung base. A thoracentesis reveals milky fluid. Subsequent laboratory workup reveals lymphocytopenia and hypoproteinemia and hypogammaglobulinemia. Which of the following features could also be expected with this condition?

(A) Abnormal peripheral lymphatics
(B) Dilated and telangiectatic lymphatic vessels in the lamina propria on small-bowel biopsy
(C) Response to lactose-free diet
(D) Response to low-fat diet supplemented by medium-chain triglycerides
(E) 1 g D-xylose in 5-h urine collection after 25 g oral D-xylose

397. A patient with newly diagnosed tropical sprue could have which of the following extragastrointestinal manifestations of malabsorption?

(A) Megaloblastic anemia
(B) Night blindness
(C) Purpura
(D) Tetany
(E) Hypochromic red cells

398. Correct statements concerning sulfasalazine therapy for inflammatory bowel disease include

(A) sulfasalazine is a drug requiring cleavage by colonic bacteria to be effective
(B) the active moiety is sulfapyridine, which inhibits the *Helicobacter* (formerly *Campylobacter*) bacteria believed to cause the colitis
(C) it must be used along with steroids to provide effective treatment for an acute attack
(D) the active moiety can be given by enema and provides an effective treatment
(E) chronic use of sulfasalazine may reduce recurrences in patients with ulcerative colitis

399. Women taking oral contraceptives have a greater likelihood of developing

(A) benign hepatic adenoma
(B) peliosis hepatis
(C) focal nodular hyperplasia of the liver
(D) hepatic angiosarcoma
(E) rhabdomyosarcoma

400. Gilbert's syndrome is characterized by which of the following statements?

(A) The serum total bilirubin is predominantly unconjugated and rarely exceeds 85 μmol/L (5 mg/dL)
(B) Fasting increases the serum bilirubin concentration
(C) It appears to be inherited in an autosomal recessive pattern
(D) Serum bilirubin concentration increases after the administration of phenobarbital
(E) Examination by light microscopy of liver biopsy specimens discloses normal results

401. Correct statements concerning the hereditary polyposis syndromes include which of the following?

(A) Gardner's syndrome is characterized by multiple hamartomatous polyps in the large and small intestines
(B) In Peutz-Jeghers syndrome adenomatous polyps in the large and small intestine have a high rate of malignant degeneration
(C) Turcot's syndrome is similar to familial colonic polyposis except that malignant brain tumors frequently accompany the polyposis
(D) Familial colonic polyposis is inherited in an autosomal dominant fashion
(E) Patients with familial colonic polyposis have a 100 percent incidence of colon cancer by age 40

402. Which of the following serologic patterns would be consistent with acute hepatitis B infection?

	HBsAg	Anti-HBs	Anti-HBc	HBeAg	Anti-HBeAg
(A)	+	−	IgM	+	−
(B)	+	−	IgG	+	−
(C)	−	−	IgM	−	−
(D)	+	−	IgG	−	+
(E)	−	+	IgG	−	−

403. Reye's syndrome often is associated with

(A) marked hyperbilirubinemia
(B) ingestion of salicylate
(C) hyperglycemia
(D) elevated serum levels of aminotransferase
(E) recent viral illness

404. True statements about hepatitis B *e* antigen (HBeAg) include which of the following?

(A) HBeAg can be detected transiently in the sera of patients ill with acute hepatitis B infection
(B) The presence of HBeAg in the serum is correlated with infectiousness
(C) The absence of HBeAg in the serum rules out chronic infection caused by the hepatitis B virus
(D) HBeAg is immunologically distinct from HBsAg, but is genetically related to HBcAg
(E) The disappearance of HBeAg from the serum may be a harbinger of resolution of acute hepatitis B infection

405. Which of the following disorders are associated with an increased incidence of hepatocellular carcinoma?

(A) Hemochromatosis
(B) α_1-Antitrypsin deficiency
(C) Long-term ingestion of aflatoxin
(D) Chronic hepatitis B virus infection
(E) Alcoholic liver disease

406. A patient undergoes a liver biopsy for chronic abnormalities on liver function tests. On pathologic review, multiple granulomas are found. Correct statements concerning this patient's condition include

(A) an empirical trial of steroids should be instituted
(B) sarcoidosis is a possible etiology
(C) a careful drug-exposure history should be obtained
(D) schistosomiasis is a possible etiology
(E) the absence of caseating granulomas rules out miliary tuberculosis

407. Which of the following patients would be suitable candidates for liver transplantation?

(A) A 35 year old with severe hepatic enlargement secondary to recently diagnosed hepatic vein thrombosis
(B) A 45-year-old man with end-stage cryptogenic cirrhosis
(C) A 6 year old with progressive cirrhosis due to α_1-antitrypsin deficiency
(D) A 45 year old with end-stage primary biliary cirrhosis
(E) A 40 year old with alcohol-related cirrhosis who has been abstinent for 3 months

408. Correct statements regarding nonsurgical therapy of gallstone disease include which of the following?

(A) Oral bile acid therapy is equally effective in dissolving cholesterol and pigment gallstones

(B) The major therapeutic effect of the two oral agents available for the dissolution of gallstones, chenodeoxycholic acid and ursodeoxycholic acid, is to alter the bile acid/cholesterol/lecithin ratio (the lithogenic index)

(C) Self-limited diarrhea and abnormalities of liver function tests are the most common side effects associated with chenodeoxycholic acid therapy

(D) Complete dissolution of gallstones occurs in over 50 percent of patients on oral bile acid therapy

(E) Extracorporeal shock wave lithotripsy is an effective therapy for some patients with large (>1.5 cm) gallstones

409. A 65-year-old man presents because his wife notes that his eyes are becoming yellow. On further questioning, the patient complains of epigastric discomfort, dark urine, light stools, and pruritus. Past medical history and physical examination are unremarkable. Laboratory tests confirm the clinical impression of an elevation in the serum level of conjugated bilirubin. Abdominal ultrasound demonstrates a mass in the head of the pancreas and enlargement of the common bile duct. Chest x-ray and abdominal-pelvic CT disclose no additional abnormalities. A CT-guided needle biopsy of the mass obtains tissue that, on pathologic examination, reveals neutrophils and fibrous elements.

Which of the following procedures would be reasonable at this point?

(A) Another attempt at CT-guided needle biopsy

(B) Endoscopic retrograde cholangiopancreatography (ERCP)

(C) Celiac angiography

(D) Repeat CT scan in 2 to 3 months

(E) Percutaneous placement of biliary stent

DIRECTIONS: The following group of questions consists of lettered headings followed by a set of numbered items. For each numbered item select the **one** lettered heading with which it is **most** closely associated. Each lettered heading may be used **once, more than once, or not at all.**

Questions 410–413

Match each of the following case histories of esophageal disease with the barium swallow x-ray with which it is most likely to be associated.

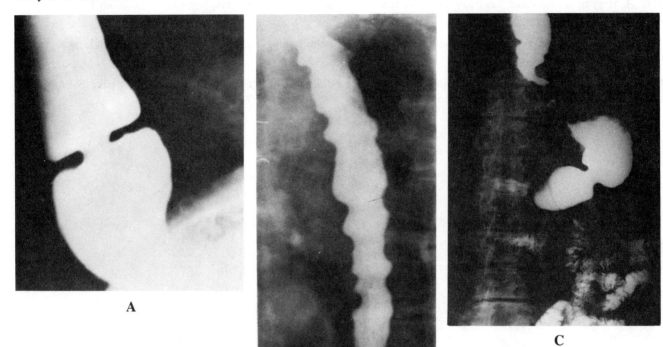

A

B

C

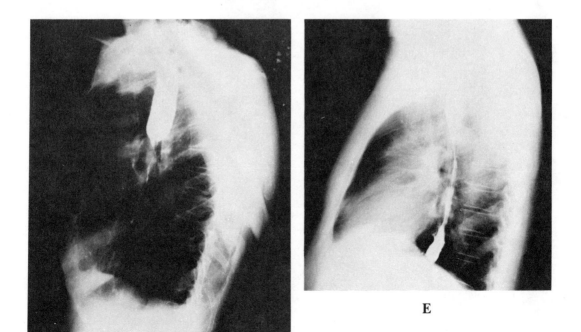

D

E

    (A)   Radiograph A
    (B)   Radiograph B
    (C)   Radiograph C
    (D)   Radiograph D
    (E)   Radiograph E

410. A 40-year-old truckdriver has had occasional dysphagia for solid foods for the last 5 years

411. A 61-year-old bartender has had frequent heartburn for the last 4 years and dysphagia for solid foods for the last 3 months

412. A 55-year-old alcoholic man has had mild dysphagia for solid foods for the last month, during which time he has lost 5 kg (11 lb)

413. A 35-year-old accountant has occasional dysphagia for solid foods and frequent retrosternal chest pain that radiates to the back, occurs at rest, and lasts several minutes

Disorders of the Alimentary Tract and Hepatobiliary System

Answers

319. The answer is A. *(Wilson, ed 12. chap 44. Shiau, Ann Intern Med 102:773, 1985.)* In the case described, the osmolality of fecal water is approximately equal to serum osmolality. Furthermore, there is no osmotic "gap" in the fecal water—the osmolality of the fecal water can be accounted for by the stool electrolyte composition: $[2 \times ([Na^+] + [K^+])] = [2 \times (39 + 96)] = 270$. A villous adenoma of the colon typically produces a secretory diarrhea. Lactose intolerance, nontropical sprue, and excessive use of milk of magnesia produce osmotic diarrheas with osmotic "gaps" caused by lactose, carbohydrates, and magnesium, respectively. Pancreatic insufficiency causes steatorrhea, not watery diarrhea.

320. The answer is D. *(Wilson, ed 12. chap 238.)* Physiologic feedback loops mediate inhibition of gastrin release, thereby inhibiting secretion of acid in the stomach; the two most important are acidic gastric pH and presence of fat or hypertonic fluids in the duodenum. Acid-induced release of somatostatin by antral endocrine cells may mediate, in a paracrine fashion, inhibition of secretion of gastrin and activity of parietal cells. Secretin is released in the presence of acid in the upper small intestine and can also inhibit secretion of gastric acid. Other peptides found in the small intestine that may play a role in the inhibition of secretion of gastric acid include gastric inhibitory peptide, vasoactive intestinal peptide, enteroglucagon, neurotensin, peptide YY, and urogastrone. Histamine, presumably released by the mast cells lying adjacent to the acid secretory parietal cells in the gastric mucosa, acts together with gastrin and acetylcholine to stimulate release of acid.

321. The answer is B. *(Wilson, ed 12. chap 238. Dooley, Ann Intern Med 108:70, 1988.)* Gastric colonization with the short gram-negative bacillus *Helicobacter* (formerly *Campylobacter*) *pylori* is thought to be the principal cause of active chronic gastritis, which is characterized by a neutrophilic exudate in the gastric mucosa, which is not in itself ulcerated. The bacteria do not invade the mucosa, but rather grow in the deep mucus gel layer and synthesize a glycoprotein-destroying protease, thereby contributing to mucosal injury. Though *H. pylori* colonization is associated with gastric and duodenal ulcers, causality remains unproven. *H. pylori* may be identified in gastric biopsy samples by histology (the bacteria are Giemsa-positive), culture, or urease activity. Colloidal bismuth compounds can eradicate the organism by unknown means; treatment with ampicillin and metronidazole is also associated with eradication of *H. pylori* with concomitant disappearance of the inflammatory changes in the gastric mucosa.

322. The answer is E. *(Wilson, ed 12. chap 46.)* The presence of "coffee-grounds" material in a nasogastric aspirate from a person with melena indicates recent upper gastrointestinal tract bleeding. In a patient with obvious signs of cirrhosis, esophageal varices must be considered in the differential diagnosis of upper gastrointestinal bleeding; other possible diagnoses include peptic ulcer, gastroduodenitis, esophagitis, and Mallory-Weiss tear. Before diagnostic procedures, such as endoscopy or upper gastrointestinal series, are undertaken, the placement of a large-bore intravenous line and commencement of volume replacement therapy are mandatory in order to prevent hypotension. Moreover, blood should be typed and cross-matched in case of further bleeding. Diagnostic angiography is indicated only when brisk bleeding prevents diagnosis by endoscopy or barium study. Specific therapy for variceal bleeding—i.e., passage of a Sengstaken-Blakemore tube and intravenous infusion of pitressin—should be considered if diagnostic studies reveal bleeding varices.

323. The answer is D. *(Wilson, ed 12. chap 237.)* A Zenker's diverticulum typically causes halitosis and regurgitation of saliva and food particles consumed several days earlier. When a Zenker's diverticulum fills with food, it may produce dysphagia by compressing the esophagus. Gastric outlet obstruction can cause bloating and regurgitation of newly ingested food. Gastrointestinal disorders associated with scleroderma include esophageal reflux, the development of wide-mouthed colonic diverticula, and stasis and bacterial overgrowth. Achalasia typically presents with dysphagia for both solids and liquids. Gastric retention caused by the autonomic neuropathy of diabetes mellitus usually results in postprandial epigastric discomfort and bloating.

324. The answer is D. *(Wilson, ed 12. chaps 236, 239.)* The x-ray presented shows a large malignant-appearing gastric ulcer on the lesser curvature of the stomach. Because the differentiation between benign and malignant gastric ulcer by x-ray is not infallible (there are as many as 25 percent false positives and negatives), the diagnosis of gastric cancer should be confirmed by fiberoptic gastroscopy with brush cytology and at least six biopsies from the ulcer margin. Gastroscopy is useful in diagnosing primary gastric lymphoma, which is associated with a much better 5-year survival rate than is adenocarcinoma. Double-contrast radiographic techniques help to detect small lesions by improving mucosal detail but do not generally improve accuracy in distinguishing benign from malignant ulcers.

325. The answer is E. *(Wilson, ed 12. chaps 48, 246.)* Chylous ascites contains thoracic or intestinal lymph and has a turbid, milky appearance. There is an increased triglyceride content, and microscopic examination reveals Sudan-staining fat globules. Chylous ascites is usually the result of lymphatic obstruction. The leading causes are trauma, tumors, tuberculosis, and filariasis. Chylous ascites is also occasionally associated with the nephrotic syndrome.

326. The answer is A. *(Wilson, ed 12. chap 242. Trotman, Gut 29:218, 1988.)* This presentation is classic for one of the three clinical variants of the irritable bowel syndrome, each associated with abnormal colonic motility. Other groups have chronic abdominal pain and constipation or alternating constipation and diarrhea. The chronic nature of the condition and the presence of formed stool militate against a workup for secretory or osmotic diarrhea. Giardiasis, while typically occult and requiring jejunal sampling for diagnosis, usually presents with belching and pain, not diarrhea of 4 years' duration. The absence of discernible significant organic pathology should not prompt a discussion with the patient that centers on a psychogenic cause of her problem; such an approach will frequently lead to alienation of the patient. Instead, an effort to effect safe symptomatic improvement of the diarrhea with antispasmodics is worthwhile. Psyllium to increase stool bulk is a good choice for patients with irritable bowel syndrome who complain of constipation.

327. The answer is A. *(Wilson, ed 12. chap 245.)* Virtually any condition that can lead to abdominal pain needs to be included in the differential diagnosis of appendicitis. Diagnostic accuracy is about 75 percent. Although acute diverticulitis, cholecystitis, perforated ulcer, pancreatitis, obstruction, renal stone, and pyelonephritis can present diagnostic difficulties, the most frequent findings at operation when appendicitis is incorrectly diagnosed are (in order of frequency) mesenteric lymphadenitis, no organic disease, acute pelvic inflammatory disease, ruptured ovarian cyst, and acute gastroenteritis.

328. The answer is C. *(Wilson, ed 12. chap 237.)* Achalasia is a motor disorder of esophageal smooth muscle in which the lower esophageal sphincter (LES) does not relax properly in response to swallowing and normal esophageal peristalsis is replaced by abnormal contractions. Manometry reveals a normal or elevated LES pressure and a reduced or absent swallow-induced relaxation. A decreased number of ganglion cells is noted in the esophageal body and LES of patients with achalasia, suggesting that defective innervation of these areas is the underlying abnormality. Dysphagia, chest pain, and regurgitation are the predominant symptoms. The chest x-ray often reveals absence of the gastric air bubble and the barium swallow reveals a dilated esophagus. Calcium-channel antagonists such as nifedipine relax smooth muscle and have been effective in treating some patients. However, the mainstay of therapy remains pneumatic dilation.

329. The answer is C. *(Wilson, ed 12. chap 239.)* Squamous cell cancer of the esophagus accounts for approximately 10,000 deaths annually in the U.S. Worldwide, incidences vary greatly, but it is particularly common in a belt from the Caspian Sea to northern China. In the United States, epidemiologic studies have linked smoking and alcohol to squamous cell cancer of the esophagus and may explain the association of this tumor with head and neck carcinoma. The long-term stasis associated with achalasia leads to chronic irritation of the esophagus, which is thought to predispose to cancer formation. Tylosis is a genetically acquired disease characterized by thickening of the skin of the hands and feet and is associated with squamous cell cancer of the esophagus. Barrett's esophagus is associated with adenocarcinoma but not squamous cell carcinoma of the esophagus.

330. The answer is C. *(Wilson, ed 12. chap 238.)* The causes of stomal (anastomotic) ulceration following peptic ulcer surgery include incomplete vagotomy, retained gastric antrum, the Zollinger-Ellison syndrome (gastrinoma), poor gastric emptying, and ingestion of ulcerogenic drugs. In the case presented, if the previous antrectomy had been complete, the serum gastrin level should not be elevated. An elevated serum gastrin level that declines after intravenous administration of secretin is characteristic of a retained gastric antrum attached to the duodenal stump. Neither frequent antacid therapy nor a total vagotomy is effective in healing a stomal ulcer; thus, resection of the retained antrum is indicated. In the Zollinger-Ellison syndrome, the serum gastrin level paradoxically increases after intravenous infusion of secretin.

331. The answer is C. *(Wilson, ed 12. chap 240.)* Eosinophilic enteritis is a disorder of the stomach, small intestine, or colon or all three in which some part of the gut wall is infiltrated by eosinophils. The diagnosis also requires the presence of peripheral blood eosinophilia. Although early reports emphasized the presence of food allergies, less than half the patients have a history of food allergies or asthma. The presence of anemia, Hemoccult-positive stools, abnormalities of the ileum and cecum on barium radiographic studies, and a favorable response to administration of steroids may make eosinophilic enteritis difficult to distinguish from Crohn's disease. Although no controlled trials of corticosteroid therapy have been performed, symptoms usually respond to short-term corticosteroid therapy.

332. The answer is C. *(Wilson, ed 12. chap 240.)* Malabsorption due to bacterial overgrowth results from bacterial utilization of ingested vitamins and the deconjugation of bile salts by bacteria in the proximal jejunum. Deconjugated bile salts do not form micelles in the jejunum, and long-chain fatty acids cannot be absorbed. The bacteria also separate ingested vitamin B_{12} from intrinsic factor, thus interfering with its absorption from the ileum. The absorption of simple carbohydrates generally is not impaired, though complex carbohydrates may be metabolized by bacteria. Thus, persons with bacterial overgrowth have steatorrhea, an abnormal Schilling test (even with administration of intrinsic factor), increased metabolism of nonabsorbable carbohydrates (e.g., lactulose), and increased bacterial concentrations in jejunal aspirates. Absorption of D-xylose, a simple carbohydrate, is often normal.

333. The answer is C. *(Wilson, ed 12. chap 240.)* Because of autonomic neuropathy, persons who have diabetes not uncommonly display clinical symptoms and radiologic findings suggestive of gastric retention. Metoclopramide, a stimulant of gastric motility, often can help relieve symptoms of retention. Poor gastric emptying that is not due to ulceration would be unlikely to respond to antacids or cimetidine. The use of propantheline might aggravate the condition, considering that anticholinergic medications tend to retard gastric emptying. Surgical treatment is rarely necessary and should not be considered unless an adequate trial of nonsurgical therapy is unsuccessful.

334. The answer is D. *(Wilson, ed 12. chap 240. Keinath, Gastroenterology 88:1867, 1985.)* The man described in the question has Whipple's disease, a bowel disorder associated with dilated gut lymphatics and characterized by weight loss, abdominal pain, diarrhea, malabsorption, and arthralgias. Electron microscopy has revealed the presence of bacilliform bodies in the lamina propria; these rod-shaped structures, which are located within or adjacent to macrophages that contain PAS-positive granules, resemble microorganisms, suggesting an infectious etiology of Whipple's disease. The treatment of choice is at least 1 year of therapy with antibiotics, with trimethoprim-sulfamethoxazole as first-line therapy. Clinical recovery is accompanied by the disappearance of the bacilliform bodies.

335. The answer is B. *(Wilson, ed 12. chap 240.)* The histologic specimen pictured in the question shows villous atrophy, crypt hyperplasia, and inflammation typical of intestinal changes in nontropical sprue (celiac disease), an illness with a high incidence in Ireland. The disease is associated with an increased incidence of histocompatibility antigens HLA-B8 and HLA-DW3. Although two-thirds of symptomatic cases present in childhood, the onset of clinical symptoms of malabsorption may occur at any age. Persons with subclinical sprue during adolescence may have mild growth retardation and may be smaller than their siblings. Because the villous absorptive surface is markedly reduced in affected persons, an acquired lactase deficiency is often present and causes symptoms of milk intolerance. A strict gluten-free diet or use of corticosteroids usually relieves symptoms and signs of malabsorption and promotes restoration of normal jejunal histology. A malabsorptive syndrome associated with abdominal pain, arthralgias, low-grade fever, and lymphadenopathy is not typical of celiac disease and should suggest another diagnosis, such as Whipple's disease or lymphoma.

336. The answer is B. *(Wilson, ed 12. chap 241.)* Sigmoidoscopic demonstration of a hyperemic mucosa studded with plaquelike lesions is characteristic of pseudomembranous (antibiotic-associated) colitis, which is caused by the enterotoxin of *Clostridium difficile*. Although symptoms commonly develop while the offending antibiotic is still being taken, the syndrome may not become evident until several days or weeks after completion of therapy. Ischemic colitis may cause bloody diarrhea but not the mucosal lesions described. Amebic or *Shigella* infestation is associated with punched-out ulcerations of the mucosa. Toxic megacolon is a complication of active colitis. Treatment is directed at either binding the toxin (cholestyramine) or eradicating the bacteria (oral vancomycin or metronidazole).

337. The answer is C. *(Wilson, ed 12. chap 241.)* Radiographic demonstration of luminal narrowing, mucosal ulceration, and cobblestoning in the ileum is compatible with a diagnosis of regional enteritis. In Whipple's disease, x-rays characteristically show marked thickening of mucosal folds in the duodenum and jejunum. On barium enema, an appendiceal abscess usually presents as a mass indenting the cecal tip. Adenocarcinoma of the small bowel usually occurs as an ulcerated mass lesion in the duodenum. Infiltrating lymphomas of the distal bowel may be difficult to distinguish from regional enteritis radiographically, but stenotic bowel segments would not suggest lymphoma.

338. The answer is E. *(Wilson, ed 12. chap 241.)* The clinical history and x-ray presented in the question are consistent with toxic megacolon in association with severe ulcerative colitis. Toxic megacolon is most likely to occur when hypomotility agents, such as diphenoxylate or loperamide, are given to persons with severe colitis, or when such persons undergo a barium-enema radiographic procedure. In the case presented, a barium enema was not only dangerous but, in fact, unnecessary, because the presence of diarrhea and signs of systemic illness indicated that the disease no longer was limited to the rectum. Colonic perforation may also be associated with severe ulcerative colitis; the presence of subdiaphragmatic air on abdominal x-rays would be suggestive.

339. The answer is E. *(Wilson, ed 12. chap 243. Vogelstein, N Engl J Med 319:595, 1988.)* The specific cause of colon cancer is unknown, although recent studies reveal an excess of genetic allele loss in advanced colonic neoplasia. However, certain diseases are known to increase the risk of development of cancer of the colon. Crohn's colitis is associated with an increased risk of colon cancer, although the risk is less than that for patients with ulcerative colitis. Colon cancer has been observed to occur with increased frequency in patients with uterine cancer. Patients with adenomatous polyps are at higher risk for the subsequent development of colon cancer than is the general population. Therefore, such patients should have periodic follow-up examinations. Despite the importance of these risk factors, only 1 percent of persons with colon cancer have an identifiable risk factor other than age. The polyps in juvenile polyposis are hamartomatous and have no malignant potential. Colonic neoplasms at a site distal to the ureteral implant have been noted to occur 15 to 30 years after uterosigmoidostomy.

340. The answer is D. *(Wilson, ed 12. chap 254.)* Primary biliary cirrhosis (PBC) is a disease of unknown etiology, but the frequent association with autoimmune disorders such as rheumatoid arthritis, CRST syndrome, scleroderma, and sicca syndrome has suggested that an abnormal immune response plays an etiologic role. The disease typically affects middle-aged women and runs a slowly progressive course, with death resulting from hepatic insufficiency occurring within 10 years of diagnosis. A positive antimitochondrial antibody test is relatively sensitive and specific for PBC, occurring in greater than 90 percent of patients. Other serum abnormalities include increased alkaline phosphatase and 5′-nucleotidase activities and the presence of cryoproteins. Treatment is entirely supportive. Neither corticosteroids nor D-penicillamine have proved to be effective. Colchicine may have a role in slowing the progression of disease.

341. The answer is C. *(Wilson, ed 12. chap 254. Crossley, Gut 26:325, 1985.)* Spontaneous bacterial peritonitis refers to the development of acute bacterial peritonitis without an obvious primary source of infection. The diagnosis can be suspected on clinical grounds and supported by an elevated leukocyte count in ascitic fluid. However, confirmation of the diagnosis can be made only by bacterial culture. In the United States, *Escherichia coli* is the leading cause of spontaneous bacterial peritonitis and is isolated from approximately 30 percent of patients. *Streptococcus pneumoniae* and *Klebsiella* species are the second and third most commonly isolated organisms. Therefore, when the diagnosis is suspected, empiric therapy with ampicillin and an aminoglycoside is frequently instituted.

342. The answer is B. *(Wilson, ed 12. chap 241.)* The x-ray presented in the question shows loss of haustrations and shortening of the colon typical of chronic ulcerative colitis. In addition, a stricture is present at the junction of the sigmoid and descending colon. The duration of the man's colitis and the presence of a stricture raise the question of colonic cancer, which necessitates colonoscopy. Air-contrast barium enema may better define mucosal detail but cannot substitute for a tissue diagnosis. The main value of serum carcinoembryonic antigen levels is to detect promptly the presence of metastases following resection of a colonic carcinoma, not to confirm the presence of a primary tumor. Therapeutic measures, such as the use of azathioprine or steroids, are not appropriate until the diagnostic workup has been completed.

343. The answer is E. *(Wilson, ed 12. chap 260.)* Purtscher's retinopathy is a relatively rare but devastating complication of acute pancreatitis. It is characterized by sudden loss of vision and the presence of cotton-wool spots and hemorrhages in the area of the optic disc and macula. The cause is thought to be occlusion of the posterior retinal artery by aggregated granulocytes.

344. The answer is B. *(Wilson, ed 12. chap 244.)* Carcinoma of the colon is the most common cause of mechanical obstruction of the colon and is followed in frequency by sigmoid diverticulitis and volvulus. These three causes account for 90 percent of cases of colonic obstruction. Adhesions and hernias cause about 75 percent of cases of small-intestine obstruction but are uncommon causes of colonic obstruction.

345. The answer is B. *(Wilson, ed 12. chap 256.)* Fatty liver refers to the infiltration of hepatocytes by triglyceride. Typically, the fat accumulates in large cytoplasmic droplets. However, in acute fatty liver of pregnancy and in Reye's syndrome, the fat is contained in small vacuoles and is termed *microvesicular fat*. The reason for the specific morphologic appearance of fat in these two disorders is unknown, but it provides a useful histologic differential point.

346. The answer is D. *(Wilson, ed 12. chap 248.)* MRI may be more sensitive than CT in evaluating hepatic mass lesions. Vascular lesions such as benign hemangiomas or malignant angiosarcomas caused by chronic exposure to vinyl chloride are well-detected by MRI. At this time the value of MRI in most diffuse hepatic parenchymal diseases, such as drug-induced or infectious hepatitis or cirrhosis, is unclear. On the other hand, MRI is quite useful for monitoring diseases characterized by the hepatic deposition of metals such as copper (Wilson's disease) or iron (hemochromatosis or conditions associated with secondary iron overload, such as thalassemia intermedia).

347. The answer is D. *(Wilson, ed 12. chap 252.)* Acetaminophen hepatotoxicity is mediated by a toxic metabolite formed by the hepatic cytochrome p450 system. Glutathione is responsible for detoxifying the metabolite, but when stores of this scavenger are depleted, hepatocyte necrosis may ensue. Thus, acetaminophen is a direct hepatotoxin; a single dose of 10 to 15 g will produce evidence of liver injury and doses above 25 g can be fatal. Such injury can be ameliorated somewhat by timely administration (<24 h after overdose) of a glutathione-restoring sulfhydryl compound such as *N*-acetylcysteine. Many other agents produce hepatic injury in an idiosyncratic fashion due to hypersensitivity (halothane, methyldopa, chlorpromazine), genetic variations in the handling of drug metabolites (isoniazid, diphenylhydantoin), or unknown mechanisms.

348. The answer is B. *(Wilson, ed 12. chaps 250, 254.)* Gastrointestinal bleeding, which causes an increase in the production of ammonia and other nitrogenous substances in the colon, is a common predisposing factor to hepatic encephalopathy in persons with cirrhosis. Hypokalemic alkalosis, caused by excessive diuresis or vomiting, may precipitate hepatic encephalopathy by increasing the ratio of ammonia to ammonium; gut and renal absorption of ammonia increases, and more ammonia enters the brain. Acidosis has the opposite effect. Deterioration of liver function, such as in viral hepatitis, can precipitate encephalopathy in cirrhotic persons. If worsening renal function produces an increase in blood urea nitrogen, there is additional availability for NH_3 production via the action of gut bacterial urease on urea.

349. The answer is E. *(Wilson, ed 12. chap 252.)* About 10 percent of persons treated with isoniazid develop mild elevations of serum aminotransferase levels during the first few weeks of therapy. These levels usually return to normal despite continued use of isoniazid. About 1 percent of persons with elevated aminotransferase levels develop symptoms of hepatitis and are at high risk for developing fatal hepatic failure. The older the patient, the higher the risk of isoniazid hepatitis; thus, because the patient described in this question is young and asymptomatic, isoniazid can safely be continued, as long as she is watched for symptoms of hepatitis. A liver biopsy would not be indicated at this time.

350. The answer is C. *(Wilson, ed 12. chaps 249, 250, 254.)* Alcohol produces impairment in the absorption of many nutrients, including vitamin K. (The use of neomycin in the treatment of hepatic encephalopathy also can lead to a decrease in vitamin K.) When hypoprothrombinemia in a person with liver disease is easily corrected by parenteral vitamin K administration, decreased intestinal absorption of vitamin K should be suspected. Coagulopathy resulting from impaired hepatic function, such as in alcoholic hepatitis, is unlikely to be corrected by exogenous vitamin K. Although the patient discussed in the question is probably deficient in folate, as evidenced by the high mean corpuscular volume, folic acid administration has no effect on prothrombin time. Exogenous vitamin K would not correct the hypoprothrombinemia associated with disseminated intravascular coagulation.

351. The answer is E. *(Wilson, ed 12. chap 251.)* Benign postoperative intrahepatic cholestasis can develop as a consequence of major surgery for a catastrophic event in which hypotension, extensive blood loss into tissues, and massive blood replacement are notable. Factors contributing to jaundice include the pigment load from transfusions, decreased liver function due to hypotension, and decreased renal bilirubin excretion due to tubular necrosis. Jaundice becomes evident on the second or third postoperative day, with bilirubin levels (mainly levels of conjugated bilirubin) peaking by the tenth day. Serum alkaline phosphatase concentration may be elevated up to tenfold, but aspartate aminotransferase (AST) levels are only mildly elevated. Hepatitis and hepatic infarct are unlikely diagnoses in the absence of abdominal pain or tenderness or a significant rise in AST levels. The incubation period of posttransfusion hepatitis is 7 weeks, making this diagnosis unlikely.

352. The answer is E. *(Wilson, ed 12. chap 253.)* Glucocorticoid therapy has been shown to prolong survival in patients with chronic active hepatitis of nonviral etiology. This patient, who has evidence of chronic hepatitis B infection as the cause of her chronic active hepatitis (this diagnosis has been made because of piecemeal necrosis on liver biopsy), would not benefit from administration of steroids. Though many agents have been tried in chronic active viral hepatitis, none have thus far been shown to be effective in the majority of patients. Small randomized studies using alpha interferon have shown promise in that improvement in liver histology has been observed.

353. The answer is D. *(Wilson, ed 12. chap 254.)* Primary erythrocytosis with organomegaly strongly suggests the diagnosis of polycythemia rubra vera. One well-recognized complication of this condition is hypercoagulability, with a particular propensity toward hepatic vein thrombosis. Such an occlusion would lead to the Budd-Chiari syndrome characterized by a grossly enlarged, tender liver with severe ascites. In addition to hepatic vein thrombosis secondary to a hypercoagulable state, such a syndrome could result from idiopathic causes, hepatic invasion by tumor, or the venoocclusive disease associated with chemotherapy or radiation. Once right-sided heart failure is excluded clinically, the diagnosis is best established by hepatic venography or liver biopsy showing sinusoidal dilatation.

354. The answer is E. *(Wilson, ed 12. chap 253.)* Although chronic active hepatitis may be associated with extraintestinal manifestations (e.g., arthritis) and the presence in the serum of autoantibodies (e.g., anti-smooth-muscle antibody), these factors are not invariably present. The distinction between chronic active and chronic persistent hepatitis can only be established by liver biopsy. In chronic active hepatitis there is piecemeal necrosis (erosion of the limiting plate of hepatocytes surrounding the portal triads) and extension of inflammation into the liver lobule, features not seen in chronic persistent hepatitis. Both diseases may be associated with serologic evidence of hepatitis B infection.

355. The answer is D. *(Wilson, ed 12. chap 258. Ranshoff, Gastroenterology 92:1588, 1987.)* The risk of subsequent complications or symptoms in a patient with silent, or asymptomatic, gallstones is less than 1 to 2 percent per year. A prolonged period of being asymptomatic suggests that the risk of subsequent gallbladder-related problems is quite low; few patients develop complications without prior warning symptoms. Thus, it is no longer recommended that diabetics with silent gallstones undergo prophylactic cholecystectomies. If symptoms of biliary colic (an aching or pressure in the epigastrium or right upper quadrant, often with vomiting) occur with a frequency or severity great enough to disrupt the patient's normal routine, then cholecystectomy should be performed. Surgery should also be undertaken in patients who have experienced a prior complication of gallstone disease, such as pancreatitis, acute cholecystitis, or gallstone fistula or ileus. Finally, certain underlying gallbladder conditions predispose to subsequent complications and should be treated with cholecystectomy. Such conditions include calcified or porcelain gallbladder, which is associated with the development of gallbladder carcinoma, cholesterolosis (lipid deposition in the lamina propria of the gallbladder wall), and adenomyomatosis (benign nodular proliferation of gallbladder surface epithelium).

356. The answer is C. *(Wilson, ed 12. chaps 259, 260.)* Approximately 75 percent of patients with acute pancreatitis will have an elevated serum amylase, which, if over 7.5 μkat/L (450 U/L), virtually confirms the diagnosis in the absence of major bowel catastrophe. However, hypertriglyceridemia can falsely depress the serum amylase in the setting of acute pancreatitis. Amylase is found in many other extrapancreatic organs, including the salivary glands, liver, and small intestine, and can be produced ectopically by certain tumors, including lung, breast, and ovarian cancer. In these situations, as well as in acidotic states and pregnancy, the amylase produced can be distinguished from that of a pancreatic source by isoenzyme analysis. In the workup of suspected acute pancreatitis, the serum lipase value offers the benefit of increased specificity.

357. The answer is C. *(Wilson, ed 12. chaps 46, 254. Chojkier, Gastroenterology 77:540, 1979.)* The value of angiography as both a diagnostic and therapeutic tool is well established in cases of gastrointestinal hemorrhage. Angiography can detect actively bleeding lesions in areas not able to be reached by an endoscope, provided the rate of blood loss is at least 0.5 to 1.0 mL/min. Hemostasis by infusion of vasoconstrictor agents through the angiography catheter has been successfully achieved in cases of duodenal ulcer and other conditions. In the control of bleeding from esophageal varices, however, intraarterial vasopressin is no more effective than peripheral intravenous vasopressin.

358. The answer is E. *(Wilson, ed 12. chap 254.)* Persons who have cirrhosis, particularly alcoholic cirrhosis and ascites, may develop acute bacterial peritonitis without a clearly definable precipitating event. The clinical presentation of spontaneous bacterial peritonitis may be subtle, such as fever of unknown origin and mild abdominal pain, and be attributed to other causes. Diagnosis is based on a careful examination of ascitic fluid obtained by paracentesis and should include cell count, Gram's stain, and culture.

359. The answer is B. *(Wilson, ed 12. chaps 46, 254.)* The x-ray presented in the question demonstrates esophageal varices, which are associated with portal hypertension. Of the diseases listed, only Laennec's cirrhosis would lead directly to portal hypertension. Although the other lesions might be associated with upper gastrointestinal bleeding, none would be expected to produce varices.

360. The answer is B. *(Wilson, ed 12. chap 258.)* Obesity, clofibrate therapy, and oral contraceptive therapy predispose to gallstone formation by increasing biliary cholesterol excretion. Extensive ileal resection leads to malabsorption of bile salts, depletion of the bile acid pool, and a more lithogenic bile, resulting in an increased risk of gallstone formation. No correlation exists between serum cholesterol concentration and biliary cholesterol secretion; consequently, hypercholesterolemia per se does not predispose to cholelithiasis.

361. The answer is B. *(Wilson, ed 12. chap 254.)* If fluid and sodium restriction is unsuccessful in the mobilization of ascitic fluid, cautious diuresis is indicated; spironolactone, rather than furosemide or acetazolamide, would be the drug of choice. Aggressive diuretic therapy can lead to volume depletion, azotemia, electrolyte disturbances, and hepatic encephalopathy. Therapeutic paracentesis is indicated only in the face of respiratory compromise and significant patient discomfort; repeated paracentesis may result in volume depletion and hypoproteinemia. The peritoneovenous (LeVeen) shunt should be reserved for cases of intractable ascites; its use is accompanied by significant complications, including infection and disseminated intravascular coagulation.

362. The answer is B. *(Wilson, ed 12. chap 255.)* The clinical constellation of tender hepatomegaly, a bruit in the right upper quadrant of the abdomen, bloody ascites, and very elevated alkaline phosphatase occurring in a patient with previously stable cirrhosis is characteristic of primary hepatocellular carcinoma. This disease typically is associated with very high levels of α-fetoprotein, a unique and specific fetal α_1-globulin. Rarely, ectopic hormones, such as chorionic gonadotropin, are found in the serum of patients with hepatocellular carcinoma. The enzyme 5'-nucleotidase may be elevated in any condition associated with hepatocellular damage.

Antimitochondrial antibodies are found in primary biliary cirrhosis and are not typical of primary hepatocellular carcinoma.

363. The answer is E. *(Wilson, ed 12. chap 260.)* Conventional therapy for acute pancreatitis includes analgesia, intravenous volume replacement, and abstinence from oral intake to "rest" the pancreas. Controlled trials have not demonstrated any benefit to symptomatic recovery or survival rate by administration of cimetidine, aprotinin (an inhibitor of pancreatic enzyme release), antibiotics, or glucagon. However, antibiotics are beneficial when secondary infection supervenes (e.g., abscess, phlegmon, or ascending cholangitis). Anticholinergic agents have not been shown to be beneficial and may worsen tachycardia, bowel hypomotility, and oliguria.

364. The answer is E. *(Wilson, ed 12. chap 258.)* The radiograph reproduced in the question shows emphysematous cholecystitis, a form of acute cholecystitis in which the gallbladder, its wall, and sometimes even the bile ducts contain gas secondary to infection by gas-producing bacteria. This condition occurs most frequently in elderly men and diabetic persons. The morbidity and mortality rates associated with emphysematous cholecystitis exceed those of acute cholecystitis. Once preoperative preparations are complete, laparotomy and cholecystectomy should be performed promptly.

365. The answer is B. *(Wilson, ed 12. chap 260.)* Vitamin B_{12} (cobalamin) malabsorption is commonly associated with chronic pancreatitis. The mechanism of vitamin B_{12} malabsorption is thought to be excessive binding of the vitamin by nonintrinsic-factor binding proteins, which normally are destroyed by pancreatic proteases. Consequently, the condition is corrected by administration of pancreatic enzymes. Gastric varices, which may bleed, are caused by splenic vein thrombosis due to inflammation of the tail of the pancreas. Pleural effusions, most notably left-sided, can result from leaking pseudocysts or a pancreatic-pleural fistula; effusion fluid has a high amylase content. Jaundice results from compression of the common bile duct caused by edema or inflammation in the head of the pancreas. Although persons with chronic pancreatitis may develop tender red nodules on the legs, these are due to subcutaneous fat necrosis and not to erythema nodosum.

366. The answer is A. *(Wilson, ed 12. chap 260.)* Serum bilirubin elevations >68 μmol/L (>4.0 mg/dL) occur in about 10 percent of patients with acute pancreatitis, are usually transient, and do not portend a poor prognosis unless accompanied by very high levels of serum lactic dehydrogenase. The finding of hypoxemia, often heralding the development of the adult respiratory distress syndrome, is ominous. Hypocalcemia (<1.96 mmol/L [<8 mg/dL]), possibly indicating intraperitoneal fatty acid saponification of calcium, is also a grave prognostic sign. Hypoalbuminemia and massive requirement for colloid replacement suggest profound peripancreatic disease as does the presence of discolored or hemorrhagic fluid obtained at paracentesis. Other risk factors for high mortality during an attack of acute pancreatitis include older age, hypotension, leukocytosis, hyperglycemia, fall in hematocrit, and azotemia.

367. The answer is B. *(Wilson, ed 12. chap 262. Feldman, Semin Oncol 14:237, 1987.)* Carcinoid tumors are the most common endocrine tumors of the gastrointestinal tract and can produce symptoms due to local effects or to secretion of serotonin, histamine, or other peptide hormones. Gastrointestinal bleeding, abdominal pain, or obstruction from serotonin-induced mesenteric fibrosis, intussusception, or tumor growth are common. The classic triad of findings in the hormone-mediated carcinoid syndrome includes cutaneous flushing, diarrhea, and valvular heart disease. The diarrhea can result from partial mechanical obstruction or mesenteric vascular insufficiency due to fibrosis, but the most common mechanism is a combination of hypersecretion and hypermotility leading to watery stools—a condition unresponsive to fasting. Steatorrhea, commonly seen with somatostatin-producing tumors, is not a feature of the carcinoid syndrome. Endocardial fibrosis causing pulmonary stenosis and tricuspid insufficiency can lead to right-sided heart failure and associated edema. Both serotonin and histamine can mediate wheezing, which is noted in about 20 percent of patients with the carcinoid syndrome.

368. The answer is B. *(Wilson, ed 12. chap 262.)* The combination of weight loss, anemia, and a bullous skin eruption in a patient with hepatic metastases and evidence of a pancreatic lesion is highly suggestive of a glucagonoma. This tumor of pancreatic alpha cells is usually malignant; metastasizes early; often occurs in middle-aged women; and is accompanied by hyperglycemia, painful stomatitis and cheilosis, hypoaminoacidemia, and a characteristic skin rash—necrolytic migratory erythema. With appropriate histologic techniques, the diagnosis of a pancreatic alpha-cell tumor can be established by liver biopsy, but marked plasma hyperglucagonemia is pathognomonic. Arteriography may demonstrate a pancreatic tumor but is not diagnostic. Treatment is early surgical removal; chemotherapy of metastatic disease is usually ineffective.

369. The answer is A-Y, B-Y, C-N, D-N, E-N. *(Wilson, ed 12. chap 252.)* The delta agent hepatitis D virus (HDV) is a recently recognized defective RNA virus that coinfects with and requires the helper function of HBV for its replication and expression. Therefore, the duration of HDV infection is determined by and limited to the duration of HBV infection. Although the delta core is encapsulated by an outer coat of HBsAg, the delta antigen has no antigenic similarity to that of any of the HBV antigens, and the RNA genome is not homologous with HBV DNA. HDV infection has a worldwide distribution and exists in two epidemiologic patterns, endemic and epidemic. In endemic areas (Mediterranean countries) HDV infection is endemic among those with HBV infection and is transmitted predominantly by nonpercutaneous routes, such as close personal contact. In nonendemic areas, such as the United States or northern Europe, HDV infection is limited to persons with frequent exposure to blood products, such as intravenous drug addicts and hemophiliacs. In general, patients with simultaneous HBV and HDV infections do not have an increased risk of development of chronic hepatitis over patients with acute HBV infection alone. HDV superinfection of patients with chronic HBV infection carries an increased risk of fulminant hepatitis and death.

370. The answer is A-Y, B-N, C-N, D-Y, E-Y. *(Wilson, ed 12. chaps 236, 238.)* Although upper gastrointestinal endoscopy is superior to radiographic techniques in its ability to identify superficial lesions of the esophagus, stomach, and duodenum, barium studies are able to detect a very high percentage of lesions that breach the mucosa. For example, most gastric and duodenal ulcers can be identified on an air-contrast upper gastrointestinal series. In contrast, erosive gastritis, the telangiectasias of Osler-Rendu-Weber syndrome, and small mucosal tears of the gastroesophageal junction (Mallory-Weiss tears) are missed with the best radiographic techniques but usually are found by routine endoscopy.

371. The answer is A-N, B-Y, C-Y, D-Y, E-Y. *(Wilson, ed 12. chaps 46, 254. Cello, N Engl J Med 316:11, 1987.)* Peripheral (intravenous) and central (superior mesenteric artery) infusions of vasopressin are equally effective in temporarily controlling variceal hemorrhage. For more permanent hemostasis, surgery may be required. Elective portacaval shunt surgery can prevent recurrent variceal bleeding, although the overall survival rate is not improved. The distal splenorenal shunt, when compared with the portacaval shunt, appears to have a lower incidence of postoperative encephalopathy; for either procedure, however, the presence of jaundice, ascites, or encephalopathy portends a less favorable operative outlook. Sclerotherapy is a promising newer technique that is an effective therapy to be employed, if available, prior to surgery.

372. The answer is A-Y, B-Y, C-N, D-Y, E-Y. *(Wilson, ed 12. chap 237.)* Chronic acid-induced (reflux) esophagitis may cause bleeding from diffuse erosions or discrete ulcerations. Peptic damage to the submucosa can result in fibrosis and subsequent stricture. Barrett's esophagus is formed as destroyed squamous epithelium is replaced by columnar epithelium, usually similar to that of the adjacent gastric mucosa. Adenocarcinoma may develop in 2 to 5 percent of persons with a Barrett's esophagus. A lower esophageal ring is a structural lesion that is not related to reflux esophagitis.

373. The answer is A-N, B-N, C-Y, D-Y, E-N. *(Wilson, ed 12. chap 252.)* The prevention of viral hepatitis is of particular importance because of the limited therapeutic options. The prophylactic approach varies with the type of hepatitis. All preparations of immune globulin (IG) contain sufficient titers of anti-HAV to prevent a clinically apparent type A hepatitis. If given early enough, infection will be prevented in approximately 80 percent of patients. For intimate contacts, 0.02 mL/kg of IG is recommended as soon as possible after exposure. The prevention of hepatitis B is based upon both passive immunoprophylaxis with hepatitis B immune globulin (HBIG) and hepatitis B vaccine. HBIG appears to be effective in reducing clinically apparent illness but does not appear to prevent infection. Hepatitis B vaccine has been shown to be highly effective in preventing HBV infection. Because only persons with HBV infection are susceptible to delta hepatitis, hepatitis B vaccine is effective in preventing delta infection in persons who are not carriers of HBsAg. There is no effective prophylaxis of HDV infection for those patients who are already HBsAg carriers. Although it has not been shown to be effective, many authorities recommend postexposure prophylaxis of non-A, non-B hepatitis with IG because it is safe and inexpensive and may be effective.

374. The answer is A-N, B-N, C-Y, D-Y, E-Y. *(Wilson, ed 12. chap 41.)* An atrophic, or "bald," tongue may be seen in association with several hematologic disorders, including iron deficiency and B_{12} deficiency as in the patient with malabsorption due to prior ileal or gastric resection. Impaired salivary production, as in the case of the patient with Sjögren's syndrome, can lead to an increased incidence of dental caries as well as to a bald tongue. The oral gummatous lesions characteristic of tertiary syphilis may also be associated with glossitis and bald tongue. An enlarged (but normally papillated) tongue is associated with Down's syndrome (which carries an increased risk for the development of acute leukemia), infiltration with lymphoma or amyloid, and acromegaly, as exemplified by the man with enlarged feet and glucose intolerance (due to the hyperglycemic effects of growth hormone).

375. The answer is A-N, B-Y, C-Y, D-N, E-N. *(Wilson, ed 12. chap 43.)* Two areas in the central nervous system control the act of vomiting. The vomiting center in the lateral reticular formation in the medulla receives input from both the gastrointestinal tract and from higher centers in the brain and controls outflow to the phrenic nerve, spinal nerve, and vagus, each of which innervates muscles involved in retching. The chemoreceptor trigger zone located near the floor of the fourth ventricle can be activated by a host of stimuli or drugs including opiates, dopaminergics, digitalis, radiation, and varied metabolic toxins and abnormalities (e.g., uremia). Pathways emanating from the chemoreceptor trigger zone lead to the vomiting center, which directly controls the act of vomiting. Dopaminergic inhibitors, such as the phenothiazine derivative prochlorperazine, inhibit the dopamine receptors in the chemoreceptor trigger zone, thereby suppressing vomiting. Phenothiazine derivatives frequently are associated with troublesome anticholinergic side effects such as sedation, dry mouth, and hypotension. Metoclopramide is another dopamine antagonist that can affect central pathways, but it has the added benefit of cholinergic effects that enhance gastric emptying. Antihistamines such as promethazine and anticholinergics such as scopolamine do not act on the chemoreceptor trigger zone, but can be helpful in the control of vomiting caused by dysfunction of the inner ear. While tetrahydrocannabinol, the active ingredient in marijuana, is an effective antiemetic after cancer chemotherapy, its mechanism of action is unknown.

376. The answer is A-Y, B-N, C-Y, D-N, E-Y. *(Wilson, ed 12. chaps 237, 240.)* Symptomatic esophageal involvement occurs in at least half of all persons who have scleroderma. Reduced lower esophageal tone leads to reflux esophagitis, and a loss of esophageal motility may cause dysphagia. Steatorrhea results both from bacterial overgrowth in an atonic small bowel and from obliteration of lymphatics by fibrosis. Pneumatosis intestinalis, which refers to radiolucent cysts or streaks in the wall of the small bowel, occurs more often than normal in association with scleroderma. There is no known predisposition to gallstones or pancreatitis in affected persons.

377. The answer is A-N, B-N, C-N, D-N, E-Y. *(Wilson, ed 12. chap 238.)* The only way to differentiate conclusively between a benign and a malignant gastric ulcer is by endoscopic or surgical biopsy. If six endoscopic biopsies of the inner margin of the ulcer crater along with brush cytologies are benign, then malignancy can be ruled out (0.95 confidence). At least 4 percent of gastric ulcers with a benign radiographic appearance prove to be malignant on biopsy. Both benign and malignant gastric ulcers occur more often on the lesser than on the greater curvature. Although ulcers greater than 3 cm in diameter are more likely to be cancerous, malignant gastric ulcers may be any size. About 70 percent of persons with gastric ulcers are not achlorhydric. Nearly three-quarters of malignant ulcers undergo significant healing, at least temporarily, during medical treatment for peptic ulcer disease.

378. The answer is A-Y, B-N, C-Y, D-N, E-N. *(Wilson, ed 12. chaps 240, 243. Haber, Semin Oncol 15:154, 1988.)* Primary intestinal lymphoma should be distinguished from secondary involvement of the intestine by lymphoma originating elsewhere in the body. Primary intestinal lymphoma originates within the lamina propria and in the lymphoid follicles of the mucosa and submucosa. Although the intestinal involvement is usually localized, it can be diffuse. In the latter case, malabsorption often occurs as a result of extensive mucosal involvement. In addition, malabsorption may be caused by lymphatic obstruction or localized narrowing of the intestinal lumen that leads to stasis of intestinal contents and bacterial overgrowth. Hepatosplenomegaly, peripheral adenopathy, and abdominal masses are unusual, but CT scans of the abdomen may reveal enlarged abdominal lymph nodes. The diagnosis is best made by laparotomy with full-thickness biopsy. Unless the duodenum or ileum is involved, the tumor is inaccessible to the endoscope. Perforation, bleeding, and intestinal obstruction are common events, especially late in the course of the disease.

379. The answer is A-N, B-Y, C-N, D-N, E-Y. *(Wilson, ed 12. chaps 47, 251.)* A simple and important method to determine whether the cause of jaundice is conjugated or unconjugated hyperbilirubinemia is measurement of urinary excretion of bilirubin. Under normal circumstances the urine contains no bilirubin since the unconjugated, water-soluble bilirubin, which accounts for 96 percent of the bilirubin in serum, is tightly bound to albumin and is not filtered by the glomeruli. Even in cases of unconjugated hyperbilirubinemia due to overproduction (as in hemolysis or the ineffective erythropoiesis characteristic of certain hemoglobinopathies) or due to decreased conjugation, there is no urinary excretion of bilirubin. Congenital deficiencies of the glucuronyl transferase enzyme responsible for converting bilirubin into its soluble form include Gilbert's syndrome and Crigler-Najjar types I and II (in type I disease, the transferase enzyme is totally absent). In cases of conjugated hyperbilirubinemia, in which more than 50 percent of the serum bilirubin is composed of the conjugated type, enough bilirubin remains unbound that filtration of this substance occurs and the urine dipstick becomes positive. In addition to extrahepatic obstruction, causes of conjugated hyperbilirubinemia include defects in hepatic excretion of a congenital (e.g., Dubin-Johnson or Rotor syndromes) or an acquired (hepatocellular disease or estrogen use) nature.

380. The answer is A-Y, B-Y, C-N, D-N, E-N. *(Wilson, ed 12. chap 238.)* Most gastrinomas are found in the pancreas, often in multiple locations. In about 25 percent of cases, gastrinomas are associated with other components of the multiple endocrine neoplasia (MEN) type I syndrome (neoplasms in the parathyroid or pituitary as well as the pancreas). The Zollinger-Ellison (Z-E) syndrome accounts for less than 1 percent of all peptic ulcers. About two-thirds of gastrinomas are malignant. The diagnosis should be suspected in cases of multiple, unusually located, recurrent, fulminant, or poorly responding peptic ulcers. On upper gastrointestinal examination, large mucosal folds are mainly noted in the stomach, but can also be observed at more distal sites. Diarrhea due to hypersecretion of acid or, less commonly, steatorrhea due to acid-mediated inactivation of pancreatic lipase may occur even in the absence of peptic ulcers. Endoscopic retrograde cholangiopancreatography (ERCP) is highly inferior to selective angiography or CT in identifying pancreatic gastrinomas, which are difficult to localize presurgically by any means. Elevated fasting levels of gastrin (>200 ng/L) are required for the diagnosis of gastrinoma; two normal levels in the absence of overwhelming evidence to the contrary essentially rule out the diagnosis. Positive responses to provocative tests include a paradoxical rise in serum gastrin by 200 ng/L after infusion of secretin, a rise in serum gastrin level by 400 ng/L after infusion of calcium gluconate, or a failure to rise above baseline after administration of a standard meal.

381. The answer is A-N, B-Y, C-N, D-Y, E-Y. *(Wilson, ed 12. chaps 238, 239.)* Although adenomatous gastric polyps may contain regions of adenocarcinoma or be associated with carcinoma elsewhere in the stomach, most gastric cancers do not begin as polyps. Atrophic gastritis may be a predisposing factor for both polyps and cancer; however, most persons who have atrophic gastritis, a common condition of the elderly, do not develop gastric cancer. Despite the fact that most persons with a malignant ulcer secrete some acid, achlorhydria after pentagastrin stimulation usually is incompatible with a diagnosis of benign peptic ulcer. Gastric cancers do not begin as benign ulcers, even if the ulcer is recurrent. Blood group A—not blood group O—is slightly increased in frequency in persons with gastric cancer. Billroth II partial gastrectomy seems to increase the risk for gastric cancer (a higher incidence of gastric cancer is being noted 10 to 20 years postoperatively). Gastric adenocarcinoma accounts for 90 percent of all malignancies of the stomach, with lymphoma representing about 7 percent and leiomyosarcoma most of the remainder.

382. The answer is A-Y, B-Y, C-N, D-Y, E-N. *(Wilson, ed 12. chap 240.)* Surgical resection of a significant portion of small intestine can result in a variety of clinical abnormalities, which are collectively referred to as the *short bowel syndrome.* By a mechanism as yet unelucidated, massive small-bowel resection can lead to transient gastric hypersecretion, which results in inactivation of pancreatic enzymes directly and in dilution of pancreatic secretions. The loss of ileal tissue causes poor absorption of bile salts; depletion of the bile acid pool results in steatorrhea, which is best managed by a low-fat diet (40 g/d). Increased passage of bile acids into the colon stimulates a secretory diarrhea. Antiperistaltic agents, such as belladonna alkaloids and diphenoxylate, presumably enhance absorption by prolonging mucosal contact time and thus can benefit patients with the short bowel syndrome.

383. The answer is A-N, B-N, C-Y, D-N, E-Y. *(Wilson, ed 12. chap 241.)* Several extraintestinal disorders are associated with both Crohn's disease and ulcerative colitis, including pericholangitis, uveitis, and a variety of skin and joint manifestations. Complications that are unique to Crohn's disease because of inflammation of the terminal ileum include hypocalcemia, which is caused by malabsorption of vitamin D, and the formation of urinary oxalate stones, which results from increased intestinal absorption of dietary oxalate. Owing to bile-salt malabsorption caused by ileal disease, cholesterol gallstones tend to form in persons having regional enteritis.

384. The answer is A-Y, B-Y, C-Y, D-N, E-N. *(Wilson, ed 12. chap 241. Summers, Gastroenterology 77:847, 1979. Ursing, Gastroenterology 83:550, 1982.)* Among the findings of the National Cooperative Crohn's Disease

Study in 1979 were that corticosteroids are more efficacious in the treatment of Crohn's disease of the small intestine than in the treatment of Crohn's disease of the colon, and that azathioprine may be a useful adjunct to corticosteroid therapy but is less effective as a single agent. Sulfasalazine was found to be effective in the therapy of active colonic disease, but neither sulfasalazine nor corticosteroids decrease the frequency of recurrence once remission has been achieved. Both drugs may be used safely in treating pregnant women. In more recent studies, metronidazole has been reported to be useful in the treatment of chronic perianal fistulas associated with Crohn's disease.

385. The answer is A-Y, B-N, C-Y, D-N, E-N. *(Wilson, ed 12. chap 241.)* Risk factors for the development of colon carcinoma in persons who have ulcerative colitis include presence of the disease for more than 10 years, extensive mucosal involvement (pancolitis), and a family history of carcinoma of the colon. The risk of cancer in persons with pancolitis is estimated to be 12 percent at 15 years, 23 percent at 20 years, and 42 percent at 24 years. Neither a history of toxic megacolon nor the prolonged use of high-dose steroids increases the risk of cancer. Pseudopolyps, although frequently associated with severe disease, are not precancerous lesions.

386. The answer is A-N, B-N, C-Y, D-Y, E-Y. *(Wilson, ed 12. chap 243.)* Carcinoembryonic antigen (CEA) is a glycoprotein present in fetal serum and in the serum of persons who have certain malignant and inflammatory conditions. As a marker, however, it is neither sensitive nor specific for gastrointestinal malignancies in general or colonic cancer in particular. Smoking, sclerosing cholangitis, and inflammatory bowel disease are associated with mild elevations of serum CEA concentration; very high serum levels suggest malignancy. Once a diagnosis of cancer is made in a person with an elevated serum CEA level, serial CEA determinations can be used to monitor the success of treatment and warn of possible recurrence.

387. The answer is A-N, B-Y, C-Y, D-Y, E-N. *(Wilson, ed 12. chap 242.)* Ischemic colitis most often occurs in elderly persons who have vascular disease. Areas of the colon with extensive collateral circulation, such as the rectum, usually are spared. Angiography of arteries and veins rarely is indicated for diagnosis or therapy, because vessel occlusions are almost never detected. Even though acute ischemic colitis may present with rectal bleeding and lower abdominal pain, most cases do not present with the severity of signs and symptoms suggestive of an acute abdomen. This disease usually does not recur, and symptoms tend to resolve in 2 to 4 weeks. Ischemic colitis is sometimes diagnosed retrospectively as the cause of a colonic stricture.

388. The answer is A-Y, B-Y, C-Y, D-N, E-Y. *(Wilson, ed 12. chap 242.)* Meckel's diverticulum is the most frequently occurring congenital anomaly of the gastrointestinal tract and is found in 2 percent of autopsied adults. The diverticulum may contain ectopic gastric mucosa, and local acid secretion may produce ileal ulceration and lower gastrointestinal bleeding. In young adults, Meckel's diverticulitis can mimic acute appendicitis. Technetium, taken up by diverticular gastric mucosa, may detect the lesion. The more common gastrointestinal barium x-rays usually do not demonstrate the diverticulum. Gastrointestinal obstruction may occur if the diverticulum intussuscepts or twists on a fibrous remnant of the omphalomesenteric duct. Surgical excision is the treatment of any significant complication of a Meckel's diverticulum.

389. The answer is A-N, B-Y, C-Y, D-N, E-Y. *(Wilson, ed 12. chap 242.)* Acute hemorrhage from colonic diverticula is the most common cause of lower gastrointestinal bleeding among elderly persons. Although diverticula are more common in the left side of the colon, bleeding tends to originate from the ascending (right) colon. Bleeding usually stops with bed rest and transfusion; however, when conservative measures fail to curb hemorrhage, intraarterial infusion of vasoconstrictive medications, introduced during angiography, can be effective. Although acute diverticulitis may be associated with occult bleeding, gross hemorrhage rarely occurs.

390. The answer is A-Y, B-N, C-Y, D-Y, E-N. *(Wilson, ed 12. chaps 44, 242.)* Demonstration of polymorphonuclear leukocytes in the stool indicates an invasive inflammatory process in the bowel mucosa. Both amebae and *Shigella* bacteria may cause such a response, as might idiopathic ulcerative colitis. Diarrhea caused by cholera is due to toxin production; mucosal invasion does not occur. Giardiasis may cause striking histologic abnormalities in the small bowel, but an exudative inflammatory response is not characteristic.

391. The answer is A-Y, B-Y, C-N, D-Y, E-N. *(Wilson, ed 12. chap 249.)* Unexplained hepatosplenomegaly and unexplained persistence of elevated liver function tests are the principal indications for percutaneous needle liver biopsy. The presence of these phenomena suggests a diagnosis either of diffuse parenchymal disease of the liver, which occurs with drug reactions and metabolic liver disease, or of multiple focal lesions, which are caused by granulomatous or metastatic disease. The diagnosis of miliary tuberculosis, for example, can often be made by liver biopsy (more than 40 percent of all cases have a positive liver biopsy). A focal defect identified on liver scan also can be evaluated by percutaneous liver biopsy, often with sonographic guidance of the needle. A percutaneous liver biopsy should never be performed, however, when a vascular lesion of the liver, such as an angioma, is suspected. Although liver biopsy can confirm the presence of suspected biliary obstruction, ultrasonography, computerized tomography, and transhepatic or endoscopic cholangiography are better techniques for determining the cause of common bile duct obstruction.

392. The answer is A-Y, B-Y, C-N, D-N, E-Y. *(Wilson, ed 12. chap 249.)* Elevated levels of serum alkaline phosphatase (of hepatic origin) generally reflect impaired hepatic excretory function. Thus, the concentration of this enzyme may be elevated in persons with incomplete extrahepatic biliary obstruction (e.g., bile duct stricture) or intrahepatic cholestasis (e.g., chlorpromazine-induced cholestasis or early primary biliary cirrhosis); in all three of these examples, serum bilirubin concentration is only slightly elevated. Both acute viral hepatitis and acetaminophen hepatotoxicity are associated with extensive hepatocellular damage and frequently produce peak serum aspartate aminotransferase levels of above 8.33 μkat/L (500 U/L).

393. The answer is A-Y, B-Y, C-Y, D-Y, E-Y. *(Wilson, ed 12. chap 243.)* Adenomatous polyps of the colon are very common in the general population, and the incidence increases with age. They are usually detected by screening barium enemas or colonoscopy which have been performed as part of an evaluation of occult gastrointestinal blood loss. A small minority of polyps cause bleeding or obstruction. The majority of polyps occur in the rectosigmoid colon. An increasing size correlates with an increased risk of malignancy. Polyps less than 1 cm have a 1 percent chance of containing malignant cells whereas 50 percent of polyps greater than 2 cm contain malignant cells. There are three histologic types of polyps: tubular, tubulovillous, and villous. Of these, villous adenomas tend to be the largest and have the greatest risk of malignancy. Because polyps with carcinoma in situ do not metastasize, colonoscopic resection is considered curative. However, affected patients must be examined carefully for synchronous lesions and followed for recurrent disease.

394. The answer is A-N, B-Y, C-Y, D-N, E-N. *(Wilson, ed 12. chap 252.)* Peak serum levels of the serum aminotransferases AST and ALT may be as high as 68 μkat/L (4000 IU) or more; however, the acute level of these enzymes is poorly correlated with the degree of hepatocellular damage. A prolonged prothrombin time, hypoalbuminemia, hypoglycemia, and marked hyperbilirubinemia portend a poor prognosis. A serum sickness–like syndrome is associated with hepatitis B infection, occurring in 5 to 10 percent of affected persons. The etiologic agent cannot be surmised accurately from the presenting symptoms and signs in most persons. Steroid therapy has no value in the treatment of acute viral hepatitis.

395. The answer is A-Y, B-Y, C-Y, D-Y, E-Y. *(Wilson, ed 12. chaps 252, 253.)* Non-A, non-B hepatitis, which is thought to be caused by a variety of agents not yet identified, accounts for 90 percent of all cases of posttransfusion hepatitis. The incubation period is variable, with a mean of approximately 50 days (mean incubation period of hepatitis A is 30 days, and hepatitis B about 75 days). In humans, the disease is spread by both percutaneous and nonpercutaneous exposure; the existence of asymptomatic chronic carrier states also has been demonstrated. There are two distinct syndromes of non-A, non-B hepatitis. One is the blood-borne variety, which accounts for transfusion-associated hepatitis. Furthermore, at least two blood-borne non-A, non-B agents exist. One of these is an RNA virus whose genome was recently cloned (hepatitis C virus) and now can be detected serologically. A water-borne non-A, non-B syndrome caused by an enteric HAV-like virus has been identified in Asia, Africa, and Central America.

396. The answer is A-Y, B-Y, C-N, D-Y, E-N. *(Wilson, ed 12. chap 240.)* Patients with intestinal lymphangiectasia—characterized by protein-losing enteropathy, hypoproteinemia, hypogammaglobulinemia, edema, chylous effusions, fat malabsorption, and lymphocytopenia—typically present in childhood or young adulthood. The generalized congenital disorder of lymphatic development includes the dilated lymph vessels typically seen on small-bowel biopsy. The abnormal lymphatics are presumed to rupture into the bowel lumen, which leads directly to hypoproteinemia and steatorrhea. Absorption of carbohydrates such as D-xylose and lactose that are not dependent upon lymphatics is typically preserved. The decreased lymph flow associated with a low-fat diet supplemented by medium-chain triglycerides (transported by the portal vein rather than the lymph) results in significant clinical improvement.

397. The answer is A-Y, B-Y, C-Y, D-Y, E-Y. *(Wilson, ed 12. chap 240.)* Tropical sprue is a malabsorptive disease of unclear etiology that may be due to a nutritional deficiency, a microorganism, or a toxin elaborated by a microorganism. Malabsorption of at least two nutrients is the rule. Patients commonly malabsorb iron, vitamin B_{12}, xylose (carbohydrates), and fat. Consequently, megaloblastic anemia and problems associated with the absorption of the fat-soluble vitamins A (night blindness), D (hypocalcemia possibly with tetany), and K (hypoprothrombinemia and purpura) may be seen. In the setting of prolonged calorie malnutrition, a state of secondary hypopituitarism may be manifested by decreased libido. The diagnosis of tropical sprue is supported by a jejunal biopsy disclosing shortened and thickened villi, increased crypt height, and infiltration of mononuclear cells in the lamina propria. Treatment with vitamin B_{12}, folate, and antibiotics should be undertaken.

398. The answer is A-Y, B-N, C-N, D-Y, E-Y. *(Wilson, ed 12. chap 241. Peppercorn, Ann Intern Med 101:377, 1984.)* Sulfasalazine (Azulfidine) as a single agent is an effective treatment for an acute attack of inflammatory bowel disease of mild-to-moderate severity. In ulcerative colitis, controlled trials have shown that chronic use can decrease subsequent attack rates. Sulfasalazine is cleaved by intestinal bacteria to the inactive moiety sulfapyridine, which is rapidly excreted in the urine, and into the active compound 5-aminosalicylate, which is thought to work via inhibition of prostaglandin synthesis in the colon. The latter agent can be administered effectively by enemas, allowing use by patients who are poorly tolerant of oral sulfasalazine.

399. The answer is A-Y, B-Y, C-Y, D-N, E-N. *(Wilson, ed 12. chap 255.)* Rare hepatic diseases that occur with increased frequency in women who use oral contraceptive agents include hepatic adenoma, which is encapsulated, and focal nodular hyperplasia, which is not. Both may regress when use of the oral contraceptive is discontinued. Peliosis hepatis (blood-filled, dilated sinusoids) has been described in users of oral contraceptives as well as in persons taking androgenic steroids. Angiosarcoma, a malignant vascular tumor, has been described in association with vinyl chloride exposure, past administration of Thorotrast (a radioactive contrast agent in wide use 30 to 40 years ago), and use of androgenic steroids, but *not* with use of oral contraceptives. A presumed association between use of oral contraceptives and primary hepatocellular carcinoma has been refuted by recent epidemiologic evidence; however, malignant transformation of hepatic adenomas has been reported. Rhabdomyosarcoma is a tumor rarely found in the liver; there is no known association with use of oral contraceptives.

400. The answer is A-Y, B-Y, C-N, D-N, E-Y. *(Wilson, ed 12. chap 251.)* Gilbert's syndrome is a benign disorder in which a partial deficiency of bilirubin glucuronyl transferase leads to mild unconjugated hyperbilirubinemia. The serum total bilirubin concentrations fluctuate between 17 μmol/L (1 mg/dL) and 51 μmol/L (3mg/dL) and rarely exceed 86 μmol/L (5 mg/dL). No clear pattern of inheritance has been identified. Fasting reliably raises the serum bilirubin concentration and is a useful diagnostic test. Phenobarbital, which enhances glucuronyl transferase activity, results in a decrease in serum bilirubin concentration. Although a liver biopsy is not required for the diagnosis, liver biopsy specimens are normal when examined by light microscopy.

401. The answer is A-N, B-N, C-Y, D-Y, E-Y. *(Wilson, ed 12. chap 243.)* Familial polyposis of the colon is a rare condition inherited in an autosomal dominant fashion. It is characterized by adenomatous polyps throughout the colon. A total proctocolectomy can eliminate the certain risk of cancer by age 40. Peutz-Jeghers syndrome is characterized by hamartomatous polyps (without risk of malignant degeneration) in the stomach and all intestinal sites. In Gardner's syndrome adenomatous polyps line the large and small intestine; in addition to a high risk of colon cancer, such patients are plagued with multiple benign tumors including osteomas, fibromas, and lipomas. Turcot's syndrome refers to the constellation of adenomatous colonic polyps and malignant brain tumors.

402. The answer is A-Y, B-N, C-Y, D-Y, E-N. *(Wilson, ed 12. chap 252.)* The diagnosis of acute hepatitis B infection can be made by the detection of HBsAg in serum, unless there is the simultaneous presence of IgG anti-HBc, which indicates chronic infection. The only exception to the latter rule is in the case of late acute (or early chronic) infection when anti-HBe is present as well as HBsAg and the anti-HBcAg has already converted from the IgM to IgG. HBeAg is a marker of infectivity, either in acute or chronic infection. Positivity for both IgG anti-HBcAg and anti-HBsAg indicates recovery from prior infection (anti-HBeAg may be positive or negative in this case). An additional caveat is the relatively uncommon situation during acute infection when the level of HBsAg is too low to be detected, but the presence of IgM anti-HBcAg establishes the diagnosis.

403. The answer is A-N, B-Y, C-N, D-Y, E-Y. *(Wilson, ed 12. chap 254.)* Reye's syndrome typically occurs in children recovering from a viral illness. There is often a history of ingestion of aspirin during the viral illness.

Marked elevations in the serum levels of aminotransferase and ammonia as well as in prothrombin time are usually present, and affected children often develop hypoglycemic episodes. Despite these biochemical and physiologic signs of deranged hepatic function, jaundice is usually minimal.

404. The answer is A-Y, B-Y, C-N, D-Y, E-Y. *(Wilson, ed 12. chap 252.)* Hepatitis B *e* antigen (HBeAg) is a protein that is associated with the HBV core particle. HBeAg is a soluble protein found only in HBsAg-positive serum and is immunologically distinct from HBsAg as well as from intact HBcAg, an antigen expressed on the hepatitis B virus nucleocapsid core. Interestingly, both HBcAg and HBeAg are encoded on the so-called C-gene of the hepatitis B genome. Owing to the close association of HBeAg and HBsAg, the presence of HBeAg in the serum is linked with infectiousness, and the antigen is present during the viremic period of acute hepatitis B. Although HBeAg correlates well with viral replication, detection of HBeAg in serum has not been found to predict the subsequent development of chronic hepatitis B infection; equally, the absence of HBeAg in serum does not preclude the development of chronic hepatitis B infection. In acute hepatitis B, the disappearance of HBeAg from serum often presages resolution of the acute infection; however, HBeAg-negative persons should be considered infectious until antibody to hepatitis B surface antigen is detected in the serum.

405. The answer is A-Y, B-Y, C-Y, D-Y, E-Y. *(Wilson, ed 12. chap 255.)* Chronic liver disease of any etiology is associated with an increased incidence of hepatocellular carcinoma (HCC). Thus, patients with alcoholic liver disease, hemochromatosis, and α_1-antitrypsin deficiency are all at increased risk of development of HCC. Worldwide, chronic hepatitis B virus infection is an important cause of chronic liver disease and subsequent HCC. Mycotoxins such as aflatoxin are found in foodstuffs in many parts of the world and are thought to be carcinogenic.

406. The answer is A-N, B-Y, C-Y, D-Y, E-N. *(Wilson, ed 12. chap 256.)* Granulomas can be found on liver biopsy in cases of fever of unknown origin or during evaluation of patients who have abnormalities of unclear etiology on liver function tests. Though mild transaminase abnormalities may occur, hepatic dysfunction is usually restricted to mild elevations of the alkaline phosphatase. In approximately 20 percent of cases it is not possible to identify a systemic cause of the hepatic granulomas. In such a situation, and only if a diagnosis of miliary tuberculosis is rigorously excluded (even including an initial empirical trial of antituberculous therapy), a trial of steroids could be considered. Though tuberculosis is the etiology in the majority of cases when caseating lesions are present, the absence of caseating granulomas does not exclude tuberculosis. Systemic granulomatous diseases other than tuberculosis that may involve the liver include schistosomiasis, histoplasmosis, brucellosis, berylliosis, sarcoidosis, and drug reactions.

407. The answer is A-N, B-Y, C-Y, D-Y, E-N. *(Wilson, ed 12. chap 257. O'Grady, Gut 29:560, 1988.)* Though replacement of a diseased liver with a healthy organ obtained from a brain-dead donor is complex and dangerous, improvements in supportive care and outcome have made this an acceptable alternative for certain patients with irreversible hepatic failure. Transplantation should be undertaken before the patient has deteriorated past the point of being a reasonable operative risk, and after the point that the liver disease has any chance of stabilizing or improving. For example, since many patients with Budd-Chiari syndrome will recanalize their occluded vena cava, transplantation in this group should be reserved for those who progress on to irreversible hepatic failure. Patients with end-stage primary biliary cirrhosis, cryptogenic (nonalcoholic, nonviral) cirrhosis, and sclerosing cholangitis are all potential candidates for liver transplantation. Results involving hepatic transplantation for alcohol-related liver disease have been disappointing.

408. The answer is A-N, B-Y, C-Y, D-N, E-N. *(Wilson, ed 12. chap 258.)* Oral bile acid therapy with chenodeoxycholic acid (CDCA) or a related compound, ursodeoxycholic acid (UDCA), serves to alter the lithogenic index, thereby decreasing the tendency to maintain and form gallstones. CDCA decreases activity of HMG-CoA reductase, the rate-limiting enzyme in cholesterol biosynthesis. UDCA directly promotes dispersion of cholesterol from gallstones. Therapy with these agents results in complete or partial gallstone dissolution in about 50 percent of patients, with complete response being achieved in one-third of responders. CDCA and UDCA are ineffective in the treatment of pigment stones, radiopaque stones, large (> 1.5 cm in diameter) stones, and stones found in patients whose gallbladders are not visualized after administration of oral contrast agents. Self-limited diarrhea and mild, transient elevations of hepatic transaminase are sometimes seen in patients on therapy with CDCA; serious hepatotoxicity occurs in less than 1 to 2 percent. Gallstone lithotripsy is emerging as effective therapy for selected patients (those with biliary colic, radiolucent stones, a visualizable gallbladder after oral contrast, or one to four stones all less than 30 mm in diameter, and those with absence of obstruction, inflammation, and pregnancy). The rate of recurrence after lithotripsy-induced complete stone resolution and the effectiveness of this modality for calcified stones are among the issues requiring definition. Application of methyl tertiary butyl ether by percutaneous transhepatic catheter can also dissolve cholesterol gallstones.

409. The answer is A-N, B-Y, C-Y, D-N, E-N. *(Wilson, ed 12. chap 261.)* The clinical history is highly suggestive of carcinoma of the head of the pancreas. The failure to obtain diagnostic tissue at needle biopsy is not unusual because of surrounding inflammation, edema, and fibrosis. Even though well over 90 percent of patients with pancreatic cancer cannot be cured surgically, an attempt at such a procedure is appropriate, particularly for lesions in the pancreatic head, which tend to present earlier because they produce extrahepatic biliary obstruction and because of the frequent confusion with other more curable lesions in this location (duodenal, ampullary, and distal bile duct tumors). Therefore, such a patient should undergo a preoperative celiac angiogram to rule out vascular invasion by tumor and ensure resectability. It would not be unreasonable to attempt a preoperative diagnosis via ERCP, although the yield will be small. Repeating a needle biopsy is unlikely to achieve diagnostic results. Neither watchful follow-up nor palliative biliary stent therapy is appropriate until a tissue diagnosis of cancer and a determination of unresectability have been made.

410–413. The answers are: 410–A, 411–E, 412–D, 413–B. *(Wilson, ed 12. chaps 42, 237.)* Dysphagia for solid food that has been present for several years indicates a benign disease and is characteristic of a lower esophageal (Schatzki) ring (radiograph A). This lesion appears as a thin, web-like constriction near the lower esophageal sphincter. Even though the ring is congenital, dysphagia, which typically is episodic, may not occur until middle age.

Dysphagia for solid foods following a long history of heartburn suggests the development of a peptic stricture (radiograph E). (However, peptic stricture can develop in persons who do not have a history of heartburn.) On barium swallow, peptic strictures usually are seen to be 1 to 3 cm long and located near the squamocolumnar junction. Longer strictures may result from persistent vomiting or prolonged nasogastric intubation.

Rapidly progressive dysphagia and weight loss are characteristic of esophageal carcinoma (radiograph D). Dysphagia begins with solid foods but may progress to include liquids. Alcohol and tobacco use can be important predisposing factors. Barium swallow may show an ulcerating, infiltrating, or polypoid lesion.

Dysphagia caused by diffuse esophageal spasm (radiograph B) may occur with or without chest pain and often involves both solids and liquids. The chest pain, which may mimic the pain of myocardial ischemia, usually occurs at rest or on swallowing. Barium swallow shows uncoordinated, simultaneous contractions that may create a "corkscrew" configuration.

Radiograph C shows features typical of achalasia. A "beak-like" tapering of the distal esophagus and proximal dilation are prominent features. Affected persons characteristically present with painless dysphagia for solids and liquids.

Immunologic, Allergic, and Rheumatic Disorders

DIRECTIONS: Each question below contains five suggested responses. Choose the **one best** response to each question.

414. The least mature cells in the B-cell lineage are the pre-B cells. These cells are best defined by the presence of

(A) surface immunoglobulin M
(B) surface immunoglobulin D
(C) surface immunoglobulin G
(D) cytoplasmic μ chains
(E) Fc receptors

415. The hyperviscosity syndrome is most characteristic of which of the following plasma cell disorders?

(A) Multiple myeloma
(B) Heavy chain disease
(C) Indolent myeloma
(D) Waldenström's macroglobulinemia
(E) Primary amyloidosis

416. A 35-year-old woman comes to the local health clinic because for the last 6 months she has had recurrent urticarial lesions, which occasionally leave a residual discoloration. She also has had arthralgias. Sedimentation rate obtained now is 85 mm/h. The procedure most likely to yield the correct diagnosis in the case would be

(A) a battery of wheal-and-flare allergy skin tests
(B) measurement of total serum immunoglobulin E (IgE) concentration
(C) measurement of C1 esterase inhibitor activity
(D) skin biopsy
(E) patch testing

417. A 23-year-old man seeks medical attention for perennial nasal congestion and postnasal discharge. He states he does not have asthma, eczema, conjunctivitis, or a family history of allergic disease. His nasal secretions are rich in eosinophils. The test most likely to yield a specific diagnosis in this setting is

(A) competitive radioimmunosorbent test
(B) elimination diet test
(C) pollen skin testing
(D) dust and mold skin testing
(E) sinus x-rays

418. A 47-year-old man has had fever, weight loss, arthralgias, pleuritic chest pain, and midabdominal pain for the last 2 months. One week ago he noticed difficulty dorsiflexing his right great toe. Blood pressure is 150/95 mmHg (he has always been normotensive), and laboratory studies reveal anemia of chronic disease, high erythrocyte sedimentation rate, and polymorphonuclear leukocytosis. The most likely diagnosis is

(A) giant cell arteritis
(B) allergic granulomatosis
(C) Wegener's granulomatosis
(D) polyarteritis nodosa
(E) hypersensitivity vasculitis

419. Which of the following statements regarding the renal involvement associated with systemic lupus erythematosus is true?

(A) Clinically apparent renal disease occurs in 90 percent of affected persons
(B) Interstitial nephritis is a rare finding on renal biopsy
(C) Renal biopsy is not initially necessary in patients with deteriorating renal function and active urine sediment
(D) Renal disease is uncommon in patients with high-titer anti–double-stranded DNA antibodies
(E) Urinalysis in affected persons usually reveals proteinuria but little sediment and no red blood cells

420. All the following are immunologic abnormalities detected in patients with acquired immunodeficiency syndrome (AIDS) EXCEPT

(A) deficient T-lymphocyte response to antigenic and mitogenic stimulation
(B) decreased serum levels of immunoglobulins
(C) depletion of T4$^+$ lymphocytes
(D) normal numbers of T8$^+$ lymphocytes
(E) defective natural killer cell function

421. All the following statements concerning the HLA-D region on the sixth human chromosome are correct EXCEPT

(A) it is located outside of the major histocompatibility gene complex
(B) it encodes proteins involved in the mixed lymphocyte response
(C) it encodes proteins expressed only on certain immune effector or closely related cells
(D) siblings matched for HLA-A, -B, and -C antigens will usually be matched at the D region
(E) it is located in close proximity to genes encoding for complement components

422. All the following statements concerning the ataxia-telangiectasia syndrome are correct EXCEPT

(A) it is inherited in an autosomal recessive manner
(B) the cause is adenosine deaminase deficiency
(C) malignancy is a common cause of death
(D) bronchiectasis may occur
(E) both humoral and cellular limbs of the immune system are affected

423. All the following statements regarding the epidemiology of HIV infection are correct EXCEPT

(A) the occupational risk of HIV infection among health-care workers is small (<0.5 percent per exposure) but real
(B) over 1 per 1000 U.S. military recruits are infected
(C) most U.S. cases of AIDS are now in the high-risk group of intravenous drug abusers
(D) the chance that a single donor blood unit will contain HIV is between 1:40,000 and 1:250,000
(E) most pediatric cases arise because of in utero transmission from an infected mother

424. A 32-year-old homosexual man complains of weight loss, sweats, diarrhea, and swollen glands for the past 3 to 4 months. Over the previous 1 to 2 months he has had increasing dyspnea and fever and a nonproductive cough. Each of the following pathogens is associated with this patient's illness EXCEPT

(A) *Pneumocystis carinii*
(B) cytomegalovirus
(C) *Mycoplasma pneumoniae*
(D) *Cryptococcus neoformans*
(E) *Mycobacterium tuberculosis*

425. All the following pharmacologic agents may be useful in the treatment of the *acute* manifestations of anaphylaxis EXCEPT

(A) corticosteroids
(B) aminophylline
(C) antihistamines (e.g., diphenhydramine)
(D) epinephrine
(E) oxygen

426. All the following are compatible with illness induced by therapeutic administration of antithymocyte globulin EXCEPT

(A) malaise and fever 2 to 3 days after beginning therapy
(B) lymphadenopathy
(C) depressed CH_{50} level
(D) positive C1q binding assay
(E) fever

427. A woman who has rheumatoid arthritis suddenly develops pain and swelling in the right calf. The most likely diagnosis is

(A) ruptured plantaris tendon
(B) pes anserinus bursitis
(C) ruptured popliteal cyst
(D) deep thrombophlebitis
(E) Achilles tendonitis

428. All the following are considered to be disease-modifying agents in the treatment of rheumatoid arthritis EXCEPT

(A) gold
(B) prednisone
(C) D-penicillamine
(D) sulfasalazine
(E) hydroxychloroquine

429. Which of the following systemic manifestations is LEAST characteristic of early adult rheumatoid arthritis?

(A) High fever
(B) Weight loss
(C) Muscle wasting
(D) Vague musculoskeletal symptoms
(E) Fatigue

430. Which of the following conditions is LEAST likely to occur in late extraarticular seropositive rheumatoid arthritis?

(A) Neutropenia
(B) Dry eyes
(C) Leg ulcers
(D) Sensorimotor polyneuropathy
(E) Hepatitis

431. In which of the following clinical situations would a diagnosis of ankylosing spondylitis most likely be correct?

(A) For the last 10 years, a 28-year-old man has had low back pain and stiffness, worse at night and relieved with activity
(B) For the last 5 years, a 32-year-old man has had low back pain made worse with activity but improved with bed rest
(C) For the last 10 years, a 34-year-old man has had intermittent bouts of mild low back pain; now, however, he suddenly is unable to dorsiflex his right great toe
(D) For the last 10 years, a 65-year-old man has had low back pain radiating down both posterior thighs to the knees
(E) For the last 15 years, a 72-year-old man has had progressive low back pain made worse with walking but improved with rest and leaning forward

432. Arthritis associated with psoriasis can be manifest in several different ways. Each of the following is characteristic of psoriatic arthritis EXCEPT

(A) asymmetrical oligoarticular arthritis
(B) rheumatoid factor–positive symmetrical polyarthritis
(C) arthritis of distal interphalangeal joints
(D) severe destructive polyarthritis (arthritis mutilans)
(E) spondylitis and sacroiliitis with or without peripheral arthritis

433. The arthropathy of inflammatory bowel disease can be characterized by all the following EXCEPT

(A) peripheral arthritis is more commonly associated with colonic than with small-bowel involvement
(B) the presence and activity of the peripheral arthritis is related to the extent and activity of bowel involvement
(C) the peripheral arthritis is usually a symmetrical small-joint polyarthritis
(D) the peripheral arthritis resolves without residual joint damage
(E) spondylitis is not related to the extent or activity of colonic involvement

434. For the last 2 years, a 27-year-old man has had recurrent episodes of asymmetrical inflammatory oligoarticular arthritis involving his knees, ankles, and elbows lasting from 2 to 4 weeks. He also states he has had recurrent, painful "canker sores" in his mouth for the last 10 years. Now, he presents with fever, arthritis, mild abdominal pain, severe headache, and superficial thrombophlebitis in the left leg. The most likely diagnosis in this man is

(A) regional enteritis
(B) systemic lupus erythematosus
(C) Behçet's syndrome
(D) Whipple's disease
(E) ulcerative colitis

435. Which of the following findings is LEAST characteristic of early disseminated gonococcal infection?

(A) Fever
(B) Skin lesions
(C) Tenosynovitis
(D) Monoarticular arthritis
(E) Negative synovial fluid cultures

436. Which of the following clinical findings would be LEAST compatible with a diagnosis of tuberculous arthritis?

(A) Normal chest x-ray
(B) Absence of fever
(C) Synovial fluid white blood cell count featuring 75 percent polymorphonuclear leukocytes
(D) Acute arthritic presentation
(E) Coexistent osteomyelitis

437. A 37-year-old woman with Raynaud's phenomenon complains of progressive weakness with inability to arise out of a sitting position without assistance. On examination, the patient has swollen "sausagelike" fingers, alopecia, erythematous patches on the knuckles, facial telangiectasias, and proximal muscle weakness. Laboratory evaluation includes a normal CBC and serum chemistries, except for creatine phosphokinase 4.5 μkat/L (270 U/L) and aldolase 500 nkat/L (30 U/L). The following serologic profile is found: rheumatoid factor is positive at 1:1600; ANA is also positive at 1:1600 with a speckled pattern and very high titers of antibodies against the ribonuclease-sensitive ribonucleoprotein component of extractable nuclear antigen. This patient probably has

(A) early rheumatoid arthritis
(B) systemic sclerosis
(C) systemic lupus erythematosus
(D) dermatomyositis
(E) mixed connective tissue disease

438. All the following physical findings may be seen in osteoarthritis EXCEPT

(A) Heberden's nodes
(B) Bouchard's nodes
(C) bony crepitus on joint movement
(D) boutonnière deformity
(E) positive ''shrug'' sign

439. A 50-year-old woman has had Raynaud's phenomenon of the hands for 15 years. The condition has become worse during the last year, and she has developed arthralgias and arthritis involving the hands and wrists as well as mild sclerodactyly and difficulty swallowing solid foods. Laboratory studies reveal a positive serum antinuclear antibody assay at a dilution of 1:160. The most likely diagnosis of this woman's disorder is

(A) systemic sclerosis
(B) mixed connective-tissue disease
(C) overlap syndrome
(D) dermatomyositis
(E) systemic lupus erythematosus

440. A 25-year-old man has had pain and swelling in the right knee for the last year. He is otherwise well and gives no history of trauma. X-rays show several erosions at the margin of the right knee joint. Aspiration of the joint yields 25 mL of dark-brown synovial fluid of good viscosity. The most likely diagnosis is

(A) atypical rheumatoid arthritis
(B) incomplete Reiter's syndrome
(C) hemangioma
(D) osteochondritis dissecans
(E) pigmented villonodular synovitis

441. A 52-year-old previously well man who has had hoarseness as well as intermittent pain and swelling in his right knee and left foot over the past few months presents now because of pain and swelling in both ears. On examination he has conjunctivitis and beefy red skin over the ears and bridge of the nose, although the earlobes appear normal. His most likely diagnosis is

(A) Cogan's syndrome
(B) Reiter's syndrome
(C) relapsing polychondritis
(D) rheumatoid arthritis
(E) squamous carcinoma

DIRECTIONS: Each question below contains five suggested responses. For **each** of the **five** responses listed with every question, you are to respond either YES (Y) or NO (N). In a given item **all, some, or none of the alternatives may be correct**.

442. True statements about human B lymphocytes include which of the following?

(A) They represent 10 percent of lymphocytes in bone marrow

(B) They play a necessary helper function in the synthesis of lymphokines

(C) Maturity is heralded by the presence of IgD on the cell surface

(D) They have membrane receptors for the Fc portion of IgG

(E) They have membrane receptors for the (activated) C3 component of complement

443. A physician working on a Hopi Indian reservation in New Mexico develops a flulike illness with the additional features of cough; conjunctivitis; painful, red lesions on his legs; and a painful, swollen right knee. Correct statements regarding this patient's arthritis include

(A) culturing the joint fluid will probably yield the diagnosis

(B) serology may be helpful in establishing the diagnosis

(C) the arthritis could have arisen from hematogenous seeding

(D) the arthritis could be a sterile manifestation of acute hypersensitivity

(E) the arthritis could have arisen from adjacent osteomyelitis

444. Correct statements regarding T-cell immunophenotype include which of the following?

(A) The T-cell antigen receptor is the earliest surface marker of T-cell lineage

(B) The expressions of CD4 (T4) and CD8 (T8) surface antigens are mutually exclusive

(C) The T-cell adhesion molecule, CD2 (T11), accounts for the ability of T cells to form rosettes with sheep red blood cells

(D) The T-cell antigen receptor complex consists of a signal-transducing moiety and an antigen-recognition moiety

(E) Mature T cells display surface proteins that are members of the immunoglobulin gene superfamily

445. True statements about human T cells include which of the following?

(A) They are the principal cells in the cortical "germinal centers" and medullary cords of lymph nodes

(B) They carry membrane-bound IgD on their surface

(C) They constitute 70 to 80 percent of circulating blood lymphocytes

(D) They arise from stem cells in the thymus

(E) They are the main effectors of antibody-dependent, cell-mediated cytotoxicity

446. Human immunoglobulin A (IgA) can be described by which of the following statements?

(A) It is the predominant immunoglobulin in plasma

(B) It exists in four subclasses, of which IgA2 is predominant

(C) It can prevent attachment of microorganisms to epithelial cell membranes

(D) It is prominent early in the immune response and is the major class of antibody in cold agglutinins

(E) It has the shortest half-life of the five classes of immunoglobulin

447. True statements about cell-mediated immunity include

(A) it is effected and amplified by the action of lymphokines

(B) cooperation between T helper cells and B cells is necessary for normal function

(C) immune competence can be assessed by skin testing with various antigens

(D) berylliosis is a pathologic expression of this form of immunity

(E) interleukin 3 directly augments this form of immunity

448. Following the activation of complement component C5, which is a protein of molecular weight 180,000, a small fragment called C5a is released. True statements regarding the biologic activity of C5a include which of the following?

(A) It can promote non-IgE-dependent release of histamine from mast cells

(B) It stimulates lysosomal enzyme release, oxidative metabolism, and aggregation of neutrophils

(C) It promotes phagocytosis by interacting with cells possessing C5a receptors

(D) It promotes release of neutrophils from the bone marrow

(E) It stimulates activation of the alternative complement pathway

449. Persons who are diagnosed as having Di George's syndrome usually have

(A) hypocalcemic tetany
(B) hypothyroidism
(C) T-cell deficiency
(D) hypogammaglobulinemia
(E) congenital heart disease

450. Correct statements about isolated immunoglobulin A deficiency include which of the following?

(A) The incidence of atopic disease is high
(B) The risk of adverse reactions to transfusions is increased
(C) The incidence of autoimmune disease is increased
(D) Secretory IgA levels usually are normal
(E) The reduced number of IgA-bearing B cells accounts for the reduced serum IgA levels

451. True statements regarding immune-complex disease include which of the following?

(A) Normally, most immune complexes are removed by the reticuloendothelial system
(B) Signs and symptoms stem from the deposition of immune complexes in tissues other than those of the reticuloendothelial system
(C) Persistence of immune complexes in the circulation seems to be a requirement for the development of renal manifestations
(D) Renal lesions depend on antigen-antibody combinations in which antigen is in slight excess
(E) The rash of cutaneous necrotizing vasculitis may be an example of immune-complex disease

452. True statements regarding HLA class I molecules include

(A) they consist of four polypeptide chains
(B) they include a beta$_2$-microglobulin subunit
(C) they share less than 25 percent homology with one another
(D) they are distributed unevenly from one racial group to another
(E) they are expressed on all cells except mature red blood cells

453. Correct statements regarding the treatment of patients with ARC/AIDS include which of the following?

(A) Zidovudine (AZT) therapy has been proved to be beneficial in those patients with <500 CD4 (T4)-positive lymphocytes, even if they are asymptomatic
(B) AZT is ineffective in treating HIV-related neurologic symptoms
(C) Myelosuppression is the most common and important side effect of AZT
(D) AZT is an antiretroviral drug by virtue of its ability to selectively inhibit viral DNA polymerase
(E) Aerosolized pentamidine is an effective prophylactic treatment for recurrent pneumocystis pneumonia, but its use has been associated with some cases of *P. carinii* infection at other sites

454. A 27-year-old woman with systemic lupus erythematosus is in remission; current treatment is azathioprine, 75 mg/d, and prednisone, 5 mg/d. Last year she had a life-threatening exacerbation of her disease. She now strongly desires to become pregnant. Her physician should

(A) advise her that the risk of spontaneous abortion is high
(B) warn her that exacerbations can occur in the first trimester and in the postpartum period
(C) tell her it is unlikely a newborn will have lupus
(D) advise that fetal loss rates are higher if anticardiolipin antibodies are detected in her serum
(E) stop the prednisone just before she attempts to become pregnant

455. A 63-year-old woman with a history of rheumatoid arthritis since her forties is seen for the first time by a new physician. The patient has been doing poorly of late. Though her joint disease has not been a problem, she has lost weight and has been plagued by chronic foul-smelling diarrhea, easy bruising, profound fatigue, and peripheral edema. On examination she has waxy skin plaques clustered in the axillary folds, a large tongue, a quiet precordium, hepatosplenomegaly, guaiac-positive stool, and peripheral neuropathy. Laboratory evaluation includes the positive findings of proteinuria (5 g/d), normal serum chemistry except slightly low albumin and slightly elevated alkaline phosphatase, and low voltage on the ECG. In order to expeditiously diagnose the problem, one could

(A) perform a bone marrow aspirate and biopsy
(B) obtain three serial sputum samples for acid-fast bacillus (AFB) culture
(C) perform an abdominal CT examination
(D) obtain an abdominal subcutaneous fat pad aspirate
(E) perform a rectal biopsy

456. Drug-induced systemic lupus erythematosus (SLE) can be characterized by which of the following statements?

(A) Twenty percent of patients receiving procainamide develop drug-induced lupus

(B) Nephritis is a frequent consequence of hydralazine-induced lupus

(C) Most patients on hydralazine develop a positive antinuclear antibody (ANA) test; however, only 10 percent suffer from lupuslike symptoms

(D) If patients with drug-induced lupus fail to respond within several weeks of discontinuing the offending agent, a trial of corticosteroids is indicated

(E) If a patient with drug-induced lupus has persistent symptoms for longer than 6 months, an anti-ds antibody and CH_{50} levels should be drawn

457. Correct statements concerning the use of nonsteroidal anti-inflammatory drugs (NSAIDs) in the treatment of rheumatoid arthritis include which of the following?

(A) The mechanism of action of NSAIDs is the blockade of 5-lipoxygenase

(B) The newer NSAIDs are more efficacious than aspirin

(C) The newer NSAIDs induce platelet dysfunction

(D) NSAIDs can exacerbate allergic rhinitis and asthma

(E) The mechanism of NSAID-induced azotemia is unrelated to these drugs' ability to disrupt arachidonic acid metabolism

458. True statements about sarcoidosis include which of the following?

(A) Accumulation of suppressor-cytotoxic T lymphocytes occurs in sites of disease activity

(B) The ratio of black to white patients in the United States may exceed 10:1

(C) Chest radiography and pulmonary function testing are sensitive means of evaluating the intensity of pulmonary inflammation

(D) Transbronchial biopsy may reveal granulomata in a high percentage of patients and is a useful means of diagnosis

(E) Asymptomatic hilar adenopathy accounts for 10 to 20 percent of cases of sarcoidosis in the United States

459. Which of the following may be features of primary Sjögren's syndrome?

(A) Dental caries

(B) Corneal ulceration

(C) Renal tubular acidosis

(D) Pseudolymphoma

(E) Palpable purpura

460. Accurate statements about rheumatoid factors include which of the following?

(A) They are antibodies to the Fc fragment of immunoglobulin G

(B) They are associated with several conditions in which there is chronic antigenic stimulation

(C) Their presence in the serum of persons with rheumatoid arthritis correlates with a worse prognosis than that for persons with seronegative disease

(D) Their presence correlates with articular manifestations of rheumatoid arthritis

(E) They frequently do not appear in the serum of persons with rheumatoid arthritis until late in the course of the illness

461. The diagnosis of many rheumatic diseases, including rheumatoid arthritis, is based entirely on clinical grounds. Clinical characteristics associated with rheumatoid arthritis include

(A) prolonged morning stiffness

(B) migratory polyarthritis

(C) arthritis involving the distal interphalangeal joints

(D) arthritis of the cervical spine

(E) carpal tunnel syndrome

462. A 27-year-old man presents because of a painful, swollen knee and ankle of 2 weeks' duration. He has never had joint disease prior to this time. The patient also complains of low back pain and a recent history of clear penile discharge. On examination he has vesicles (some of which have crusted over) on the palms, soles, and glans penis; injected conjunctivae; a swollen right index finger; and arthritis of the right knee and left ankle. Correct statements regarding this patient include

(A) he will probably benefit from indomethacin

(B) his joint disease will probably improve after a course of tetracycline

(C) he is probably HLA-B27 positive

(D) x-ray of the pelvis would probably demonstrate blurring of the sacroiliac joint

(E) his erythrocyte sedimentation rate is likely to be elevated

463. A 40-year-old woman presents with purulent nasal discharge, cough, hemoptysis, and dyspnea. Chest x-ray reveals bilateral nodules; creatinine and erythrocyte sedimentation are elevated; urinalysis reveals hematuria and proteinuria. Accurate statements regarding this woman's condition include

(A) she probably has circulating anti-basement membrane antibodies
(B) she probably has circulating antineutrophil antibodies
(C) necrotizing granulomatous vasculitis would probably be found if a lung biopsy was carried out
(D) glucocorticoids and cyclophosphamide should be administered
(E) even with appropriate therapy, her prognosis is poor

464. Development of the x-ray findings shown below is linked on occasion to the presence of which of the following disorders?

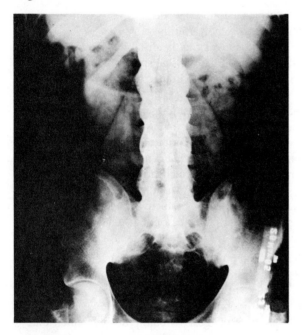

(A) Kidney stones
(B) Aortic insufficiency
(C) Peripheral neuropathy
(D) Uveitis
(E) Quadriplegia

465. A strong association exists between the HLA-B27 histocompatibility antigen and ankylosing spondylitis. This association may be characterized by which of the following statements?

(A) A positive HLA-B27 determination in a person with low back pain can verify a diagnosis of ankylosing spondylitis
(B) Half of all HLA-B27–positive persons have sacroiliitis or spondylitis
(C) Persons who are black or of Asian heritage have a higher prevalence of both ankylosing spondylitis and HLA-B27 antigen
(D) Up to 10 percent of cases of ankylosing spondylitis are not associated with HLA-B27 antigen
(E) The concordance rate in identical twins is nearly 100 percent

466. Reiter's syndrome follows certain venereal and dysenteric illnesses. Reiter's syndrome following *dysenteric* illness is associated with infection by

(A) enteropathogenic *Escherichia coli*
(B) *Salmonella*
(C) *Shigella*
(D) *Yersinia*
(E) *Campylobacter*

467. The arthritis associated with the deposition of calcium pyrophosphate dihydrate crystals is accurately described by which of the following statements?

(A) Calcium pyrophosphate dihydrate crystals are thought to form from supersaturated solutions of calcium phosphate in synovial fluid
(B) Calcium pyrophosphate dihydrate crystals appear under polarized light as elongated rods with strong negative birefringence
(C) Clinical manifestations usually are limited to the knee joints
(D) Most affected persons have radiographic evidence of chondrocalcinosis
(E) Clinical syndromes caused by deposition of calcium pyrophosphate dihydrate crystals can mimic degenerative joint disease

468. True statements describing septic arthritis include which of the following?

(A) Hematogenous spread from a primary infection elsewhere, and not direct extension from infected bone or soft tissue, is the usual mode of joint seeding

(B) A septic joint cavity can be irrigated with sterile saline to enhance the removal of inflammatory debris

(C) Intraarticular infusion of antibiotics is a useful adjunct to intravenous antibiotic therapy

(D) To minimize the chance of joint destruction, surgical drainage is usually preferred over needle aspiration

(E) Gonococci isolated from patients whose joint involvement is due to disseminated gonococcemia are more resistant to penicillin than those strains involved in uncomplicated genitourinary infection

469. Acute sarcoidosis is characterized by which of the following syndromes?

(A) Cough, hemoptysis, and interstitial pulmonary involvement

(B) Myopathy, keratotic skin lesions on the palms and soles, and arthralgias

(C) Fever, pulmonary stenotic murmur, and nailbed lesions

(D) Erythema nodosum, arthralgias, and hilar adenopathy

(E) Fever, parotid enlargement, uveitis, and facial nerve palsy

470. Familial Mediterranean fever (FMF) is correctly characterized by which of the following statements?

(A) Fifty percent of patients have no family history of the disease

(B) Chest pain is unusual

(C) Colchicine is likely to be beneficial

(D) Levels of dopamine beta-hydroxylase are increased

(E) Amyloidosis is a common complication throughout the world

471. A 52-year-old woman presents with nasal discharge and stuffiness, difficulty in breathing through the nose, and sinus pain. ENT examination reveals ulcers on the nasal septum and perforation of the soft palate. There is no history of prior illness or drug abuse. Biopsy of involved material under anesthesia reveals noncaseating granulomatous inflammation with necrotic debris. No malignant cells, vasculitis, or microorganisms are noted. Correct statements concerning this patient's condition include which of the following?

(A) The history and findings are consistent with Wegener's granulomatosis

(B) If she is not appropriately treated, the disease will probably be fatal

(C) The treatment of choice is radiation therapy

(D) The disease, if unchecked, can progress to involve the mediastinum and lungs

(E) Optimal treatment should involve surgical debridement

DIRECTIONS: Each group of questions below consists of five lettered headings followed by a set of numbered items. For each numbered item select the **one** lettered heading with which it is **most** closely associated. Each lettered heading may be used **once, more than once, or not at all**.

Questions 472–476

For each clinical situation presented, select the complement profile with which it is most likely to be associated.

(A) Deficiency of C2; other components normal
(B) Deficiency of C3; other components normal
(C) Deficiency of C8; other components normal
(D) Absence of C1 inhibitor; low C4 and C2; other components normal
(E) Reduced C3 and factor B; low CH_{50}; normal C4

472. A 29-year-old man has had episodic abdominal pain and angioedema of the lips, tongue, and larynx

473. A 20-year-old woman has had severe, recurrent bacterial infections, including streptococcal pharyngitis, pneumococcal pneumonia, and bacterial sinusitis

474. A 23-year-old woman develops proteinuria, hematuria, hypertension, and nephrotic syndrome

475. A 21-year-old man, with no current medical problems, donates blood to an immunology laboratory for complement testing

476. A 23-year-old woman presents with fever, arthralgias, and a rash; her serum lacks bactericidal activity against *Neisseria gonorrhoeae*

Questions 477–480

For each clinical setting described below, select the associated autoantibody.

(A) Antihistone
(B) Anticentromere
(C) Anti-Ro (SSA)
(D) Anticardiolipin
(E) None of the above

477. A young woman with a history of nephritis gives birth to a child with congenital heart block

478. A 37-year-old woman with a history of recurrent arterial thrombosis is found to have a prolonged partial thromboplastin time and a false-positive result on the Venereal Disease Research Laboratory (VDRL) test

479. A 60-year-old man has a rash, arthritis, and pleuritis occurring after antihypertensive therapy with hydralazine

480. A young woman has the CREST syndrome (*c*alcinosis, *R*aynaud's phenomenon, *e*sophageal hypomotility, *s*clerodactyly, and *t*elangiectasias)

Questions 481–484

For each diagnosis that follows, select the synovial-fluid findings with which it is most likely to be associated.

(A) Fluid, clear and viscous; white blood cell count, 400/mm^3; no crystals
(B) Fluid, cloudy and watery; white blood cell count, 8000/mm^3; no crystals
(C) Fluid, dark brown and viscous; white blood cell count, 1200/mm^3; no crystals
(D) Fluid, cloudy and watery; white blood cell count, 12,000/mm^3; crystals, needlelike and strongly negatively birefringent
(E) Fluid, cloudy and watery; white blood cell count, 4800/mm^3; crystals, rhomboidal and weakly positively birefringent

481. Pigmented villonodular synovitis

482. Calcium pyrophosphate deposition disease

483. Gout

484. Degenerative joint disease

Immunologic, Allergic, and Rheumatic Disorders

Answers

414. The answer is D. *(Wilson, ed 12. chap 13.)* Lymphoid cells, including both T and B lymphocytes, arise from hematopoietic stem cells. Those cells destined to enter the B-cell lineage arise continuously in the bone marrow. The earliest cells destined to become B cells express surface CD10 (CALLA, J-5) protein, an endopeptidase thought to inactivate certain peptide hormones. These pre-B cells are large lymphoid cells containing cytoplasmic μ chains, the heavy chain of immunoglobulin M (IgM), as detected by immunofluorescence. Cytoplasmic light chains are not present, and pre-B cells lack membrane-bound IgM or immunoglobulin of any other class. In the process of B-cell maturation, smaller lymphoid cells will appear that bear a narrow rim of cytoplasmic IgM; later, cells with membrane-bound IgM develop.

415. The answer is D. *(Wilson, ed 12. chap 265.)* Plasma cell diseases are a group of conditions in which a clone of cells capable of synthesizing and secreting immunoglobulins, or the heavy or light chain component of these molecules, proliferates abnormally. IgG immunoglobulins are the most common class produced in such diseases. Also, free light chains usually are produced in excess and are detected in urine as Bence Jones protein. Multiple myeloma is the most common plasma cell neoplasm. Its classic presentation includes bone pain, anemia, hypercalcemia, renal failure, and recurrent infections in an elderly person. Diagnosis is best made by looking for a homogeneous globulin peak on electrophoresis of serum, urine, or both. Waldenström's macroglobulinemia is a related condition in which the monoclonal immunoglobulin is of the IgM class. Because IgM is so large (it circulates as a pentamer), it is restricted to the bloodstream and in high concentrations tends to cause hyperviscosity of the blood. Other features differentiating Waldenström's macroglobulinemia from multiple myeloma are enlargement of lymph nodes and spleen and occasional transformation to chronic lymphocytic leukemia or lymphocytic lymphoma.

416. The answer is D. *(Wilson, ed 12. chap 267.)* Urticaria and angioedema are common disorders, affecting approximately 20 percent of the population. In acute urticarial angioedema, attacks of swelling are of less than 6 weeks' duration; chronic urticarial angioedema is by definition more long-standing. Urticaria usually is pruritic and affects the trunk and proximal extremities. Angioedema is generally less pruritic and affects the hands, feet, genitalia, and face. The woman described in the question has chronic urticaria, which probably is due to a cutaneous necrotizing vasculitis. The clues to the diagnosis are the arthralgias, presence of residual skin discoloration, and elevated sedimentation rate—these would be uncharacteristic of other urticarial diseases. Diagnosis can be confirmed by skin biopsy. Chronic urticaria is rarely of allergic cause; hence, allergy skin tests and measurement of total immunoglobulin E levels are not helpful. Measurement of C1 esterase inhibitor activity is useful in diagnosing hereditary angioedema, a disease not associated with urticaria. Patch tests are used to diagnose contact dermatitis.

417. The answer is D. *(Wilson, ed 12. chap 267. Jacobs, J Allergy Clin Immunol 67:253–262, 1981.)* There are three common types of rhinitis: allergic, vasomotor, and eosinophilic nonallergic (intrinsic). Allergic rhinitis can be either seasonal as a result of pollen exposure or perennial as a result of exposure to dust or mold spores (or both). In these IgE-mediated reactions to inhaled foreign substances, nasal eosinophilia is common. Vasomotor rhinitis is a chronic, nonallergic condition in which vasomotor control in the nasal membranes is altered. Irritating stimuli, such as odors, fumes, and changes in humidity and barometric pressure, can cause nasal obstruction and discharge in affected persons, and nasal eosinophilia is not noted. Eosinophilic nonallergic rhinitis causes perennial nasal congestion and discharge. Although it is nonallergic in etiology, it is associated with the presence of numerous eosinophils in nasal secretions. Because the man described in the question has either perennial allergic rhinitis due to dust or mold-spore allergy or eosinophilic nonallergic rhinitis, skin testing for responses to suspected allergens should be diagnostic. The competitive radioimmunosorbent test measures total serum IgE but would not be diagnostic (only 40 percent of patients with allergic rhinitis have elevated serum IgE levels). Pollen skin tests are unlikely to be helpful because of the perennial nature of the condition described. An elimination diet can be used diagnostically or therapeutically in persons with suspected food allergy; however, food allergy rarely causes rhinitis. Sinus x-rays, whether positive or negative, would not reveal the underlying cause of the rhinitis.

418. The answer is D. *(Wilson, ed 12. chap 276.)* Polyarteritis nodosa is a vasculitis of medium-sized vessels. Early systemic features include fever, weakness, anorexia, weight loss, myalgias, and arthralgias (though severe and persistent arthritis is uncommon). Pericarditis and pleuritis also can occur. Mononeuritis multiplex develops because of involvement of the vasa nervorum; it is reflected in the man described by the sudden loss of the ability to dorsiflex his right great toe. Abdominal pain occurs in 60 to 70 percent of affected persons and is related to disease involvement of mesenteric arteries. Hypertension develops from arterial occlusion and occurs before renal involvement. Laboratory findings of elevated erythrocyte sedimentation rate, anemia of chronic disease, and polymorphonuclear leukocytosis all occur with polyarteritis nodosa. Pulmonary involvement is unusual and serves to distinguish this entity clinically from allergic granulomatosis and Wegener's granulomatosis. Hypersensitivity vasculitis is a term applied to small-vessel vasculitides associated with a range of findings—from purely cutaneous disease to minimal skin disease but life-threatening involvement of major organs. Giant cell arteritis involves the aorta and other great vessels, producing constitutional symptoms and large-vessel occlusion in young women (Takayasu's disease) and in the elderly (temporal arteritis, polymyalgia rheumatica).

419. The answer is C. *(Wilson, ed 12. chap 269. Balow, Ann Intern Med 106:79, 1987.)* Renal disease is clinically evident in about half those persons with systemic lupus erythematosus (SLE). However, nearly all persons with SLE have some evidence of renal disease on renal biopsy. Renal disease associated with SLE includes both glomerulonephritis and interstitial nephritis. Glomerular disease has been classified into membranous nephritis and mesangial, focal, and diffuse glomerulonephritis. Immune-complex interstitial nephritis occurs most commonly in persons who have diffuse glomerulonephritis. Urinalysis performed for persons with active renal disease usually reveals microscopic hematuria, red cell casts, and proteinuria; the exception is membranous lupus nephritis, in which proteinuria is the dominant finding. Drug-induced lupus rarely leads to renal disease. Anti-dsDNA antibodies at high titer put the patient at risk for severe nephritis. Renal biopsy is not necessary in SLE patients whose renal function is rapidly deteriorating when they have an active sediment. If such patients fail to respond to the prompt initiation of glucocorticoid therapy demanded in such a situation, then biopsy should be undertaken. Patients with mild clinical disease should have a biopsy to determine if they have active, severe, inflammatory lesions, which might respond to therapy.

420. The answer is B. *(Wilson, ed 12. chap 264.)* AIDS is characterized by the infection of T4$^+$ lymphocytes by the AIDS retrovirus (HTLV-III/LAV), with subsequent deficiency in numbers and functions of this T-cell subpopulation, which includes the important helper-inducer cells necessary for production of a variety of immune responses. Thus, there is a defect in the response of T cells to soluble antigen and to mitogenic substances such as phytohemagglutinin and concanavalin A. Natural killer cell function is abnormal and may be augmented in vitro by addition of the lymphokine interleukin 2. There is polyclonal activation of B lymphocytes, with a resultant increase in serum immunoglobulin levels and occasional production of autoantibodies.

421. The answer is A. *(Wilson, ed 12. chap 14.)* The major histocompatibility gene complex (MHC), located on the short arm of chromosome 6, contains genes involved in the recognition of self, antigen presentation to T and B cells, and the rejection of tissue allografts. Ubiquitously expressed class I molecules are the products of the HLA-A, -B, and -C genes. Also in the MHC, the HLA-D region, separated from the ABC genes by an area responsible for certain complement components (C2, C4B, Bf, C4A) and tumor necrosis factor, codes for class II molecules, which are only expressed on T cells, B cells, and monocytes (and their derivatives, such as Langerhans' skin cells). Class II molecules are responsible for the mixed lymphocyte reaction (MLR), which is important in determining compatibility of donor and host tissues in a potential transplant situation. Because the ABC and D regions are closely linked, recombination between these two areas is uncommon (approximately 2 percent). Thus, an ABC-matched sibling is usually, but not always, matched at the D locus as well. In addition to a recombination event, another reason for a positive MLR in an HLA-ABC matched sibling pair is histoincompatibility at minor loci, which are located throughout the genome.

422. The answer is B. *(Wilson, ed 12. chap 263. Rosen, N Engl J Med 311:235, 1989.)* Ataxia-telangiectasia is an autosomal recessive primary immunodeficiency disorder associated with abnormal thymic development, progressive cerebellar ataxia, and oculocutaneous telangiectasia. The responsible gene, located on chromosome

11, leads to a generalized defect in the ability to repair damage to DNA. Such a defect accounts for the frequent occurrence of malignancies, particularly lymphomas, and the exquisite sensitivity to therapeutic irradiation. There is evidence for both humoral and cellular immunodeficiency; most patients have depressed IgA and IgE levels as well as cutaneous anergy. Sinopulmonary infections are common with severe resultant respiratory insufficiency, often associated with bronchiectasis. Adenosine deaminase deficiency is associated not with ataxia-telangiectasia, but with severe combined immunodeficiency.

423. The answer is C. *(Wilson, ed 12. chap 264. Curran, Science 239:610, 1988.)* Among the U.S. cases of AIDS in adults, 60 percent are in homosexual men who do not use intravenous drugs; however, attack rates have precipitously declined in the homosexual community, probably owing to behavior modification. On the other hand, infections continue to rise among intravenous drug users. Because of blood donor screening and heat treatment of factor VIII concentrates, the rate of seroconversion in hemophiliacs is dropping. Blood donor screening reduces the risk of exposure to HIV in a single unit of blood to between 1/40,000 and 1/250,000. Pediatric AIDS arises mainly in infants born to mothers who are intravenous drug users or sexual partners of intravenous drug users. The remainder of pediatric AIDS patients are hemophiliacs or recipients of blood transfusions. The overall prevalence of HIV infection is quite low: about 0.04 percent of blood donors, who are a low-risk group because of the voluntary exclusion of high-risk individuals, to 0.15 percent of U.S. military recruits, a group relatively high in risk because of sexual activity and socioeconomic status. There is a small but real risk of seroconversion in those who are exposed to HIV-contaminated materials at the work place; less than 0.5 percent of those who have sustained penetrating injuries or whose mucosae have been splashed with blood from AIDS patients have become infected.

424. The answer is C. *(Wilson, ed 12. chap 264.)* The clinical situation suggests the diagnosis of the acquired immunodeficiency syndrome (AIDS). *M. pneumoniae,* while a frequent cause of mild community-acquired pneumonia in the otherwise normal host, is not commonly associated with AIDS. *P. carinii,* a protozoal pathogen, is the most frequent cause of respiratory disease in the AIDS patient; it affects approximately 60 percent of such patients some time during the course of their illness. Both cytomegalovirus and *C. neoformans* are less common but significant respiratory pathogens in this patient population. Tuberculosis must always be considered in an AIDS patient with pulmonary symptoms. Tuberculous dissemination occurs frequently.

425. The answer is A. *(Wilson, ed 12. chap 267.)* Anaphylaxis is a systemic reaction to the sudden release of mediators from sensitized mast cells triggered by interaction with specific antigen. Manifestations of anaphylaxis include: (1) cutaneous—pruritus, urticaria, and angioedema; (2) vascular collapse; (3) respiratory distress; and (4) gastrointestinal—nausea, vomiting, pain, and diarrhea. Therapeutic efforts in anaphylaxis should be directed toward preventing further mediator release and reversing the effects of mediators already released. Corticosteroids do not have any acute effect in anaphylaxis, though they may be necessary to control persistent bronchospasm or hypotension, or both. Onset of action of steroids requires several hours. Aminophylline may help ameliorate bronchospasm, while antihistamines (usually injectable diphenhydramine) will work to block histamine effects on the skin, vasculature, and airways. Epinephrine should be administered subcutaneously or intravenously, or both, in appropriate concentrations to control minor problems such as pruritus and urticaria as well as to reverse vascular instability. Oxygen should be given to combat the hypoxemia associated with bronchospasm and may be combined with inhaled bronchodilators such as isoproterenol.

426. The answer is A. *(Wilson, ed 12. chap 268. Lawly, N Engl J Med 311:1407, 1984.)* The administration of horse antithymocyte globulin (ATG) to patients with aplastic anemia or as an immunosuppressant after bone marrow transplant can lead to a clinical syndrome identical to that of classic serum sickness and one that approximates animal models of immune complex disease. Eight to thirteen days after beginning therapy with ATG, the clinical features begin with fever, malaise, rash (often urticarial), arthralgias, nausea, melena, lymphadenopathy, and proteinuria. There are high levels of circulating immune complexes; more precise quantitation rests on one of a number of generally inconclusive assays, including the Raji cell assay (lymphoblastoid line that binds to C3) and C1q binding assay (first complement subcomponent). With all these immune complexes and their Fc receptors, the complement system is overactivated, so there are accompanying decreases in C3, C4 and CH_{50}.

427. The answer is C. *(Wilson, ed 12. chap 270.)* Persons who have rheumatoid arthritis can develop popliteal cysts as a complication of synovitis of the knee. Popliteal cysts can expand upward into the thigh or downward into the calf. Rupture of a popliteal cyst produces sudden pain and swelling; because these symptoms resemble those of thrombophlebitis—though perhaps more dramatic in onset—an arthrogram may be needed to confirm the diagnosis. Although rupture of the plantaris tendon can occur in persons exposed to mechanical trauma, it would not be the most likely diagnosis for the woman described in the question. The anserine bursa is located on the medial aspect of the knee joint and not in the calf. Achilles tendonitis should not cause pain and swelling of the calf.

428. The answer is B. *(Wilson, ed 12. chap 270. Pinals, Semin Arthritis Rheum 17:246, 1988.)* The so-called disease-modifying drugs used in the treatment of rheumatoid arthritis include gold compounds, D-penicillamine, sulfasalazine, and antimalarials. They are minimally anti-inflammatory and take weeks or months to induce a remission; therefore, nonsteroidals must be continued during their administration. Toxicities of these drugs, which are substantial, mandate careful consideration prior to their use and careful followup during maintenance. The indications to employ one of these disease-modifying agents are unclear, but one should consider these agents when symptoms cannot be controlled after several months' trial of nonsteroidals. Glucocorticoids have not been shown to modify the course of rheumatoid arthritis and have substantial long-term side effects, although they clearly can provide short-term control.

429. The answer is A. *(Wilson, ed 12. chap 270.)* Systemic manifestations in early rheumatoid arthritis may be severe, but are frequently nonspecific. Such nonspecific constitutional symptoms require a period of observation before synovitis supervenes and the diagnosis becomes clear. Weight loss and muscle wasting may be as severe as in persons who have a malignancy or primary muscle disease. In about 10 percent of patients, the disease begins in a more fulminant fashion with the rapid onset of polyarthritis associated with fever, lymphadenopathy, and splenomegaly.

430. The answer is E. *(Wilson, ed 12. chap 270.)* Many of the systemic manifestations of late rheumatoid arthritis are related to the presence of rheumatoid factors in high titer in the serum. Joint disease, paradoxically, may not be active during this stage of the illness. Nail-fold thrombi, leg ulcers, and sensorimotor polyneuropathy are all manifestations of rheumatoid vasculitis and presumably are related to the effect of immune complexes containing rheumatoid factors. High levels of immune complexes are detected by immune-complex assays done at this stage of disease. Felty's syndrome, characterized by neutropenia and splenomegaly, occurs late in the course of rheumatoid arthritis and is related to the presence of high titers of rheumatoid factors. Many affected persons also have rheumatoid vasculitis. Fifteen to twenty percent of patients with rheumatoid arthritis develop Sjögren's syndrome with associated dry eyes. Hepatitis is not a common feature of late extraarticular seropositive rheumatoid arthritis.

431. The answer is A. *(Wilson, ed 12. chap 274.)* The diagnosis of ankylosing spondylitis is made on clinical grounds. Historical features suggesting inflammatory back disease include pain and prolonged stiffness that are worse at night and during rest periods and characteristically relieved with activity. In contrast, mechanical low back pain usually is eased with bed rest and made worse with activity, such as sitting, standing, walking, and lifting. Signs of nerve-root compression are not part of the clinical spectrum of ankylosing spondylitis. Ankylosing spondylitis usually presents before the age of 40 years; on the other hand, degenerative joint disease and degenerative disk disease are common causes of back pain in the elderly. Back pain made worse with walking and improved with rest and lumbar flexion is characteristic of the pseudoclaudication syndrome associated with lumbar spinal stenosis.

432. The answer is B. *(Wilson, ed 12. chap 283.)* Five different clinical syndromes of psoriatic arthritis have been described. The most common (70 percent of cases) is an asymmetrical, oligoarticular arthritis. A second group produces arthritis mainly in distal interphalangeal joints and is associated with severe psoriatic nail changes. Psoriatic spondylitis is similar to the spondylitis of Reiter's syndrome. Rheumatoid factor–negative symmetrical polyarthritis also is associated with psoriasis, and this condition can look very much like rheumatoid arthritis. About 5 percent of patients with psoriatic arthritis have a destructive variety called "arthritis mutilans." Persons who have psoriasis and rheumatoid factor–positive symmetrical polyarthritis are thought to have both psoriasis and rheumatoid arthritis.

433. The answer is C. *(Wilson, ed 12. chap 241.)* Peripheral arthritis and spondyloarthropathy can be associated with inflammatory bowel disease. The characteristic peripheral arthritis, which is more commonly associated with colonic disease than with small-bowel involvement alone, involves a few joints in the lower extremities, usually in an asymmetrical fashion, and resolves in a few months without residual joint damage. The presence and activity of peripheral arthritis are related to the extent and activity of colonic involvement. In contrast, the presence and activity of spondylitis are not related to the activity of bowel disease. This form of spondyloarthropathy behaves very much like ankylosing spondylitis and may even precede the emergence of bowel disease by many years.

434. The answer is C. *(Wilson, ed 12. chap 275.)* Behçet's syndrome, a recurrent disease of unknown cause, is characterized by painful oral and genital ulcers, eye inflammation, arthritis, central nervous system symptoms, thrombophlebitis, fever, and abdominal symptoms. The combination of fever, aphthous ulcers, arthritis, and abdominal pain may mimic inflammatory bowel disease, although central nervous system involvement (e.g., severe headache) and thrombophlebitis would make this diagnosis less likely. Whipple's disease is associated with arthritis, abdominal pain, and central nervous system disease, but not with aphthous ulcers and thrombophlebitis; also, Whipple's disease usually affects middle-aged men. Fever, arthritis, abdominal pain, and headache would be compatible with a diagnosis of systemic lupus erythematosus. However, the mucosal lesions of lupus are painless and occur on the hard and soft palate, and thrombophlebitis is not a characteristic feature.

435. The answer is D. *(Wilson, ed 12. chap 96.)* Gonococcal arthritis is the most common cause of bacterial arthritis in young adults. Persons with disseminated gonococcal infection usually present with fever, vesiculopustular skin lesions, tenosynovitis, and polyarthralgias. The polyarthritis may evolve in a few days to a monoarticular septic arthritis, heralding the change from the bacteremic to the septic joint phase of the disease. The clinical picture, however, may be quite variable—on occasion, affected persons present only with monoarticular purulent arthritis and no systemic features. Cultures of synovial fluid are positive in less than half the cases of gonococcal joint infection. Disseminated gonococcal infection occurs more commonly in women who are menstruating or pregnant or in those with terminal complement deficiency.

436. The answer is D. *(Wilson, ed 12. chap 96.)* Tuberculous arthritis is produced by direct hematogenous spread or extension from disease in adjacent bone. The process tends to be chronic and without significant constitutional symptoms, although low-grade fever and night sweats may be present. The synovial fluid white blood cell count is usually greater than 10,000/mm^3 with polymorphonuclear leukocytes predominating. Many persons who have skeletal tuberculosis do not have radiographic evidence of pulmonary disease.

437. The answer is E. *(Wilson, ed 12. chap 272.)* Mixed connective tissue disease (MCTD) is a syndrome characterized by high titers of circulating antibodies to the ribonucleoprotein component of extractable nuclear antigen in association with clinical features similar to those of SLE, systemic sclerosis, polymyositis, and rheumatoid arthritis. The average patient with MCTD is a middle-aged woman with Raynaud's phenomenon who also has polyarthritis, sclerodactyly (including swollen hands), esophageal dysfunction, pulmonary fibrosis, and inflammatory myopathy. Cutaneous manifestations include telangiectasias on the face and hands, alopecia, a lupuslike heliotropic rash, and erythematous patches over the knuckles. Myopathy may involve severe weakness of proximal muscles associated with high levels of creatine phosphokinase and aldolase. Both pulmonary involvement and esophageal dysmotility are common, but frequently asymptomatic until quite advanced. Almost all patients have high titers of rheumatoid factor and antinuclear antibodies. Such antibodies are directed toward the ribonuclease-sensitive ribonucleoprotein component of the extractable nuclear antigen.

438. The answer is D. *(Wilson, ed 12. chap 281.)* Osteoarthritis, the most common joint disease, is diagnosed on the basis of clinical and laboratory features. One of the earliest x-ray findings is joint space narrowing as periarticular cartilage is lost. A joint involved with osteoarthritis may be tender or slightly swollen; significant effusions are rare. The sensation of bone rubbing against bone (bony crepitus) may be elicited upon movement of an affected joint. Bony prominences on both the distal interphalangeal joints (Heberden's nodes) and the proximal interphalangeal joints (Bouchard's nodes) are commonly seen. Osteoarthritis in the patellofemoral joint may manifest as a positive "shrug" sign, i.e., pain when the patella is manually compressed against the femur when the quadriceps contract. In contrast, rheumatoid arthritis (RA) commonly involves the proximal interphalangeal joint. Moreover, destruction of ligaments and tendons seen in RA may result in characteristic hand changes such as hyperextension of the proximal interphalangeal joints with compensatory flexion of the distal interphalangeal joints (swan-neck deformity) or flexion deformity of the proximal interphalangeals and extension of the distal interphalangeals (boutonnière deformity).

439. The answer is A. *(Wilson, ed 12. chaps 271, 272. Kelly, chap 76, pp 1211–1230.)* Systemic sclerosis can be classified into two variants depending on whether scleroderma is present only in the fingers (sclerodactyly) or whether it is also present proximal to the metacarpophalangeal joints. The former disorder is associated with a constellation of findings labeled the *CREST syndrome: c*alcinosis, *R*aynaud's phenomenon, *e*sophageal dysmotility, *s*clerodactyly, and *t*elangiectasia. Although once thought not to be associated with significant internal organ involvement, the CREST variant of systemic sclerosis has occurred in association with involvement of the lungs, heart, and kidneys, in this respect resembling systemic sclerosis associated with proximal scleroderma. The fluorescent antinuclear antibody (ANA) test is positive in 40 to 80 percent of persons with systemic sclerosis. Antibodies are produced to deoxyribonucleoprotein, nucleolar, centromere, and topoisomerase 1 antigens.

Mixed connective-tissue disease is the overlap of three rheumatic disease syndromes: systemic lupus erythematosus (SLE), polymyositis, and the CREST variant of systemic sclerosis. It is associated with high titers of antinuclear antibodies directed against the extractable nuclear antigen ribonucleoprotein. Arthritis and a positive ANA are not sufficient to make a diagnosis of SLE. Overlap syndromes are diseases that fulfill diagnostic criteria for two rheumatic diseases. In the case described, symptoms and signs were insufficient to fulfill the diagnostic criteria for more than one rheumatic syndrome.

440. The answer is E. *(Wilson, ed 12. chap 284.)* Pigmented villonodular synovitis, the cause of which is unknown, is a disorder of young adults that usually affects one joint only, frequently a knee. There is recurrent bleeding into the affected joint; the synovial fluid of that joint often contains blood and typically is dark brown in color, an indication of past bleeding from the synovium. The enlarged villi covering the synovium are made up of large numbers of round and polyhedral cells. Hemosiderin granules and cholesterol crystals can be identified in synovial cell cytoplasm as well as in interstitial spaces. Bone adjacent to the affected synovium can show evidence of erosion; however, invasion of other tissues does not occur. The synovial fluid findings in the case presented are incompatible with the diagnoses of atypical rheumatoid arthritis, incomplete Reiter's syndrome, and osteochondritis dissecans. Hemangioma usually presents in childhood.

441. The answer is C. *(Wilson, ed 12. chap 284. Michet, Ann Intern Med 104:74, 1986.)* Relapsing polychrondritis is an inflammatory disorder that affects cartilage in the ear, nose, larynx, and tracheobronchial tree. This intermittent, yet sometimes progressive disorder can also be associated with ocular manifestations, aortic regurgitation, and premonitory asymmetric oligoarthritis affecting some large and small peripheral joints. Diagnosis of relapsing polychrondritis can be made in the presence of the aforementioned clinical features; biopsy of affected tissues displaying cartilage destruction would be confirmatory, but is usually unnecessary. Patients with Wegener's granulomatosis may have nasal, but not auricular involvement. Cogan's syndrome may include ocular and auditory problems, but does not involve the external ear. There was no urethritis or skin lesions in this case to suggest Reiter's syndrome. The arthritis in rheumatoid disease tends to be symmetric and erosive. Squamous cell carcinoma would be unlikely to involve both ears and the larynx simultaneously.

442. The answer is A-Y, B-N, C-Y, D-Y, E-Y. *(Wilson, ed 12. chap 13.)* The lymphoid system can be divided into two functionally distinct compartments: the thymus-dependent T-cell compartment, and the "bursal-equivalent" B-cell compartment. B cells are the precursors of plasma cells; their role is to produce immunoglobulins. B lymphocytes in humans and most other mammalian species are characterized by the presence of readily detectable surface immunoglobulins. Most B cells have a receptor specific for the Fc portion of immunoglobulin, and some B cells have receptors for complement proteins, including the activated fragments C3b and C3d. Pre-B cells arise in the bone marrow continuously throughout life. Such pre-B cells, which mature in an antigen-independent fashion, are characterized by the presence of cytoplasmic IgM. Upon further development immature B cells, which express IgM on their cell surface, occur. Mature B cells migrate out of the bone marrow and express surface IgD as well as either IgM, IgG, IgA, or IgE. Mature B cells comprise about 15 percent of peripheral blood lymphocytes, 50 percent of splenic lymphocytes, and 10 percent of bone marrow lymphocytes. Lymphokines, which are nonantibody mediators of cellular immunity, usually are produced by T cells, and their synthesis does not require interaction with B cells.

443. The answer is A-N, B-Y, C-Y, D-Y, E-Y. *(Wilson, ed 12. chaps 96, 151.)* The patient has desert fever, a syndrome caused by coccidioidomycosis infection, which is endemic in the southwest United States. This syndrome is largely an acute hypersensitivity reaction to the primary pulmonary infection, which is symptomatic in only 40 percent of affected persons. Manifestations of hypersensitivity may include erythema nodosum, erythema multiforme, arthralgia, arthritis, conjunctivitis, and episcleritis. However, disseminated coccidioidomycosis may occur during the primary infection and could result in osteomyelitis (which may seed an adjacent synovium directly), fungal arthritis, skin lesions, or CNS disease. Even in the case of hematogenously derived joint infection, synovial fluid cultures will rarely be positive; synovial biopsy for culture and histology may be required. Serologic tests, while possibly acutely negative in a patient with primary pulmonary infection only, can be quite helpful, particularly when there is disseminated involvement.

444. The answer is A-N, B-N, C-Y, D-Y, E-Y. *(Wilson, ed 12. chap 13. Royer, N Engl J Med 274:1171, 1987.)* T-cell precursors leave the yolk sac, fetal liver, or bone marrow and migrate to the thymus, where they undergo further maturation. Even before T-cell receptor gene rearrangements occur, pre-T cells express the CD7 antigen, the earliest marker of T-cell lineage. After the CD2 adhesion molecule, which functions as the receptor for sheep red blood cells, is expressed on the cell surface, assembly of the T-cell receptor complex begins. This complex consists of the five proteins that make up the CD3 signal transduction moiety plus the two antigen-recognizing heterodimer molecules that form the actual T-cell antigen receptor. The four proteins that can function as part of the T-cell antigen receptor all have a variable (produced by V-J recombination) and constant region and bear homology to the immunoglobulin heavy and light chains. Along with the histocompatibility proteins and the CD2, CD4, and CD8 molecules, the T-cell antigen receptor chains are members of the immunoglobulin gene superfamily, which provides the immunological diversity required to distinguish self from nonself and recognize an inordinate number of foreign antigens. After CD3 T-cell receptor expression, but before suppressor or helper phenotype is determined, there is a thymic stage wherein both CD4 and CD8 antigens are expressed. Some lymphoblastic lymphomas arise from this stage of T-cell development.

445. The answer is A-N, B-N, C-Y, D-N, E-N. *(Wilson, ed 12. chap 13.)* T lymphocytes are the principal mediators of cellular immunity and also serve important helper and suppressor functions in the regulation of antibody synthesis by B lymphocytes. In humans, they have the property of forming rosettes with sheep erythrocytes (E-rosettes), and they lack readily detectable immunoglobulin of any class on their membranes. Although the maturation of T cells is thymus-dependent, the cells arise from precursors in bone marrow. T cells constitute about 70 to 80 percent of blood lymphocytes; they comprise greater than three-quarters of thymus lymphocytes but less than one-quarter of bone marrow lymphocytes. In lymph nodes, they are found in paracortical areas. Specific monoclonal antibodies have been developed to characterize various subsets of T cells—cells that carry a CD4$^+$ surface antigen are helper cells, and those with a CD8$^+$ antigen function as cytotoxic-suppressor cells. Antibody-dependent cell-mediated cytotoxicity is a property of a class of non-B, non-T lymphocytes called large granular lymphocytes (LGL cells). Antibody-dependent cell-mediated cytotoxicity can also be mediated by monocyte-macrophages and neutrophils.

446. The answer is A-N, B-N, C-Y, D-N, E-N. *(Wilson, ed 12. chap 13.)* Immunoglobulin A is the predominant immunoglobulin in body secretions (IgG is predominant in serum). Each secretory IgA molecule is a dimer consisting of a secretory component and a J chain. The secretory component, a protein of molecular weight 70,000, is synthesized by epithelial cells and facilitates IgA transport across mucosal tissues. The J chain is a small glycopeptide that aids the polymerization of immunoglobulins. IgA exists as two subclasses: IgA1 (75 percent of the total) and IgA2 (25 percent). IgA provides defense against local infections in the respiratory, gastrointestinal, and genitourinary tracts and prevents access of foreign substances to the general systemic immune system. It also can prevent attachment of microorganisms to epithelial cells. IgM, not IgA, is the principal immunoglobulin in the primary immune response and is the usual antibody in cold agglutinins. The half-life of IgA is about 6 days; IgE has the shortest half-life, approximately 2 to 2.5 days.

447. The answer is A-Y, B-N, C-Y, D-Y, E-N. *(Wilson, ed 12. chap 13.)* Cellular immunity, also known as delayed hypersensitivity, is a nonhumoral form of immunity effected by sensitized T lymphocytes through the production of biologic mediators known as lymphokines. These factors recruit and activate phagocytes and nonsensitized lymphocytes. Cellular immunity protects the host against tumor cells and intracellular microorganisms, such as *Mycobacterium tuberculosis,* fungi, and certain viruses and protozoa. Competency of the cellular immune system is best tested by delayed hypersensitivity skin tests to a battery of recall antigens, such as tuberculin, *Candida albicans,* and mumps. Contact eczema, nickel allergy, and poison ivy dermatitis are pathologic expressions of cellular immunity. Other examples of diseases in which delayed hypersensitivity plays a major role include reactions to toxins, such as beryllium, and to organic dusts, as in the case of hypersensitivity pneumonitis. Interleukins 1, 2, and 4 are important in inducing activation and proliferation of T cells and other cells involved in cell-mediated immunity. Interleukin 3 is a hematopoietin that differentiates erythroid, myeloid and multipotent progenitor cells. Antigens with repeating polymeric structures are thymus-independent, which means they stimulate B cells directly without requiring the presence of T helper cells. B cells are not required for the expression of cellular immunity.

448. The answer is A-Y, B-Y, C-N, D-N, E-N. *(Wilson, ed 12. chap 13.)* Complement component C5a (molecular weight 11,200) is a cleavage product of C5. It possesses potent biologic activity, including the ability to stimulate non-IgE-dependent mediator release from mast cells, to increase vascular permeability, and to induce smooth muscle contraction (agents with these properties are known as anaphylatoxins). C5a is also a potent chemotactic agent for neutrophils, monocytes, and eosinophils, and it stimulates lysosomal enzyme release, oxidative metabolism, and aggregation of phagocytic cells. C3a (molecular weight 9000) is a cleavage product of C3 and, like C5a, is an anaphylatoxin. C3b, not C5a, is the complement fragment with opsonic activity; it also plays a positive feedback role in the activation of the alternative complement pathway. C3e, a degradation product of C3b, is responsible for promoting the release of neutrophils from bone marrow.

449. The answer is A-Y, B-N, C-Y, D-N, E-Y. *(Wilson, ed 12. chap 263. Rosen, N Engl J Med 311:235, 1984.)* Di George's syndrome, also called *congenital thymic aplasia,* is caused by abnormal development of the third and fourth pharyngeal pouches during the sixth to eighth weeks of intrauterine life. The structures arising from these pharyngeal evaginations are the thymus, the tissues of the lips and central portion of the face, the ear tubercle, the aortic arch, and the parathyroid glands. Consequently, a child demonstrating the classic presentation of Di George's syndrome has the following abnormalities: hypocalcemic tetany; congenital heart disease involving aortic arch structures; cellular immunodeficiency with a T lymphopenia, absence of a thymus, and failure of blood lymphocytes to respond to phytohemagglutinin and allogeneic cells; and an abnormal facies with low-set ears, "fish-shaped" mouth, and hypertelorism. Thyroid function is normal, and B-cell immunity as measured by immunoglobulin levels and antibody response to immunization usually is unimpaired. Treatment of Di George's syndrome is by transplant of a fetal thymus.

450. The answer is A-Y, B-Y, C-Y, D-N, E-N. *(Wilson, ed 12. chap 263.)* Isolated IgA deficiency is the most common immunodeficiency disorder, with an incidence between 1:600 and 1:800. Affected persons have a normal or reduced number of B cells with surface IgA, but seem to have overabundant immature cells that coexpress IgA and IgM, suggesting a block in B-cell terminal differentiation. This presumption is substantiated by in vitro studies showing that lymphocytes from IgA-deficient persons can synthesize but are unable to secrete IgA. Both serum IgA and secretory IgA usually are reduced. Although IgA deficiency need not be associated with clinical disease, it frequently is. Recurrent sinopulmonary infection is most common. Allergy occurs with an incidence of 1:200 to 1:400, compared with 1:600 to 1:800 in the general population. Approximately 30 to 40 percent of IgA-deficient persons have antibodies directed against IgA, thus predisposing them to anaphylactoid reactions following the infusion of blood products. Persons with isolated IgA deficiency are also at greater risk for developing autoimmune diseases, including lupus and rheumatoid arthritis.

451. The answer is A-Y, B-Y, C-Y, D-Y, E-Y. *(Wilson, ed 12. chap 268.)* Most antigen-antibody complexes are cleared by cells of the reticuloendothelial system. It appears that in some conditions the reticuloendothelial system can be overwhelmed by immune complexes, thereby impeding the removal and leading to the deposition of immune complexes. Deposition of these complexes in tissues other than those of the reticuloendothelial system is responsible for the signs and symptoms of immune-complex disease. In animal models, the persistence of complexes is necessary for the development of renal disease; also, slight antigen excess has been found to predispose to the formation of antigen-antibody complexes, which persist in the circulation and lead to inflammatory illness. Immune complex–mediated vascular damage can lead to cutaneous necrotizing vasculitis. Electron microscopy reveals subendothelial immune complexes that presumably incite an array of inflammatory cells to migrate toward the vessel.

452. The answer is A-N, B-Y, C-N, D-Y, E-Y. *(Wilson, ed 12. chap 14.)* Class I HLA antigens are encoded at the A, B, and C loci of the human major histocompatibility complex on chromosome 6. Each such antigen consists of an 11.5-kilodalton (kd) $beta_2$-microglobulin subunit (also encoded in the HLA region) and a 44-kd chain with three separate domains that contain the antigenic specificity. Only certain areas of the heavy chain are diverse, so individual molecules share greater than 80 percent sequence homology. Class I molecules are expressed on all cells except mature red blood cells. These antigens are defined serologically and are useful in predicting results for organ transplants. Because class I antigens are not distributed evenly from one racial group to another, it can be more difficult for a person of African descent, for example, to procure a bone marrow donor from a registry where most of the potential donors descend from Northern Europe.

453. The answer is A-Y, B-N, C-Y, D-N, E-Y. *(Wilson, ed 12. chap 264. Fischel, N Engl J Med 317:185, 1987.)* AZT inhibits viral reverse transcriptase, the enzyme required in all retroviruses because it converts viral RNA into DNA, which can then be integrated into the host's genome. AZT has been a major advance in the treatment of patients with ARC and AIDS. Both asymptomatic and symptomatic patients with AIDS or ARC whose peripheral CD4+ (T4+) T-cell counts are less than 500 cells per microliter benefit from treatment with 200 mg AZT every 4 h. AZT treatment is associated with limited prolongation of survival and retardation of progression of disease in those with early disease. Moreover, impressive improvements in HIV-associated neurologic sequelae have been observed. The most common side effect, other than myelosuppression resulting in anemia and neutropenia, is gastrointestinal intolerance. Preliminary reports suggest that the myelosuppressive side effects may be ameliorated by the concomitant use of the recombinant growth factors erythropoietin and GM-CSF. Once a patient contracts *P. carinii* pneumonia, aerosolized pentamidine 300 mg/month is effective prophylaxis, but does result in an increased incidence of extrapulmonary infections.

454. The answer is A-Y, B-Y, C-Y, D-Y, E-N. *(Wilson, ed 12. chap 269.)* Although most clinicians believe that women with systemic lupus erythematosus should not become pregnant if they have active disease or advanced renal or cardiac disease, the presence of SLE itself is not an absolute contraindication to pregnancy. The outcome of pregnancy is best for those women in remission at the time of conception. Even in women with quiescent disease, exacerbations may occur (usually in the first trimester and in the immediate postpartum period), and 25 to 40 percent of pregnancies end in spontaneous abortion. Fetal loss rates are higher in patients with lupus anticoagulant or anticardiolipin antibodies. Flare-ups should be anticipated and vigorously treated with steroids. Steroids given throughout pregnancy also usually have no adverse effects on the child. In the case presented, the fact that the woman had a life-threatening bout of disease a year ago would argue against stopping her drugs at this time. Neonatal lupus, which is manifested by thrombocytopenia, rash, and heart block, is rare but can occur in mothers with anti-Ro antibodies.

455. The answer is A-N, B-N, C-N, D-Y, E-Y. *(Wilson, ed 12. chap 266.)* This patient has many of the hallmarks of systemic amyloidosis. An abdominal fat pad aspirate or a rectal biopsy is the best way to make the diagnosis, although biopsy of any affected organ may be carried out. A positive Congo red histologic stain helps to establish the diagnosis. The classification of amyloid protein fibrils that are deposited in the tissues is based on their biochemical type. AL amyloid residues bear homology to immunoglobulin light chains and are seen in primary or myeloma-associated situations. The AA type of amyloid, made up of 76 amino acid residues, is seen as a secondary problem in a host of chronic inflammatory conditions, including long-standing rheumatoid arthritis, tuberculosis, bronchiectasis, familial Mediterranean fever, and leprosy. Other types of amyloid proteins are seen in familial amyloid polyneuropathy (AF; 14 kd), medullary carcinoma of the thyroid (AE), and Alzheimer's disease (AS; the beta, or A4, protein). Amyloidosis should be suspected in any patient with an underlying chronic inflammatory disease who develops hepatomegaly, splenomegaly, malabsorption, cardiac disease, or proteinuria. Cardiac disease usually consists of congestive heart failure with low QRS-complex voltage, arrhythmias, and exquisite sensitivity to digitalis. Waxy papules or plaques in the axillary folds may signal the deposition of amyloid in the skin; purpura after minor trauma is not uncommon. Gastrointestinal lesions caused by amyloid include macroglossia, malabsorption, and bleeding. In addition to amyloid-induced synovitis, peripheral neuropathy and carpal tunnel syndrome may be seen.

456. The answer is A-Y, B-N, C-N, D-Y, E-Y. *(Wilson, ed 12. chap 269.)* The most common cause of drug-induced SLE is procainamide, which produces a positive ANA in 75 percent of those who take it and a 20 percent incidence of clinical lupus. In contrast, hydralazine induces an ANA in 25 percent and a clinical lupus syndrome in 10 percent. Slow acetylators seem to have more problems with drug-induced autoimmune phenomena. Though up to 50 percent of those with drug-induced lupus have arthralgias, pleuropericarditis, or both, renal disease is rare. In an effort to distinguish drug-induced lupus (which should last less than 6 months) from de novo lupus (a disease uniquely positive for anti-dsDNA), a complete ANA panel should be sent. Most patients will respond initially to withdrawal of the offending drug; if not, then a brief trial of steroids is indicated.

457. The answer is A-N, B-N, C-Y, D-Y, E-N. *(Wilson, ed 12. chap 270.)* NSAIDS, including aspirin, are effective agents in the treatment of symptomatic rheumatoid arthritis. However, none of the newer agents have been shown to be more effective than aspirin, though some do have fewer gastrointestinal side effects. All of these agents induce platelet dysfunction. Their mechanism of action is the blockage of the activity of the enzyme cyclooxygenase, which converts arachidonic acid into the inflammation-mediating prostaglandins. 5-Lipoxygenase, which is not inhibited by NSAIDS, converts arachidonic acid into leukotrienes. It may be the dysregulation of normal arachidonic acid metabolism that leads to the occasional NSAID-induced worsening of allergic rhinitis and asthma. The absence of renal vasodilatory prostaglandins normally produced by the action of cyclooxygenase can lead to renal insufficiency, particularly in those with underlying renal vascular disease.

458. The answer is A-N, B-Y, C-N, D-Y, E-Y. *(Wilson, ed 12. chap 277.)* Sarcoidosis is a systemic granulomatous inflammatory disorder that frequently involves the lungs, where it causes a typical interstitial lung disease that may be asymptomatic, may cause transient respiratory difficulties with or without hilar adenopathy, or may progress to end-stage pulmonary fibrosis. Extrapulmonary sarcoidosis may involve the eyes, skin, liver, bones, gastrointestinal tract, kidneys, nervous system, and heart. In the United States, 10 to 20 percent of cases consist of asymptomatic hilar adenopathy detected on chest radiographs taken for other reasons; these cases may constitute a higher fraction of the total in other countries where routine preemployment chest radiography is more widely practiced. The disease occurs more frequently among blacks than whites by a substantial margin. At sites of disease activity, such as the lung, there is an accumulation of activated helper-inducer (CD4+) lymphocytes, with release of immunologic mediators such as interleukin 2 and gamma-interferon, and resultant granuloma formation. In contrast to other interstitial lung diseases, the diagnosis may frequently be made by the demonstration of the characteristic granulomatous inflammation in tissue obtained by transbronchial biopsy. Prognosis depends on the risk of progression to advanced pulmonary fibrosis, and those persons with intense pulmonary inflammation may benefit from treatment with corticosteroids. Chest radiography and pulmonary function testing cannot distinguish accurately between active inflammation and established fibrosis; hence, most clinicians familiar with the disease utilize procedures such as bronchoalveolar lavage or gallium-67 scanning, or both, to assess the intensity of the alveolitis present. These procedures may be performed serially during the course of the patient's illness to follow the progress of the disease and response to therapy.

459. The answer is A-Y, B-Y, C-Y, D-Y, E-Y. *(Wilson, ed 12. chap 273. Fox, Semin Arthritis Rheum 14:77, 1984.)* Sjögren's syndrome, an autoimmune destruction of the exocrine glands, can be primary or it can be secondary and associated with rheumatoid arthritis, SLE, or systemic sclerosis. A mononuclear cell infiltrate, which can be seen in virtually any organ, is pathognomonic if found in the salivary gland in association with keratoconjunctivitis sicca (conjunctival and corneal dryness) and xerostomia (lack of salivation). Since minor salivary glands will be obtained in a lip biopsy, such a procedure can be diagnostic. Severe dryness of the mouth can lead to an increased incidence of dental caries. Corneal dryness may be severe enough to result in ulceration. The most common form of renal involvement (seen in 40 percent of patients with primary Sjögren's) is an interstitial nephritis resulting in renal tubular acidosis. Hypersensitivity vasculitis, manifested by palpable purpura of the lower extremities, is not uncommon. Sensory neuropathies, interstitial pneumonitis, and autoimmune thyroid disease may also accompany primary Sjögren's syndrome. Finally, pseudolymphoma, characterized by lymphadenopathy and enlargement of the parotid gland, and frank non-Hodgkin's lymphoma may occur.

460. The answer is A-Y, B-Y, C-Y, D-N, E-N. *(Wilson, ed 12. chap 270.)* Rheumatoid factors are antibodies to the Fc fragment of immunoglobulin G. They may be of the IgG, IgA, or IgM class; the widely used latex and sheep-cell agglutination tests detect rheumatoid factors primarily of the IgM class. Chronic antigenic stimulation is one of the processes important in the production of rheumatoid factors. Rheumatoid factors are associated not only with rheumatoid arthritis and other autoimmune diseases but also with lymphoreticular malignancies and chronic infections, such as subacute bacterial endocarditis. Rheumatoid factors are usually present within the first year of onset of rheumatoid arthritis; their presence correlates with the extraarticular manifestations of the disease. Patients with rheumatoid arthritis who have positive serologic tests for IgM rheumatoid factor have a worse prognosis than those who are seronegative.

461. The answer is A-Y, B-N, C-N, D-Y, E-Y. *(Wilson, ed 12. chap 270.)* Joint stiffness in the morning or after periods of inactivity lasting more than 30 min is characteristic of inflammatory rheumatic disease. Arthritis characteristic of rheumatoid arthritis is persistent, remaining in the same joints for months. Migratory arthritis, in which short-lived arthritic symptoms in one joint subside as symptoms begin in another joint, is not characteristic of rheumatoid arthritis. Persons who have rheumatoid arthritis can have involvement of the cervical spine, the wrist joints, and all the small joints of the hand except the distal interphalangeal joints. Wrist-joint arthritis can lead to median-nerve entrapment (carpal tunnel syndrome).

462. The answer is A-Y, B-N, C-Y, D-N, E-Y. *(Wilson, ed 12. chap 274.)* This patient has an acute inflammatory asymmetric polyarthritis associated with ocular (conjunctivitis, occasionally anterior uveitis) and cutaneous (keratoderma blennorrhagicum on palms and soles; circinate balanitis on the glans penis) disease. Moreover, he has had a recent episode of urethritis, possibly caused by chlamydia. He therefore has so-called reactive arthritis, also known as Reiter's syndrome. This entity can follow certain infectious illnesses, most notably dysentery or venereal disease usually in patients who are HLA-B27 positive. The constitutional symptoms associated with the acute illness can be severe. The erythrocyte sedimentation rate is frequently elevated. Sacroiliitis and spondyloarthropathy may be seen as late sequellae. Patients will respond to nonsteroidal agents, but there is little evidence to support the benefit of antibiotics, other than in eradicating chlamydia, if present.

463. The answer is A-N, B-Y, C-Y, D-Y, E-N. *(Wilson, ed 12. chap 276. Fauci, Ann Intern Med 98:76, 1983.)* This patient presents with findings characteristic of Wegener's granulomatosis. Sinus disease (manifested by bloody or purulent nasal discharge), pulmonary disease, and glomerulonephritis are seen in greater than 80 percent of affected patients. Sinus involvement would be unlikely in Goodpasture's syndrome, which is associated with anti-basement membrane antibodies. Other findings characteristic of Wegener's include ocular involvement, skin lesions, and nervous system manifestations (including cranial neuritis or mononeuritis multiplex), as well as elevated ESR, anemia, leukocytosis, and hypergammaglobulinemia. The diagnosis can be made by finding necrotizing granulomatous vasculitis in an involved site. Although the immunopathogenesis of this entity is unclear, antibodies to a neutrophil protein (found in the azurophilic granules) can be frequently found. This disease can be successfully treated in over 90 percent of patients with the use of glucocorticoids and cyclophosphamide. The glucocorticoids are gradually tapered and the cyclophosphamide, the mainstay of treatment, should be continued for about 1 year after complete remission.

464. The answer is A-N, B-Y, C-N, D-Y, E-Y. *(Wilson, ed 12. chap 274.)* The x-ray shown in the question is compatible with a diagnosis of ankylosing spondylitis. Early radiographic evidence of sacroiliitis includes blurring of joint margins, irregular subchondral erosions, and sclerosis affecting both sides of the sacroiliac joint. With progression of the disease, the joint is lost completely. Radiographic findings of early spondylitis include straightening of the lumbar spine and squaring of the lumbar and thoracic vertebrae. Later, syndesmophytes appear along the lateral and anterior surfaces of the intervertebral disks and bridge adjacent vertebrae, creating the so-called bamboo spine. Complications of ankylosing spondylitis include uveitis (in 30 percent of affected persons) and aortic insufficiency (3 percent). The rigid spine is subject to fracture, most commonly in the cervical area, and this creates the potential for quadriplegia even after relatively minor trauma.

465. The answer is A-N, B-N, C-N, D-Y, E-N. *(Wilson, ed 12. chap 274.)* The diagnosis of ankylosing spondylitis is based on a characteristic history and physical examination. A determination of HLA-B27 status does not help in the diagnosis of ankylosing spondylitis. Seven percent of the normal white population in the United States are positive for HLA-B27, and 5 to 10 percent of persons with bona fide ankylosing spondylitis are negative for HLA-B27. It has been shown that 20 percent of HLA-B27-positive persons who are first-degree relatives of cases have evidence of ankylosing spondylitis. Blacks and Asians have a lower prevalence of HLA-B27 antigenicity and a lower prevalence of ankylosing spondylitis. The concordance rate in identical twins is 60 percent or less, indicating that environmental factors also play a role in disease pathogenesis.

466. The answer is A-N, B-Y, C-Y, D-Y, E-Y. *(Wilson, ed 12. chap 274.)* In the United States and Great Britain, postdysenteric Reiter's syndrome occurs much less frequently than postvenereal Reiter's syndrome. *Salmonella, Shigella, Yersinia,* and, more recently, *Campylobacter* enteric infections have been associated with the development of the disorder. Urethritis occurs in both forms of the disease, though it is more common in the postvenereal type. It is interesting that Reiter's initial description of the disease was in patients who had the postdysenteric variety.

467. The answer is A-N, B-N, C-N, D-Y, E-Y. *(Wilson, ed 12. chap 282.)* Synovial deposition of calcium pyrophosphate dihydrate crystals occurs in pseudogout, an inflammatory disorder producing arthritis in older persons. Crystals are thought to form on the surface of articular cartilage (chondrocalcinosis) and then are shed into synovial fluid; in gout, on the other hand, crystals are thought to arise from a supersaturated solution of sodium urate. Under polarized light, calcium pyrophosphate dihydrate crystals have a weak positive birefringence and can be difficult to see if not looked for carefully. Most affected persons have radiographic evidence of chondrocalcinosis. Common sites of involvement are the menisci of the knees, articular disk of the distal radioulnar joint, the symphysis pubis, and the annulus fibrosis of the intervertebral disks. Clinical syndromes other than pseudogout, among them pseudorheumatoid arthritis and pseudodegenerative joint disease, also involve deposition of calcium pyrophosphate crystals.

468. The answer is A-Y, B-Y, C-N, D-N, E-N. *(Wilson, ed 12. chap 96. Goldenburg, N Engl J Med 312:764, 1985.)* Septic arthritis, which usually results from hematogenous spread of a primary infection at another site, is considered a medical emergency. Drainage of an infected joint is an important component of treatment and usually can be performed adequately by needle aspiration; open surgical drainage is necessary in only a few circumstances, such as when septic arthritis involves a hip joint. Systemic infusion of antibiotics produces sufficient intraarticular bactericidal activity; consequently, intraarticular administration of antibiotics is unwarranted, especially in view of the fact that it can cause a chemical synovitis. Irrigation of a septic joint cavity with sterile saline can be useful in removing inflammatory debris. Bacteria commonly causing septic arthritis include *Neisseria gonorrhoeae, Staphylococcus aureus,* and *Streptococcus pneumoniae;* gonococcal organisms associated with disseminated infection are usually very sensitive to penicillin.

469. The answer is A-N, B-N, C-N, D-Y, E-Y. *(Wilson, ed 12. chap 277.)* While 10 to 20 percent of patients with sarcoidosis present with asymptomatic disease found incidentally on chest x-ray and 40 to 70 percent have the characteristic insidious development of disease, the remainder present over the span of a few weeks. Constitutional and respiratory symptoms dominate the acute presentation. Two distinct patterns of acute sarcoidosis are recognized. Löfgren's syndrome, seen in Scandinavian, Irish, and Puerto Rican females, is characterized by erythema nodosum, arthralgias, and bilateral hilar lymphadenopathy. The constellation of findings in the Heerfordt-Waldenström syndrome consists of fever, parotid enlargement, anterior uveitis, and facial nerve palsy. Interstitial pulmonary involvement would be rare in acute sarcoidosis. Myopathy and skin lesions are most consistent with dermatomyositis. Although 5 percent of patients with sarcoidosis have cardiac abnormalities, valvular heart disease—other than occasional instances of papillary muscle dysfunction—is rare.

470. The answer is A-Y, B-N, C-Y, D-Y, E-N. *(Wilson, ed 12. chap 278.)* Familial Mediterranean fever (FMF), or familial paroxysmal polyserositis, is an inherited disorder of unknown etiology. There is no pathognomonic finding, although evidence of serosal inflammation should be documented. Recently, elevated levels of the enzyme dopamine beta-hydroxylase have been found in patients with this disorder. The relationship of such a finding to the pathophysiology of FMF is unknown; however, levels of this enzyme decline after therapy with colchicine, an agent that remarkably retards the frequency and severity of attacks. Attacks typically consist of fever and abdominal pain, although 75 percent of patients also have pleuritic chest pain or joint pain or both at some time. FMF-associated drug addiction is a more worrisome problem in the United States than is amyloidosis, which is reported in the Middle East. The reason for the unequal geographic incidence of amyloidosis is unknown. The disease is more frequently found in non-Ashkenazic Jews, Italians, and Arabs; however, approximately 50 percent of patients give no family history.

471. The answer is A-N, B-Y, C-Y, D-N, E-N. *(Wilson, ed 12. chap 279.)* Patients with midline granuloma, characterized by local inflammation and destructive mutilation of head and neck tissues, may present with nasal and sinus symptoms. Ulcerations of the nasal septum and soft and hard palates are harbingers of very destructive processes in any area in the neck or above. Granulomatous infiltration and necrosis will be noted on pathologic examination of the involved areas. Radiation therapy is the treatment of choice and is successful in averting the almost certainly fatal course in untreated patients. Midline granuloma can be difficult to distinguish from cocaine-induced septal perforation, malignant lymphoma, and a host of chronic infections including histoplasmosis, blastomycosis, coccidioidomycosis, leprosy, tuberculosis, syphilis, and leishmaniasis. While Wegener's granulomatosis is associated with similar upper airway findings, the absence of vasculitis on biopsy, the absence of pulmonary and renal disease, and the presence of palatal perforation make the diagnosis of midline granuloma much more likely. Midline granuloma never involves structures below the neck.

472–476. The answers are: 472-D, 473-B, 474-E, 475-A, 476-C. *(Wilson, ed 12. chap 13.)* Hereditary angioedema is characterized by recurrent attacks of angioedema of the hands, feet, perioral and periorbital regions, and upper airway. The condition causes abdominal pain as the result of small-bowel edema and may be fatal if laryngeal obstruction is severe. In hereditary angioedema, C1 inhibitor is absent, which leads to uncontrolled activation of the early complement proteins C4 and C2. This disease has an autosomal dominant pattern of inheritance. Treatment with danazol, an attenuated androgen, has been very effective.

Deficiency of complement component C3 is a rare condition that exists in two forms: in type I, C3 is deficient as a result of a C3 inactivator; and in type II, the reduced level of C3 is associated with decreased synthesis as well as increased destruction caused by the serum enzyme C3 convertase. By virtue of its central position in both the classic and alternative complement pathways, C3 is essential for normal host defense against pyogenic bacteria. Thus, C3-deficient persons suffer from recurrent and severe infections, usually involving the upper and lower respiratory tract and the genitourinary tract.

Membranoproliferative glomerulonephritis, a disease of children and young adults, often progresses to chronic renal failure. Histologically, the kidney shows mesangial proliferation and hypertrophy and thickened glomerular basement membranes. Many patients are found to have a serum substance labeled *C3 nephritic factor (C3NeF)*, which is an autoantibody directed against the alternative pathway. Such patients would have a complement profile featuring normal levels of C1, C4, and C2 components of the classic pathway but low levels of C3 and factor B; the overall hemolytic activity (CH_{50}) of the complement system would be depressed.

C2 deficiency is the most common hereditary deficiency of complement. It is inherited as an autosomal recessive trait; both homozygous and heterozygous forms exist, with heterozygotes possessing approximately half-normal serum levels of C2. Deficiency of C2 has been associated with systemic lupus erythematosus, chronic glomerulonephritis, and polymyositis. However, it also occurs in healthy persons. The absence of functional and immunochemically detectable C2 in affected persons is caused by an inability of macrophages to make the C2 protein.

Disseminated gonococcal infection is characterized by fever, arthralgias, and skin lesions ranging from maculopapular to pustular and hemorrhagic in appearance. Although disseminated gonococcal infection can occur in persons who have normal complement activity, it has been reported to occur with unusual frequency in association with homozygous deficiencies of C6, C7, and C8. Although sera from persons deficient in these factors possess normal opsonic activity, they lack bactericidal activity against *Neisseria* organisms, and, as a result, these persons have a greater likelihood of contracting neisserial meningitis. This phenomenon suggests that phagocytosis is insufficient to kill these organisms and that complement-mediated lysis is required.

477–480. The answers are: 477-C, 478-D, 479-A, 480-B. (*Wilson, ed 12. chaps 269, 271.*) Autoantibodies to nuclear antigens and other antigenic determinants are features common to systemic lupus erythematosus (SLE) and other so-called connective tissue disorders. Screening tests for antinuclear antibodies (ANA) may use human cell line substrates or murine tissues to detect multiple antibodies with different specificities. Autoantibodies reacting with specific nuclear antigens have been found to characterize certain disorders and clinical situations. Antihistone antibodies, reacting with nuclear histone proteins, are found in approximately 95 percent of patients with drug-induced lupus syndromes, while anticentromere antibodies are present in most patients with the CREST variant of progressive systemic sclerosis. Anti-Ro (SSA) antibodies recognize an RNA polymerase, are present in approximately 30 percent of patients with SLE (including a subset who may be ANA-negative), and have been associated with congenital heart block in infants born to women who carry this antibody. Antibodies that react with cardiolipin, a phospholipid, may be found in some 50 percent of patients with SLE. These antibodies also bind phospholipids in the prothrombin activator complex, prolong the partial thromboplastin time, and may be associated with a heightened tendency to thrombosis of the veins or arteries, or both. These antibodies also produce a false-positive reaction in the VDRL test for syphilis.

481–484. The answers are: 481-C, 482-E, 483-D, 484-A. (*Wilson, ed 12. chaps 280, 284.*) The analysis of synovial fluid begins at the bedside. When fluid is withdrawn from a joint into a syringe, its clarity and color should be assessed. Cloudiness or turbidity is caused by the scattering of light as it is reflected off particles in the fluid; these particles are usually white blood cells, although crystals may also be present. The viscosity of synovial fluid is due to its hyaluronate content. In inflammatory joint disease, synovial fluid contains enzymes that break down hyaluronate and reduce fluid viscosity. In contrast, synovial fluid taken from a joint in a person with degenerative joint disease, a noninflammatory condition, would be expected to be clear and have good viscosity. The color of the fluid can indicate recent or old hemorrhage into the joint space. Pigmented villonodular synovitis is associated with noninflammatory fluid that is dark brown in color (''crankcase oil'') as a result of repeated hemorrhage into the joint. Gout and calcium pyrophosphate deposition disease produce inflammatory synovial effusions, which are cloudy and watery. In addition, these disorders may be diagnosed by identification of crystals in the fluid—sodium urate crystals of gout are needlelike and strongly negatively birefringent, whereas calcium pyrophosphate crystals are rhomboidal and weakly positively birefringent.

Disorders of the Hematopoietic System

DIRECTIONS: Each question below contains five suggested responses. Select the **one best** response to each question.

485. All the following conditions impair the release of oxygen to body tissues EXCEPT

(A) methemoglobinemia
(B) carbon monoxide poisoning
(C) hyperventilation
(D) hypophosphatemia
(E) acidosis

486. A 28-year-old man with newly diagnosed acute myelogenous leukemia spikes a temperature to 38.7°C (101.7°F) on the sixth day of induction therapy. He feels well and has no physical complaints. His only medicine is intravenous cytosine arabinoside, 140 mg every 12 h. Physical examination is unrevealing. His white blood count is 900/mm^3, of which 10 percent are granulocytes and the rest mostly lymphocytes; platelet count is 24,000/mm^3. Findings on chest x-ray and urinalysis are normal.

After obtaining appropriate cultures, the man's physician should

(A) observe closely for the development of a clinically evident source of fever
(B) begin antibiotic therapy with gentamicin, carbenicillin, and a cephalosporin
(C) begin granulocyte transfusion and antibiotic therapy with gentamicin, carbenicillin, and a cephalosporin
(D) begin gammaglobulin treatment and antibiotic therapy with gentamicin, carbenicillin, and a cephalosporin
(E) begin antibiotic therapy with amphotericin, gentamicin, carbenicillin, and a cephalosporin

487. All the following statements about the acute leukemias are true EXCEPT

(A) the majority of cases of acute lymphocytic leukemia (ALL) express both T-cell antigens and surface immunoglobulin
(B) leukemic cells in most cases of ALL contain terminal deoxynucleotidyl transferase (Tdt), an enzyme only rarely present in cells in acute myelogenous leukemia (AML)
(C) the T-cell form of ALL occurs typically in adolescent males; it is frequently associated with an increased leukocyte count and an anterior mediastinal mass
(D) the cells of B-cell ALL frequently contain the t(8;14) chromosomal abnormality characteristic of Burkitt's lymphoma
(E) patients with the acute promyelocytic (M3) subtype of AML frequently present with disseminated intravascular coagulation (DIC)

488. Coumarin-induced skin necrosis is occasionally associated with the institution of oral anticoagulants in patients with

(A) antithrombin III deficiency
(B) protein C deficiency
(C) protein S deficiency
(D) plasminogen deficiency
(E) dysfibrinogenemias

489. A 26-year-old woman has painful mouth ulcers. Six weeks ago, she was started on propylthiouracil for hyperthyroidism. She is afebrile, and physical examination is unremarkable except for several small oral aphthous ulcers. White blood cell count is 200/mm³ (15 percent neutrophils, 80 percent lymphocytes, 5 percent monocytes); hemoglobin concentration, hematocrit, and platelet count are normal. The woman's physician should stop the propylthiouracil and

(A) schedule a follow-up outpatient appointment
(B) arrange for HLA typing of her siblings in preparation for bone marrow transplantation
(C) prescribe oral prednisone, 1 mg/kg
(D) hospitalize her for broad-spectrum antibiotic therapy
(E) hospitalize her for white blood cell transfusion

490. All the following may be found in the blood as a consequence of splenectomy EXCEPT

(A) erythrocytic Heinz bodies
(B) erythrocytic target forms
(C) erythrocytic Howell-Jolly bodies
(D) spherocytic red blood cells
(E) nucleated red blood cells

491. A 25-year-old, previously healthy woman presents with jaundice, confusion, and fever. Initial physical examination is unremarkable except for scattered petechiae on the lower extremities, scleral icterus, and disorientation on mental status examination. Laboratory examination discloses the following: hematocrit, 27 percent; white cell count, 12,000/μL; platelet count, 10,000/μL; bilirubin, 85 μmol/L (5 mg/dL); direct bilirubin, 10 μmol/L (0.6 mg/dL); urea nitrogen, 21 mmol/L (60 mg/dL); creatinine, 400 μmol/L (4.5 mg/dL). Red blood cell smear discloses fragmented red blood cells and nucleated red blood cells. Prothrombin, thrombin, and partial thromboplastin times are all normal.

The most effective and appropriate therapeutic maneuver is likely to be

(A) plasmapheresis
(B) administration of aspirin
(C) administration of high-dose glucocorticoids
(D) administration of high-dose glucocorticoids plus cyclophosphamide
(E) splenectomy

492. Paroxysmal nocturnal hemoglobinuria is associated with all the following conditions EXCEPT

(A) elevation of leukocyte alkaline phosphatase levels
(B) aplastic anemia
(C) iron-deficiency anemia
(D) venous thrombosis
(E) acute leukemia

493. Iron deficiency is LEAST likely to be associated with

(A) lead poisoning
(B) hemodialysis
(C) chronic heart-valve hemolysis
(D) hereditary hemorrhagic telangiectasia
(E) idiopathic pulmonary hemosiderosis

494. A 72-year-old man who has become progressively more fatigued is found to be anemic. Hematologic laboratory values are as follows:

Hemoglobin: 100 g/L (10 g/dL)
Hematocrit: 27.5 percent
Mean corpuscular volume (MCV): 101 fL
Mean corpuscular hemoglobin (MCH): 30 pg
Mean corpuscular hemoglobin concentration (MCHC): 340 g/L (34 g/dL)
Reticulocyte count: 0.5 percent
White blood cell count: 7300/mm³ (65 percent neutrophils)
Platelet count: 210,000/mm³

The most likely diagnosis is

(A) acute leukemia
(B) aplastic anemia
(C) autoimmune hemolytic anemia
(D) iron-deficiency
(E) myelodysplastic syndrome

495. Which of the following procedures would be most sensitive in detecting early iron overload?

(A) Quantitative iron determination in a liver biopsy specimen
(B) Urinary iron excretion in response to a test dose of desferrioxamine
(C) Serum ferritin concentration
(D) Serum iron concentration, total iron-binding capacity, and calculated transferring saturation
(E) Iron stain of a bone marrow aspirate

496. Which of the following statements concerning the diagnosis of pernicious anemia is true?

(A) The presence of antiparietal-cell antibodies is diagnostic of pernicious anemia
(B) Hematologic response to folate therapy alone rules out pernicious anemia as the cause of megaloblastic anemia
(C) Hyperkalemia may be a consequence of vitamin B_{12} therapy
(D) Bone marrow examination would be expected to reveal marked depletion of erythrocyte precursors in persons with untreated pernicious anemia
(E) Serum gastrin levels usually are elevated in persons with pernicious anemia

497. A 45-year-old woman with long-standing rheumatoid arthritis is diagnosed as having "anemia of chronic disease." The predominant mechanism causing this type of anemia in persons with chronic inflammatory disorders is

(A) defective porphyrin synthesis
(B) impaired incorporation of iron into porphyrin
(C) intravascular hemolysis
(D) depressed erythroid maturation due to decreased erythropoietin production
(E) impaired transfer of reticuloendothelial storage iron to marrow erythroid precursors

498. Which of the following groups would be most likely to develop acute leukemia?

(A) Persons who have Wiskott-Aldrich syndrome
(B) Persons who have hereditary sideroblastic anemia
(C) Persons who have paroxysmal nocturnal hemoglobinuria
(D) Persons who have Hodgkin's disease and are treated with radiation therapy
(E) Persons receiving immunosuppressive therapy following renal transplantation

499. Which of the following statements best characterizes the hemolysis associated with glucose 6-phosphate dehydrogenase (G6PD) deficiency?

(A) It is more severe in affected blacks than in affected persons of Mediterranean ancestry
(B) It is more severe in females than in males
(C) It causes the appearance of Heinz bodies on Wright staining of a peripheral smear
(D) It most often is precipitated by infection
(E) The best time to perform the diagnostic test is during a hemolytic crisis

500. Most persons who have hemoglobin variants with high oxygen affinity will

(A) adapt poorly to hypoxic conditions
(B) demonstrate abnormal hemoglobin electrophoresis
(C) have erythrocytosis
(D) have abnormal morphology of red blood cells
(E) have increased 2,3-diphosphoglycerate (2,3-DPG) concentrations in red blood cells

501. Evaluation of a person who has pure red blood cell aplasia would be expected to reveal

(A) markedly hypocellular bone marrow
(B) normochromic, normocytic red blood cells
(C) increased iron turnover on ferrokinetic studies
(D) a reticulocyte count greater than 2.0 percent
(E) decreased urinary erythropoietin content

502. A 21-year-old woman who has had severe menorrhagia is referred by her gynecologist for evaluation of a possible systemic coagulopathy. A younger sister has been noted to bleed excessively after trauma. She takes no medications; physical examination is unremarkable. Initial laboratory results include the following: platelet count, 252,000/mm^3; prothrombin time, 23.6 s (control 11.6 s); and partial thromboplastin time, 26.9 s (control 33.3 s). Further laboratory testing should consist of

(A) determination of factor VIII level
(B) screening for inhibitors
(C) determination of bleeding time
(D) determination of factor VII level
(E) determination of alpha$_2$-antiplasmin level

503. Thrombocytosis would be LEAST likely to occur in persons who have

(A) polycythemia vera
(B) hemolytic-uremic syndrome
(C) sickle cell (SS) disease
(D) iron-deficiency anemia
(E) ulcerative colitis

504. A feature of idiopathic thrombocytopenic purpura common to both children *and* adults is

(A) occurrence after an antecedent viral illness
(B) presence of antibodies directed against target antigens on the glycoprotein IIb-IIIa complex
(C) absence of splenomegaly
(D) persistence of thrombocytopenia for more than 6 months
(E) necessity of splenectomy to ameliorate thrombocytopenia

505. A 16-year-old boy presented with deep vein thrombophlebitis and pulmonary embolism. There is no familial history of thromboembolic disease. The platelet count on admission was 325,000/mm^3; prothrombin time, 13.1 s (control 11.4 s); partial thromboplastin time, 55.0 s (control 27.9 s); and thrombin time, 14.5 s (control 15 s). The most likely reason for the thrombotic diathesis in this patient is the presence of

(A) dysfibrinogenemia
(B) congenital antithrombin III deficiency
(C) lupus anticoagulant
(D) factor XI deficiency
(E) protein C deficiency

506. A young woman presents with bleeding after a dental extraction. She is found to have a bleeding time of greater than 20 min along with a normal prothrombin time and partial thromboplastin time. There is a familial history of bleeding, and the patient's laboratory evaluation reveals a normal platelet count. The factor VIII coagulant activity is 54 percent of normal, von Willebrand factor (vWF) antigen is 48 percent of normal, and ristocetin cofactor is 13 percent of normal. The abnormal vWF multimer pattern of the patient's plasma on SDS-agarose electrophoresis is caused by

(A) defective release of vWF from endothelial cells
(B) inappropriate binding of vWF to platelets
(C) reduced synthesis of vWF by endothelial cells
(D) an inability to assemble high-molecular-weight multimers or premature catabolism of vWF
(E) an alteration in the platelet receptor for vWF

507. A 1-year-old boy bleeds significantly after an inguinal hernia repair. The patient has no siblings, and there is no familial history of a bleeding diathesis. Platelet count, bleeding time, prothrombin time, and partial thromboplastin time are all normal. The most likely diagnosis is

(A) prekallikrein deficiency
(B) factor XII deficiency
(C) factor XIII deficiency
(D) thrombasthenia
(E) protein Ś deficiency

508. A 75-year-old man presents with ischemic changes of the distal lower extremities. Physical examination reveals the presence of an abdominal mass. Laboratory evaluation discloses a hematocrit of 28 percent; platelet count, 90,000/mm^3; prothrombin time, 16 s (control 12 s); and partial thromboplastin time, 55 s (control 30 s). The fibrinogen level was reduced to 1.0 g/L (100 mg/dL) and the level of fibrin split products was elevated to 160 mg/L (160 μg/mL). Which of the following is the most appropriate therapy?

(A) Plasma exchange transfusion
(B) Administration of cryoprecipitate
(C) Administration of aminocaproic acid (Amicar)
(D) Platelet transfusions
(E) Administration of fresh frozen plasma

509. Persons with polycythemia vera and a hematocrit greater than 45 percent generally have

(A) increased levels of urinary erythropoietin
(B) increased bone marrow iron stores
(C) decreased carotid blood flow
(D) hypocellular bone marrow
(E) myelophthisic changes in their peripheral blood smear, including teardrop-shaped red blood cells and normoblasts

DIRECTIONS: Each question below contains five suggested responses. For **each** of the five responses listed with every question, you are to respond either YES (Y) or NO (N). In a given item **all, some, or none of the alternatives may be correct.**

510. True statements about hairy cell leukemia include which of the following?

(A) Palpable splenomegaly is present in only a minority of cases
(B) In approximately 30 percent of patients, an associated vasculitic disorder will develop, with erythema nodosum, other cutaneous nodules, or visceral involvement similar to that of polyarteritis nodosa
(C) Virtually all treated patients have exhibited a positive response to administration of α-interferon
(D) Infectious complications are unusual
(E) The disorder results from expansion of neoplastic B-lymphocytes, which sometimes produce a monoclonal immunoglobulin

511. Macrocytosis of red blood cells, in the absence of megaloblastic changes in the bone marrow, may be due to

(A) hypothyroidism
(B) malabsorption
(C) acute hemolysis
(D) total gastrectomy
(E) liver disease

512. Defective neutrophil chemotaxis occurs in association with

(A) chronic granulomatous disease
(B) glucocorticosteroid therapy
(C) alcoholism
(D) hereditary neutrophil hyposegmentation (Pelger-Huët anomaly)
(E) deficiency of complement component C3

513. Which of the following findings would distinguish β thalassemia trait from iron deficiency?

(A) Microcytic red blood cells
(B) Absence of anemia
(C) Elevated hemogloblin A_2 level
(D) Normal transferrin saturation
(E) Normal serum ferritin concentration

514. Which of the following laboratory results would be expected in a patient who had a splenectomy for hereditary spherocytosis 6 months ago?

(A) Elevated platelet count
(B) Elevated reticulocyte count
(C) Decreased serum haptoglobin concentration
(D) Predominance of microspherocytic red blood cells on peripheral blood smear
(E) Increased osmotic fragility of red blood cells

515. Persons who have sickle cell trait (AS hemoglobinopathy) have which of the following characteristics?

(A) Impaired growth and development in childhood
(B) Increased incidence of hematuria
(C) Impaired ability to concentrate urine
(D) Increased mortality rate in pregnant women
(E) Increased incidence of splenic infarction with high-altitude hypoxia

516. Methemoglobinemia is associated with

(A) cyanosis
(B) a shift to the left of the oxyhemoglobin dissociation curve
(C) oxidation of heme iron
(D) hemoglobinuria
(E) microcytic anemia

517. For the last 2 weeks, a 28-year-old previously healthy man has had progressive fatigue and spontaneous bruising. During the last 3 days, his temperature has risen to 38.9°C (102°F) and he has had shaking chills. Hemoglobin concentration is 72 g/L (7.2 g/dL); hematocrit, 18.0 percent; reticulocyte count, 0.1 percent; white blood cell count, 350/mm³; and platelet count, 8000/mm³. A bone marrow biopsy specimen is markedly hypocellular and consists primarily of nests of lymphocytes. Management at this point should include

(A) hospitalization
(B) androgen therapy
(C) empiric antibiotic therapy
(D) platelet transfusions from an HLA-compatible donor
(E) immediate preparation for bone marrow transplantation if an HLA-matched donor is identified

518. Adhesion of platelets to walls of injured blood vessels involves which of the following?

(A) Collagen
(B) Platelet glycoprotein Ia-IIa
(C) Platelet glycoprotein Ib
(D) Platelet glycoprotein IIb-IIIa
(E) von Willebrand factor

519. A patient being treated for refractory anemia has required monthly transfusions of two units of packed red blood cells over the past several months. Three days after receiving two units of packed red blood cells for a hematocrit of 22 percent, the patient's hematocrit was 27 percent. One week after the transfusion the hematocrit is 22 percent; the patient feels ill, has a low-grade fever, and is mildly jaundiced. Correct statements about this situation include which of the following?

(A) This problem is probably due to leukocyte alloimmunization
(B) Intravascular hemolysis has probably occurred
(C) The Rh status of donor and recipient should be rechecked
(D) If the patient is Rh-negative, one should look for anti-Kell or anti-Duffy antibodies in the patient's serum
(E) A positive direct Coombs test is likely

520. True statements regarding *both* hemophilia A (factor VII deficiency) and hemophilia B (factor IX deficiency) include

(A) the defective gene is located on the X chromosome
(B) the affected factors require vitamin K for biologic activity
(C) the partial thromboplastin time is elevated, but the prothrombin time is normal
(D) joint bleeding is common
(E) the optimal therapy is fresh frozen plasma

521. The absence of ristocetin-induced platelet aggregation is associated with which of the following clinical disorders?

(A) Glanzmann's thrombasthenia
(B) Bernard-Soulier syndrome
(C) Aspirin ingestion
(D) Storage pool disease
(E) von Willebrand's disease

522. Myeloproliferative disorders characteristically are associated with which of the following potential complications?

(A) Opportunistic infection
(B) Carcinoma
(C) Excessive bleeding
(D) Thromboembolism
(E) Acute myelogenous leukemia

523. Stable-phase chronic myelogenous leukemia (CML) is associated with which of the following?

(A) Splenomegaly
(B) Eosinophilia
(C) Elevated leukocyte alkaline phosphatase
(D) Diagnostic bone marrow findings
(E) Favorable response to hydroxyurea, busulfan, or α-interferon

524. Acute graft-versus-host disease after allogeneic bone marrow transplantation is typically associated with involvement of the

(A) gastrointestinal tract
(B) heart
(C) lung
(D) liver
(E) skin

DIRECTIONS: The group of questions below consists of five lettered headings followed by a set of numbered items. For each numbered item select the **one** lettered heading with which it is **most** closely associated. Each lettered heading may be used **once, more than once, or not at all.**

Questions 525–529

For each case history that follows, select the peripheral blood smear pictured in Color Plates T through X with which it is most likely to be associated.

(A)   Color Plate B
(B)   Color Plate C
(C)   Color Plate D
(D)   Color Plate E
(E)   Color Plate F

525. A 68-year-old man complains of painful and discolored fingers. Physical examination reveals acrocyanosis and mild scleral icterus. Hematocrit is 26 percent, and reticulocyte count 9 percent

526. A 48-year-old woman is found to be anemic 3 years after mastectomy for breast carcinoma

527. A 39-year-old man presents with abdominal pain and is found to have gallstones. Physical examination reveals splenomegaly. Hematocrit is 33 percent, and reticulocyte count 8 percent

528. A previously healthy 50-year-old woman is brought to the hospital after a focal motor seizure. Hematocrit is 22 percent; reticulocyte count, 11 percent; white blood cell count, 12,200/mm^3; platelet count, 25,000/mm^3; blood urea nitrogen, 16 mmol/L (45 mg/dL); prothrombin time, normal; and partial thromboplastin time, normal

529. A healthy 22-year-old black man is found to be slightly anemic on routine screening. Physical examination is normal. Hemoglobin is 122 g/L (12.2 g/dL), and MCV is 64.7 fL

Disorders of the Hematopoietic System

Answers

485. The answer is E. *(Wilson, ed 12. chaps 290, 295.)* The affinity of the hemoglobin molecule for oxygen is altered primarily by blood pH, temperature, red blood cell concentration of 2,3-diphosphoglycerate (2,3-DPG), and arterial carbon dioxide tension. Increased affinity, such as is produced by a rise in pH or a drop in 2,3-DPG, temperature, or P_{CO_2}, favors the transport of oxygen to body tissue. That is, under these conditions, at a given P_{O_2} a greater percentage of hemoglobin will be saturated with oxygen and more oxygen can be carried by the blood. Reduced affinity for oxygen favors unloading of oxygen from the hemoglobin molecule to the tissues—or, at a given P_{O_2} less oxygen will be bound to hemoglobin. Carbon monoxide causes hemoglobin to bind oxygen more avidly. Hyperventilation, by lowering P_{CO_2} and raising pH, and hypophosphatemia, by reducing levels of 2,3-DPG, both increase affinity. Methemoglobin binds oxygen more avidly than hemoglobin, therefore impairing the release of oxygen to the tissues.

486. The answer is B. *(Wilson, ed 12. chap 296. Pizzo, Am J Med 76:436, 1984.)* If not attacked promptly, infection in neutropenic patients can be quickly fatal. Often, these patients display neither the signs nor the symptoms of infection. Fever should be regarded as an indication of infection, and antibiotic therapy should begin immediately after appropriate cultures are obtained. An effective initial antibiotic regimen would consist of a cephalosporin, carbenicillin, and gentamicin. Gammaglobulin is of little benefit in the treatment of cancer patients. Granulocyte transfusions and amphotericin administration may be of benefit in selected cases.

487. The answer is A. *(Wilson, ed 12. chap 296. Henderson, ed 5. chap 15.)* Approximately 60 percent of cases of ALL are termed *common ALL*. The cells are positive for terminal deoxynucleotidyl transferase (Tdt), express the common ALL antigen, and express neither T-cell antigens nor surface immunoglobulin. About 20 percent of cases of ALL are of the T-cell type and occur typically as described above. Less than 5 percent of cases of ALL are of the B-cell type. The cells in this form of the illness frequently express a monoclonal surface immunoglobulin, are Tdt-negative, and have the cytogenetic abnormalities also associated with Burkitt's lymphoma, another B-cell neoplasm. While there are only subtle clinical differences among the subtypes of AML, the DIC associated with the M3 (promyelocytic) variant may be profound, is typically present at the time of diagnosis, and may be exacerbated markedly during chemotherapy.

488. The answer is B. *(Wilson, ed 12. chap 289.)* Several reports have recently described the association of coumarin-induced skin necrosis in patients with congenital protein C deficiency. The skin lesions occur on the breasts, buttocks, legs, and penis. They appear to be a result of diffuse thrombosis of the venules with interstitial bleeding. This condition is presumed to result from an imbalance in hemostatic mechanism activity favoring thrombosis during the early phases of coumarin administration; a rapid drop in the effective concentration of protein C, which has a relatively short half-life within the circulation (about 14 h) compared with that of some of the procoagulant vitamin K–dependent procoagulant clotting factors (factor X and prothrombin), could produce such a situation.

489. The answer is A. *(Wilson, ed 12. chap 64. Young, Clin Haematol 9:483, 1980.)* Severe neutropenia is a rare idiosyncratic reaction to certain drugs, including propylthiouracil. In addition to having sore throat and oral and anal mucosal ulcerations, affected persons are susceptible to overwhelming, life-threatening infections. However, in the absence of fever or clinical signs of infection, they should be followed as outpatients, saving them exposure to nosocomial pathogens in the hospital. Empirical use of broad-spectrum antibiotics without fever or other signs of infection is not advisable, and corticosteroid therapy is not useful. White blood cell transfusion can be accompanied by serious morbidity (particularly, pulmonary leukostasis) and should be reserved for persons with transient neutropenia and documented septicemia. Because severe drug-induced neutropenia is generally self-limited once use of the offending drug has been stopped, consideration of bone marrow transplantation is not justified.

490. The answer is D. *(Wilson, ed 12. chap 63.)* The spleen is responsible for removing senescent red blood cells from the circulation. The older, less deformable red blood cells cannot pass through the slitlike passages in splenic sinuses and are phagocytosed by red pulp macrophages. In the absence of a spleen, particulate matter of the red blood cells, such as nuclear material (Howell-Jolly bodies) or hemoglobin (Heinz bodies), that is normally pinched off during passage of red blood cells through the spleen remains visible on examination of the peripheral smear. Red cells that escape the marrow with a nucleus still present and target forms with excess membrane are normally handled by the spleen as well. The spherocytic red cells characteristically produced by extravascular antibody-mediated hemolysis and splenic conditioning would not likely be observed after splenectomy.

491. The answer is A. *(Wilson, ed 12. chap 294. Byrne, Clin Haematol 15:413, 1986.)* This young women is suffering from a combination of hemolytic anemia with fragmented red cells in the absence of disseminated intravascular coagulation (DIC), thrombocytopenia, fever, mental status changes, and renal dysfunction, which is essentially pathognomonic of thrombotic thrombocytopenic purpura (TTP). The etiology of TTP is unknown, though immunologic and primary vasculopathic phenomena have been associated with this disorder. Pathologically, arteriolar hyalinization, which is also seen in DIC, may be noted. Seventy percent of patients with TTP improve with exchange transfusion or plasmapheresis. Glucocorticoids, antiplatelet agents, splenectomy, and vincristine have been of benefit to subsets of patients, but each is less effective and probably associated with a greater risk than therapeutic plasmapheresis.

492. The answer is A. *(Wilson, ed 12. chap 294. Schreiber, N Engl J Med 309:723, 1983.)* Paroxysmal nocturnal hemoglobinuria (PNH) is an acquired disease caused by injury to or mutation in the bone marrow stem-cell pool. PNH can develop following recovery from aplastic anemia, and pancytopenia becomes evident in many affected persons sometime during the course of their illness. Iron deficiency, resulting from urinary iron loss, is a frequent complication of the chronic, intermittent, intravascular hemolysis associated with PNH. Thrombosis is a major cause of morbidity and mortality. In a minority of affected patients, PNH transforms into acute myelogenous leukemia. Functional leukocyte defects have been demonstrated in the disease, and the leukocyte alkaline phosphatase level is typically reduced (as in chronic myelogenous leukemia). Deficiency of a complement regulatory protein in cell membranes is believed to account for the sensitivity to intravascular hemolysis.

493. The answer is A. *(Wilson, ed 12. chap 291.)* Lead poisoning causes defective heme synthesis by interfering with a number of steps in the heme synthetic pathway. In severe cases, a hypochromic, microcytic anemia results. However, iron deficiency is not present, and serum iron levels may actually be increased in affected adults. Iron deficiency results from chronic, recurrent gastrointestinal bleeding in persons with hereditary hemorrhagic telangiectasia and from pulmonary bleeding in persons with idiopathic pulmonary hemosiderosis. Chronic heart-valve hemolysis leads to intravascular liberation of hemoglobin and iron depletion through hemoglobinuria and hemosiderinuria. Iron deficiency can occur from recurrent blood loss during hemodialysis.

494. The answer is E. *(Wilson, ed 12. chap 291. Henderson, ed 5. chap 24.)* A slightly increased mean corpuscular volume and an inappropriately low reticulocyte count are characteristic of a macrocytic, hypoproliferative anemia. Iron-deficiency anemia is accompanied by microcytic red blood cell indices, and autoimmune hemolytic anemia typically is associated with reticulocytosis, unless a coexisting process, such as folate deficiency, interferes with the bone marrow erythropoietic response. Aplastic anemia and acute leukemia are unlikely diagnoses if white blood cell count and platelet count are normal. A macrocytic, hypoproliferative anemia in the older man described in the question would most likely be due to a myelodysplastic syndrome. A bone marrow examination with iron stain would be required to define the precise subtype of this heterogeneous disorder, which is characterized by a stem cell defect leading to disordered hematopoietic maturation. Given the normal platelet count and white blood cell count, either refractory anemia or refractory anemia with ringed sideroblasts is the most likely subtype. Certain acquired primary sideroblastic anemias, especially those without associated dysplastic changes in white cells or platelets, can be thought of as a defect in iron incorporation into heme and present with microcytosis.

495. The answer is A. *(Wilson, ed 12. chap 291. Bothwell, Semin Hematol 19:54, 1982.)* Serum iron and transferrin saturation, ferritin level, and desferrioxamine challenge are comparably sensitive, noninvasive tests of iron stores. They may all be normal in the early stages of iron overload, such as in precirrhotic affected family members of persons with idiopathic hemochromatosis. The most sensitive test for detecting early iron overload is a quantitative iron analysis, usually determined by atomic absorption spectroscopy, of a liver biopsy specimen.

496. The answer is E. *(Wilson, ed 12. chap 292.)* Antiparietal-cell antibodies are detected in 90 percent of persons with pernicious anemia but also in persons with atrophic gastritis and 10 to 15 percent of an unselected patient population. Although folate in large doses can correct the megaloblastic anemia of pernicious anemia, it does not correct the neurologic abnormalities. Megaloblastic anemias are characterized by ineffective erythropoiesis and bone marrow erythroid hyperplasia. Hypergastrinemia accompanies the achlorhydria of pernicious anemia. Marrow morphology begins to improve within hours of parenteral B_{12} therapy; reticulocytosis peaks in 1 week. Life-threatening hypokalemia may occur early in the course of therapy.

497. The answer is E. *(Wilson, ed 12. chap 293. Lee, Semin Hematol 20:61, 1983.)* A mild-to-moderate degree of anemia often accompanies chronic infectious, inflammatory, or neoplastic diseases. Typically, the anemia of chronic disease is normochromic and normocytic to microcytic. Bone marrow examination reveals normal erythroid maturation. Neither significant disturbance of hemoglobin synthesis nor hemolysis occurs in this type of anemia. Affected persons usually have a low serum iron concentration and a low total transferrin level (resulting in essentially normal or only slightly decreased fractional transferrin saturation). Even though storage iron is abundant, there is a decreased amount of iron in erythroblasts, reflecting a defect in the transfer of reticuloendothelial iron to developing red blood cells.

498. The answer is C. *(Wilson, ed 12. chap 294. Rosse, Clin Haematol 14:105, 1985.)* Paroxysmal nocturnal hemoglobinuria, an acquired disorder of the bone marrow stem cell, affects not only red blood cells but also platelets and granulocytes. Like related myeloproliferative disorders (e.g., chronic myelogenous leukemia, essential thrombocythemia, polycythemia vera, myeloid metaplasia, and myelofibrosis), paroxysmal nocturnal hemoglobinuria may lead to acute myelogenous leukemia. Lymphoma, particularly involving the central nervous system, may develop in renal transplant recipients on immunosuppressive therapy as well as in persons with Wiskott-Aldrich syndrome. Persons who have Hodgkin's disease and have been treated with both radiation therapy and chemotherapy are at risk for developing leukemia. Acquired idiopathic refractory sideroblastic anemia leads to acute leukemia in about 10 percent of cases, but this phenomenon does not occur in hereditary forms of sideroblastic anemia.

499. The answer is D. *(Wilson, ed 12. chap 294. Jandl, chap 11.)* The gene for glucose 6-phosphate dehydrogenase (G6PD) is located on the X chromosome; thus, G6PD deficiency is a sex-linked trait. Hemolytic anemia occurs much more commonly in males than in heterozygote female carriers, who usually are asymptomatic. Of the more than 100 variants of G6PD, the most commonly encountered variant of clinical significance in the United States is the A− type, which is found in about 15 percent of black males. It generally causes less severe hemolysis than the Mediterranean variant. Hemolysis usually is precipitated by an environmental oxidant stress, most commonly viral or bacterial infection. Certain drugs, such as antimalarial agents, sulfonamides, phenacetin, and vitamin K, also can trigger hemolysis. These oxidant stresses cause precipitation of hemoglobin, because affected persons are unable to maintain adequate intracellular levels of reduced glutathione. Precipitated hemoglobin forms Heinz bodies that are visualized only with supravital stains; these inclusions cause premature destruction of the red cells. The diagnosis should be considered in any person experiencing a hemolytic episode. However, since decreased G6PD levels are found mainly in older cells, a false negative test may be obtained during a hemolytic crisis, and the test should be repeated upon recovery.

500. The answer is C. *(Wilson, ed 12. chap 295.)* Several hemoglobin variants have an increased affinity for oxygen. This abnormality causes defective oxygen unloading to tissues, leading to erythropoietin-mediated erythrocytosis. Because reduced tissue oxygen delivery usually is compensated for fully by the development of erythrocytosis, levels of red-cell 2,3-diphosphoglycerate (2,3-DPG) are normal. Routine hemoglobin electrophoresis often is normal with these variants, and red blood cell morphology is not altered. Affected persons are not at a disadvantage when exposed to hypoxic conditions.

501. The answer is B. *(Wilson, ed 12. chap 298.)* Pure red blood cell aplasia is characterized by a normochromic, normocytic anemia and little production of reticulocytes. Erythroblasts are selectively absent from the bone marrow of affected persons; white blood cell and platelet production is preserved. In contrast to aplastic anemia, the bone marrow in persons with pure red blood cell aplasia is normocellular or even hypercellular. Iron kinetic studies reveal prolonged plasma iron clearance and reduced iron turnover. Erythropoietin levels usually are markedly elevated.

502. The answer is D. *(Wilson, ed 12. chaps 62, 288.)* A marked prolongation of the prothrombin time with a normal partial thromboplastin time localizes the hemostatic defect to the extrinsic limb of the coagulation cascade. Congenital factor VII deficiency is a rare, autosomal recessive disorder. Factor VIII deficiency and the presence of specific inhibitors directed towards a coagulation factor (most commonly factor VIII) would be associated with a prolongation of the partial thromboplastin time. Nonspecific inhibitors (lupus anticoagulants) most commonly are associated with prolongation of the partial thromboplastin time and occasionally with prolongation of the prothrombin time (particularly when hypoprothrombinemia is present). Patients with alpha$_2$-antiplasmin deficiency have a bleeding disorder associated with accelerated clot lysis. Both the prothrombin time and the partial thromboplastin time are normal in these persons.

503. The answer is B. *(Wilson, ed 12. chaps 287, 297.)* The hemolytic-uremic syndrome occurs predominantly in children and is related to thrombotic thrombocytopenic purpura. It is characterized by microangiopathic hemolytic anemia and thrombocytopenia. Polycythemia vera, as well as the other myeloproliferative disorders, often is associated with thrombocytosis. Thrombocytosis also is a long-term sequela of splenectomy or splenic infarction (e.g., in sickle cell disease) and chronic inflammatory states (e.g., inflammatory bowel disease). For reasons that are unclear, thrombocytosis frequently is associated with iron deficiency.

504. The answer is C. *(Wilson, ed 12. chap 287.)* The onset of severe thrombocytopenia after an antecedent viral illness is common in children with a diagnosis of idiopathic thrombocytopenic purpura (ITP). Unlike childhood ITP, adult ITP tends to be a chronic disease in which spontaneous remissions are rare, and a majority of patients will have a fall in their platelet count after the withdrawal of corticosteroids, necessitating elective splenectomy. The presence of antibodies directed against target antigens on the glycoprotein IIb-IIIa complex has been noted in some adults with chronic ITP but not in children. Splenomegaly is not a feature of ITP; it is a common finding in patients with secondary thrombocytopenia.

505. The answer is C. *(Wilson, ed 12. chap 288.)* The presence of nonspecific anticoagulants (lupus type) may predispose patients to thrombosis and is also associated with habitual abortions in some women. Patients with congenital dysfibrinogenemias may have variable results on screening coagulation tests. They often have slight prolongations in the prothrombin times or partial thromboplastin times, prolonged thrombin times, and a disparity between functional and immunologic assays of fibrinogen. Despite these abnormalities, patients may have either no symptoms or moderate bleeding, and a few dysfibrinogenemias have been associated with hypercoagulability. Congenital deficiencies of antithrombin III and protein C are familial thrombotic disorders and are not associated with abnormalities of the various clotting times. Factor XI deficiency is an autosomal recessive disorder often associated with bleeding following trauma or during the perioperative period.

506. The answer is A. *(Wilson, ed 12. chap 287.)* Electrophoretic analysis has allowed the delineation of three major types of defects in von Willebrand's disease (vWD). The most common abnormality (type I disease) is characterized by a moderate decrease in the plasma level of von Willebrand factor (vWF antigen) resulting from defective release of the protein from endothelial cells. There are usually concordant reductions in antihemophilic factor or factor VIII coagulant activity as well as ristocetin cofactor activity.

The various forms of type II disease are characterized by normal or near normal levels of dysfunctional protein. In both types IIa and IIb, there is a loss in high-molecular-weight multimers on SDS-agarose electrophoresis. In type IIa patients, the pattern is caused by either an inability to assemble the larger multimers or by premature catabolism in the circulation. In contrast, patients with type IIb have inappropriate binding of the abnormal, larger vWF forms to platelets, which results in the formation of intravascular platelet aggregates. These are rapidly cleared from the circulation, which causes mild, cyclic thrombocytopenia.

A severe recessive form of vWD (type III disease) results from reduced synthesis of vWF by endothelial cells. A hyperactive platelet receptor (glycoprotein Ib) with increased affinity for larger vWF multimers is the defect in so-called platelet-type vWD, or pseudo-vWD. The gene encoding vWF has been cloned and localized to chromosome 12.

507. The answer is C. *(Wilson, ed 12. chaps 62, 288.)* Factor XIII deficiency may be inherited or acquired and frequently causes severe bleeding problems. In this disorder, the bleeding time, prothrombin time, and partial thromboplastin time (PTT) are all normal. The screening test for factor XIII deficiency is a clot solubility assay. Persons with deficiencies of factor XII (Hageman factor) or prekallikrein often have dramatic prolongations of the PTT, but do not have bleeding problems even with surgery or trauma. The presence of a normal bleeding time excludes thrombasthenia, an inherited disorder in which there is defective-platelet aggregation in response to agonists that require fibrinogen binding, such as adenosine diphosphate, thrombin, or epinephrine. Protein S is a vitamin K–dependent plasma protein and a cofactor for the expression of the anticoagulant activity of activated protein C. Familial protein S deficiency is associated with a thrombotic diathesis.

508. The answer is E. *(Wilson, ed 12. chap 288.)* This patient has chronic disseminated intravascular coagulation in association with an abdominal aortic aneurysm. The prothrombin time and partial thromboplastin time are prolonged and the fibrinogen level is decreased on the basis of consumption. Appropriate therapy would include administration of fresh frozen plasma, while cryoprecipitate, a source of only factor VIII and fibrinogen, would be inadequate. Plasma exchange transfusions are the treatment of choice for thrombotic thrombocytopenic purpura. Aminocaproic acid (Amicar) is contraindicated in this setting, because it inhibits fibrinolysis and can therefore potentially induce thrombosis. The degree of thrombocytopenia is not of sufficient severity to require platelet transfusions.

509. The answer is C. *(Wilson, ed 12. chap 297.)* Persons with polycythemia vera and a hematocrit greater than 45 percent usually have diminished cerebral blood flow and are particularly at risk for developing thrombotic complications. Functional platelet abnormalities may cause both thrombotic and bleeding problems (the gastrointestinal tract is a common site of bleeding), and affected persons frequently are iron-deficient even at the time of presentation. Erythropoietin production is suppressed in polycythemia vera, a disease characterized by loss of normal control of erythroid stem-cell proliferation. The bone marrow is hypercellular, with hyperplasia of all marrow elements. Therapy is aimed at reducing the hematocrit below 45 percent.

510. The answer is A-N, B-Y, C-Y, D-N, E-Y. *(Wilson, ed 12. chap 296. Golomb, Blood 69:979, 1987.)* More than 75 percent of patients with hairy cell leukemia (HCL) will have clinically apparent splenomegaly, which in some cases may be massive. The cornerstone of therapy is splenectomy, which may ameliorate the disease in most patients. Associated vasculitis is relatively common in patients with HCL, in contrast to other leukemias. Therapy with α-interferon has been shown to be effective in a large fraction of patients and is generally quite well tolerated. Infection is the most common cause of death in patients with HCL, and common infecting organisms include *Legionella,* atypical mycobacteria, *Nocardia, Toxoplasma,* and the more usual pyogenic organisms. The malignant cell is a B lymphocyte with the characteristic cytoplasmic projections from which the disorder derives its name. The cells stain positively for tartrate-resistant acid phosphatase (TRAP) and frequently produce a monoclonal immunoglobulin.

511. The answer is A-Y, B-N, C-Y, D-N, E-Y. *(Wilson, ed 12. chaps 61, 292.)* Macrocytosis of red blood cells may be caused by defective DNA synthesis (i.e., megaloblastic anemias), among other factors. Reticulocytosis due to either blood loss or hemolysis may be associated with macrocytic indices, because reticulocytes are about 20 percent larger than mature red blood cells. Increased red-cell membrane surface area due to increased membrane cholesterol incorporation occurs in liver disease and obstructive jaundice. In hypothyroidism, nonmegaloblastic macrocytic anemia develops; the cause is unclear. Vitamin B_{12} and folate deficiency states, following total gastrectomy or accompanying malabsorption syndromes, cause megaloblastic anemia.

512. The answer is A-N, B-Y, C-Y, D-N, E-Y. *(Wilson, ed 12. chap 64.)* The stages of neutrophil defense against bacterial invasion include chemotaxis, phagocytosis, and microbicide. Accumulation of neutrophils in response to inflammation (chemotaxis) is impaired by alcohol and glucocorticosteroids. Neutrophil dysfunction may occur with various complement abnormalities; C3 deficiency, for example, results in both defective chemotaxis and defective phagocytosis. In chronic granulomatous disease, bacterial infections occur owing to failure of the normal metabolic burst following phagocytosis as well as to impaired generation of bactericidal free oxygen radicals; chemotaxis and phagocytosis are normal. Hereditary neutrophil hyposegmentation (Pelger-Huët anomaly) is not associated with abnormal neutrophil function.

513. The answer is A-N, B-N, C-Y, D-Y, E-Y. *(Wilson, ed 12. chaps 291, 295.)* Iron deficiency frequently is confused with thalassemia trait, both α and β, in that all three of these conditions are characterized by a microcytic anemia. Iron stores, as reflected by transferrin saturation, serum ferritin level, and bone marrow iron staining, are depleted in iron deficiency but normal in both types of thalassemia trait. Hemoglobin electrophoresis reveals an increased hemoglobin A_2 level in β-thalassemia trait but subnormal levels in iron deficiency and α-thalassemia trait. (In the presence of concomitant iron deficiency, hemoglobin A_2 levels may be normal in persons with β-thalassemia, but levels rise once iron stores are replenished.)

514. The answer is A-Y, B-N, C-N, D-Y, E-Y. *(Wilson, ed 12. chap 294.)* Because the spleen is the primary site of destruction of abnormal red blood cells in persons with hereditary spherocytosis, splenectomy generally restores hematologic laboratory indices to normal. Reticulocyte count decreases, and serum haptoglobin concentration, which may be low as a result of extravascular as well as intravascular hemolysis, also returns to normal following splenectomy. Although hemolysis is ameliorated by splenectomy, the intrinsic erythrocyte membrane defect is unaffected, as reflected by the persistence of increased osmotic fragility and the presence of microspherocytes on peripheral blood smear. Postsplenectomy thrombocytosis may persist for years.

515. The answer is A-N, B-Y, C-Y, D-N, E-Y. *(Wilson, ed 12. chap 295.)* Hematuria and hyposthenuria both are increased in incidence in sickle-cell trait; the mechanism of both abnormalities probably is related to the relatively hypertonic, acidotic, and hypoxic conditions of the renal medulla, which predispose to local sickling. Splenic infarction may develop at altitudes above approximately 3000 meters (10,000 feet) during flights in unpressurized airplanes. A prospective study of matched pairs of individuals has shown no deficits in standard measurements of growth and development in children with sickle cell trait when compared with other children. Mortality rates during pregnancy are not affected appreciably by sickle cell trait.

516. The answer is A-Y, B-Y, C-Y, D-N, E-N. *(Wilson, ed 12. chap 295.)* Methemoglobin is the type of hemoglobin in which iron has been oxidized to the ferric form. It accumulates in excess when red blood cells are exposed to oxidant stress and when they are deficient in enzymatic reduction mechanisms. Methemoglobin cannot bind oxygen, and excessive concentrations of methemoglobin lead to a progressive increase in oxygen affinity of the remaining functioning heme residues on the hemoglobin tetramer (i.e., shift to the left of the oxyhemoglobin dissociation curve). A methemoglobin level greater than 15 g/L (1.5 g/dL) causes visible cyanosis. Methemoglobinemia is not associated with hemolysis or red-cell morphologic changes.

517. The answer is A-Y, B-N, C-Y, D-N, E-Y. *(Wilson, ed 12. chaps 298, 299.)* Severe aplastic anemia is defined as marked pancytopenia: neutrophil count less than 500/mm^3; platelet count less than 20,000/mm^3; and anemia accompanied by a reticulocyte count less than 1 percent. Affected persons have a poor prognosis for spontaneous recovery, with bleeding and infection as the major causes of morbidity and mortality. A febrile, neutropenic patient should be hospitalized; potential sources of infection should be sought promptly by culture, and empiric broad-spectrum antibiotic therapy should begin immediately, to be modified subsequently according to culture results. Androgens do not appear to be beneficial in treating severe aplastic anemia but may stimulate the marrow in milder cases. In severe aplastic anemia occurring in younger persons having an HLA-matched donor, prompt bone marrow transplantation is the treatment of choice. If a bone marrow transplant is considered, HLA-compatible family members should not be used as blood donors; this avoids sensitization of the potential recipient to minor transplantation antigens.

518. The answer is A-Y, B-Y, C-Y, D-N, E-Y. *(Wilson, ed 12. chap 62.)* The formation of a platelet plug at the site of vascular injury (i.e., primary hemostasis) requires adhesion of platelets, release of granules, and aggregation of platelets. The first of these three processes depends on the binding of platelets to deepithelialized vessel walls through an interaction between basement membrane collagen and the collagen receptor, composed of platelet glycoproteins Ia and IIa. This link is stabilized by the binding of von Willebrand factor, a multimeric adhesive glycoprotein, to platelet glycoprotein Ib. The adherent platelets then release a host of mediators that serve to promote secretion of granules of platelets, aggregation of platelets, and activation of the coagulation cascade. Dense granules of platelets release adenosine diphosphate, which allows fibrinogen to serve as a bridge between platelets via platelet glycoprotein IIb-IIIa so that aggregation may occur.

519. The answer is A-N, B-N, C-Y, D-Y, E-Y. *(Wilson, ed 12. chap 286.)* The clinical scenario is consistent with a delayed transfusion reaction. Immediate transfusion reactions, which are most commonly due to ABO incompatibility and result from clerical error, are associated with intravascular hemolysis (anti-A and anti-B antibodies fix complement) manifested by lumbar pain, hemoglobinemia, and shock. Fever, malaise, and a drop in hematocrit with findings compatible with extravascular hemolysis (microspherocytes, indirect hyperbilirubinemia) 1 week after red-cell transfusion are typical of a delayed transfusion reaction, which is usually mediated by antibodies to Rh (or if the recipient is Rh-negative, by anti-Duffy, anti-Kidd, or anti-Kell antibodies). A previous transfusion may have been the precursor of the clinically relevant anamnestic response. These antibodies likely coat the donor red cells, thereby producing a positive direct Coombs test. Less commonly the donor's plasma could contain antibodies that would react with the recipient's cells. Sensitization to the alloantigens on donor leukocytes transfused along with the red cells could account for fever, but not hemolysis.

520. The answer is A-Y, B-N, C-Y, D-Y, E-N. *(Wilson, ed 12. chap 288.)* Hemophilia A and B are clinically indistinguishable, X-linked disorders that cause bleeding into soft tissues, muscles, and weight-bearing joints. In both disorders, all tests of coagulation are normal except for an elevation of the partial thromboplastin time. Specific-factor assays are required to define a specific disorder. Factor VIII is a 265-kilodalton protein that regulates the activation of factor X by intrinsic pathway proteases. Factor IX, which unlike factor VIII requires vitamin K–dependent, posttranslational modification, is a 55-kilodalton proenzyme converted to activated factor IXa by factor XIa. Factor IXa activates factor X with the participation of factor VIII. The distinction between these two entities is important because the therapy is different. The therapy of choice in hemophilia A (without a serum inhibitor) is factor VIII concentrate or cryoprecipitate. Recently developed heat-treated or monoclonally purified (or recombinantly derived, if available) formulations of factor VIII should be used to minimize the risk of AIDS. Either fresh frozen plasma or prothrombin complex proteins should be used to treat hemophilia B. The latter product carries the special risk of unbridled activation of the coagulation system and thrombotic complications.

521. The answer is A-N, B-Y, C-N, D-N, E-Y. *(Wilson, ed 12. chap 287.)* The interaction of von Willebrand's factor (vWF) with the platelet is most readily studied in vitro by measuring the effect of the antibiotic ristocetin on platelet aggregation. Patients whose platelets are not aggregated by ristocetin either lack vWF activity (most persons with von Willebrand's disease except those with the type IIb variant) or the platelet receptor for vWF (glycoprotein Ib). The latter situation is found in the Bernard-Soulier syndrome, a rare clinical condition also characterized by reduced levels of several other platelet membrane proteins, mild thrombocytopenia, and large, lymphocytoid platelets. Platelets from patients with Glanzmann's thrombasthenia are deficient in the glycoprotein IIb-IIIa complex. This receptor serves as the binding site for fibrinogen in platelet-platelet interactions. Hence, thrombasthenic platelets adhere normally and will agglutinate with ristocetin but will not aggregate with any of the agonists that require fibrinogen binding, such as adenosine diphosphate (ADP), thrombin, or epinephrine. Aspirin specifically acetylates the platelet cyclooxygenase enzyme and decreases the production of thromboxane A_2. This results in a defect in secondary platelet aggregation in response to agonists such as ADP and epinephrine. A similar situation is found in persons with storage pool disease whose platelet granules lack releasable stores of ADP and serotonin.

522. The answer is A-N, B-N, C-Y, D-Y, E-Y. *(Wilson, ed 12. chap 297.)* The myeloproliferative disorders (polycythemia vera, essential thrombocythemia, chronic myelogenous leukemia, myeloid metaplasia, and myelofibrosis) are a group of related diseases of the bone marrow stem cell. All cell lines—erythroid, myeloid, and megakaryocytic—are affected. Several functional platelet defects have been identified in these disorders and result paradoxically in both bleeding and thromboembolic complications, which are the major causes of morbidity and mortality. All myeloproliferative disorders may develop into acute leukemia, especially if alkylating agents are used in treatment. Although abnormal white blood cell function also may be associated with these disorders, opportunistic infections generally are not encountered.

523. The answer is A-Y, B-N, C-N, D-N, E-Y. *(Henderson, ed 5. chap 22. Wilson, ed 12. chap 297.)* Chronic myelogenous leukemia (CML), a myeloproliferative disorder in which bone marrow stem cells are affected, can be diagnosed on clinical grounds alone. A bone marrow examination disclosing myeloid hyperplasia with basophilia would be supportive but not diagnostic. Every patient with CML has a Philadelphia chromosome (translocation between the long arms of chromosomes 22 and 9), which may be identified by either cytogenetic or molecular analysis. In addition to the cytogenetic abnormality, stable-phase CML is characterized by leukocytosis with a left shift, basophilia, splenomegaly, and a low leukocyte alkaline phosphatase (high in reactive leukocytosis and in agnogenic myeloid metaplasia). The duration of the stable phase is variable, but the disease always progresses on to blast crisis, unless interrupted by an allogeneic bone marrow transplant. The leukocytosis and metabolic symptoms of stable-phase CML can be controlled with a number of agents, including hydroxyurea, busulfan, and α-interferon. Except in preliminary results with certain patients treated with α-interferon, cells containing the Philadelphia chromosome remain.

524. The answer is A-Y, B-N, C-N, D-Y, E-Y. *(Wilson, ed 12. chap 299.)* An immunologic reaction of engrafted donor T cells against host tissues results in a clinically significant syndrome in about half of those receiving marrow from an HLA-identical sibling. Acute graft-versus-host disease (AGVHD) typically initially involves the skin. Diarrhea due to intestinal involvement is the most common symptom. A combined cholestatic and hepatic picture is seen as a consequence of liver disease. AGVHD can be treated successfully with cyclosporine, methotrexate, or steroids, or a combination of these agents. In an effort to abrogate AGVHD, trials using T-cell purging of donor marrows are underway. It is unknown whether such an effort will result in the deleterious consequences of increased rates of graft failure or leukemic relapse.

525–529. The answers are: 525-D, 526-E, 527-B, 528-A, 529-C. *(Wilson, ed 12. chap 61.)* In cold agglutinin disease (Color Plate E), cold-active IgM antibodies react against red blood cell antigens. Cold agglutinins may arise secondary to infections (particularly viral and *Mycoplasma* infections), in association with lymphoproliferative disorders (e.g., lymphoma), or in idiopathic cold agglutinin disease. Symptoms are due to vasoocclusion in cold-exposed regions of the circulation; fresh blood specimens may dramatically agglutinate during withdrawal into a cooler syringe.

Myelophthisic anemia occurs in situations in which bone marrow has been invaded by nonmarrow elements, such as granulomas, fibrous tissue (myelofibrosis), or metastatic tumor. The peripheral smear (Color Plate F) typically shows marked anisocytosis and poikilocytosis of the red blood cells, with "teardrop" forms, nucleated red cells, and sometimes a "leukoerythroblastic reaction," which is characterized by leukocytosis and immature white blood cells. The diagnosis is made by bone marrow biopsy.

Hereditary spherocytosis is a relatively common hemolytic anemia, in which intrinsically defective red blood cells are prematurely destroyed in a normally functioning spleen. Adults frequently develop gallstones from increased bilirubin production. Peripheral smears (Color Plate C) typically show a predominance of microspherocytes and variable polychromatophilia (reticulocytosis).

Thrombotic thrombocytopenic purpura is characterized by microangiopathic hemolytic anemia (with marked red-cell fragmentation in the peripheral smear—Color Plate B), thrombocytopenia, and widely variable and fluctuating neurologic abnormalities. Disseminated intravascular coagulation is not present, and prothrombin and partial thromboplastin times usually are normal. The typical pathologic lesion responsible for these changes is hyaline occlusion of small vessels.

α-Thalassemia trait and β-thalassemia trait usually are asymptomatic conditions, characterized by mild anemia and markedly microcytic red-cell indices. The blood smear (Color Plate D) typically reveals variable degrees of anisocytosis and poikilocytosis, target cells, cell fragments, misshapen cells, and basophilic stippling.

Neoplasia

DIRECTIONS: Each question below contains five suggested responses. Select the **one best** response to each question.

530. Distant systemic cancer most likely would produce which of the following neurologic syndromes?

(A) Myasthenia gravis
(B) Noninflammatory myopathy
(C) Cranial nerve palsies
(D) Generalized neuropathy
(E) Grand mal seizures

531. A 70-year-old man of Irish extraction returns to his physician for a routine check of his blood pressure. He is a vigorous, retired executive who except for mild hypertension is healthy. After his examination, as he is getting dressed, he states that his wife has been nagging him to mention a spot on his nose (as shown in Color Plate G). He is certain that this lesion, which has been present for several years, is of no significance. The most likely diagnosis for this lesion is

(A) dermal nevus
(B) sebaceous hyperplasia
(C) clear cell acanthoma
(D) xanthoma
(E) basal cell carcinoma

532. A 52-year-old woman sees her physician for an "insurance physical." Physical examination reveals only a pigmented lesion (as shown in Color Plate H) present on one foot. The woman states that the lesion apparently was present at birth and does not itch or bleed; it is, however, not as homogeneous in color as it used to be. Which of the following statements about the condition described is true?

(A) Bleeding and tenderness would be the first signs of malignant degeneration
(B) It is unlikely that the lesion, present since birth, is malignant
(C) It would be dangerous to perform an incisional biopsy of this lesion
(D) Change in color of the lesion is a suspicious sign for potential malignancy
(E) Early diagnosis of this lesion would not affect prognosis

533. All the following procedures for the detection of cancer for those over age 40 are recommended by the American Cancer Society EXCEPT

(A) yearly mammography (every 1 to 2 years for those 40 to 49 years old)
(B) yearly pelvic examination (with reduction in frequency after three consecutive normal examinations)
(C) yearly Pap smear (with reduction in frequency after three consecutive normal examinations)
(D) yearly digital rectal examination
(E) colonoscopy every 3 years

534. All the following hereditary syndromes are associated with the development of malignancies EXCEPT

(A) neurofibromatosis
(B) chronic granulomatous disease of childhood
(C) ataxia-telangiectasia
(D) familial polyposis coli
(E) Fanconi's anemia

535. Metabolic derangements associated with neoplastic diseases and their treatment can best be described by which of the following statements?

(A) Secondary gout is a common concomitant of lymphoproliferative neoplasms
(B) Acidification of the urine may help promote renal excretion of uric acid and prevent urate nephrolithiasis
(C) Cytotoxic therapy of highly drug-sensitive tumors may result in serious hyperphosphatemia, hypocalcemia, and hyperkalemia
(D) Lactic acidosis may be a complication of treatment of leukemia and Burkitt's lymphoma
(E) The excessive toxicity of mithramycin makes it an undesirable agent for the treatment of tumor-associated hypercalcemia

536. All the following statements describe characteristics of the superior vena cava (SVC) syndrome EXCEPT

(A) clinical features of the syndrome include conjunctival suffusion, lower extremity edema, and pulsus paradoxus
(B) administration of corticosteroids and diuretics may be useful as temporizing measures until a diagnosis is established
(C) carcinoma of the lung is the most common neoplasm associated with the syndrome
(D) the SVC syndrome is rarely a cause of death in patients in whom it develops
(E) definitive therapy should include local irradiation and, if possible, systemic chemotherapy for the neoplasm in question

537. Which of the following characteristics is more apt to be associated with Hodgkin's disease than with non-Hodgkin's lymphoma?

(A) ''B'' symptoms
(B) Involvement of Waldeyer's ring
(C) Extralymphatic presentation
(D) Dissemination at the time of diagnosis
(E) Most common type (60 percent) of lymphoma

538. In persons who have chronic myelogenous leukemia, the Philadelphia chromosome most commonly is found in

(A) all cells of the body
(B) all three hematopoietic cell lines but not in nonhematopoietic cells
(C) all cells of the granulocytic cell line but not in nongranulocytic cells
(D) all morphologically abnormal (malignant-appearing) granulocytes
(E) occasional malignant-appearing granulocytes

539. Which of the following statements describes the relationship between testicular tumors and serum markers?

(A) Pure seminomas produce α-fetoprotein (AFP) or β-human chorionic gonadotropin (β-HCG) in more than 90 percent of cases
(B) More than 40 percent of nonseminomatous germ cell tumors produce no cell markers
(C) Both β-HCG and AFP should be measured in following the progress of a tumor
(D) Measurement of tumor markers the day following surgery for localized disease is useful in determining completeness of the resection
(E) β-HCG is limited in its usefulness as a marker, because it is identical to human luteinizing hormone

540. The cytotoxic action of anticancer agents is thought to be defined by first-order kinetics, which means that these agents

(A) kill a constant fraction of tumor cells
(B) kill a constant number of tumor cells
(C) kill a number of tumor cells directly proportional to the time of exposure to the agent
(D) kill a number of tumor cells directly proportional to the molar concentration of the agent
(E) act directly on cells and do not require metabolism to an intermediate

541. All the following statements regarding toxic effects of chemotherapy are correct EXCEPT

(A) of all the antineoplastic agents, anthracyclines suppress bone marrow stem cells to the greatest degree
(B) vincristine is a relatively weak myelosuppressive agent and can be administered during periods of low blood counts
(C) cisplatin-induced nausea and vomiting can be controlled by metoclopramide or dexamethasone or both
(D) the use of melphalan (phenylalanine mustard) has been associated with secondary leukemia
(E) cisplatin can produce hypocalcemia by inducing renal electrolyte wasting

542. All the following predispose patients to an increased risk of developing malignant lymphoma EXCEPT

(A) Chédiak-Higashi syndrome
(B) AIDS
(C) rheumatoid arthritis
(D) multiple sclerosis
(E) phenytoin

543. The use of tamoxifen, an antiestrogen agent, in treating women with metastatic breast cancer is LEAST likely to cause

(A) hot flashes
(B) nausea
(C) virilization
(D) fluid retention
(E) acute hypercalcemia

544. A 59-year-old postmenopausal woman underwent radical mastectomy 3 years ago for carcinoma of the breast. All nodes biopsied were negative, and the estrogen receptor status of the tumor was positive at 150 fmol/mg of cytosol protein. No further therapy was ordered. Now the woman presents with right upper leg pain. Plain films reveal a 3-cm lytic lesion in the right upper femur, and a bone scan shows not only the femoral lesion but also three separate lesions in her ribs, two in her skull, and one in her pelvis. Chest x-ray is unremarkable, and liver function tests are normal.

The most appropriate therapeutic option now would be

(A) tamoxifen, 10 mg twice daily
(B) tamoxifen, 10 mg twice daily, plus CMF combination chemotherapy (cyclophosphamide, methotrexate, and 5-fluorouracil)
(C) tamoxifen, 10 mg twice daily, plus external-beam radiation to the femoral lesion
(D) tamoxifen, 10 mg twice daily, plus prophylactic internal fixation of the right femur followed by external-beam radiation
(E) tamoxifen, 10 mg twice daily, plus both CMF and external-beam radiation to the femoral lesion

545. A 27-year-old man has a testicular mass. Chest x-ray reveals six discrete tumor nodules, and an abdominal CT scan shows enlarged paraaortic nodes. Serum α-fetoprotein level is elevated. He undergoes transinguinal orchiectomy, which reveals teratocarcinoma. Treatment is started with three cycles of combination chemotherapy consisting of bleomycin, vinblastine, and cis-platinum; he tolerates the chemotherapy well. Four of the six lung nodules resolve completely, the paraaortic nodes disappear, and α-fetoprotein levels return to normal. The two remaining pulmonary nodules, one in each lung, have diminished in size to about 2 cm. The man receives a fourth cycle of the same drugs with no change in his clinical status.

At this stage, his physician should

(A) continue the same chemotherapy for one more cycle but increase the dosage of drugs by 50 percent
(B) switch to a new drug regimen
(C) perform thoracotomy in order to biopsy and remove the nodule on one side
(D) administer low-dose, whole-lung radiation
(E) administer high-dose spot radiation to the individual lung nodules

546. A 60-year-old man with known lung cancer has recently developed lower back pain. Physical examination, including careful neurologic examination, is normal. Plain films of the back reveal several blastic lesions around T12 and L1. The next step in the man's management should be

(A) careful observation and frequent neurologic examinations
(B) electromyography with nerve conduction studies
(C) lumbar puncture
(D) CT scan of the spine
(E) corticosteroid therapy

547. The Health Insurance Plan of New York evaluated mammography as a screening tool for breast cancer in 62,000 persons. After an 18-year follow-up period, it was found that the screened population

(A) showed a reduction in mortality when all age groups were analyzed together
(B) showed a 30 percent reduction in mortality from breast cancer, compared with a control group, for women 35 to 50 years of age
(C) showed a 30 percent reduction in mortality from breast cancer for women at high risk for the development of breast cancer (i.e., women having prior breast cancer or an affected first-degree relative)
(D) demonstrated no change in mortality from breast cancer for women of any age group, despite the stage of cancer at diagnosis
(E) had an increased mortality from breast cancer probably due to the carcinogenic effects of radiation delivered during mammography

548. All the following statements concerning risk factors for breast cancer are true EXCEPT

(A) irregularity of the menstrual cycle increases a woman's chance of developing breast cancer
(B) late menopause (after 55 years of age) increases a woman's chance of developing breast cancer
(C) artificial menopause before 35 years of age diminishes a woman's chance of developing breast cancer
(D) bearing a first child before 18 years of age diminishes a woman's chance of developing breast cancer
(E) the effects of childbearing and menstruation are unimportant in determining the risk of breast cancer in women past the age of 75 years

549. A 38-year-old premenopausal woman has a 3-cm mass in her left breast. Breast biopsy reveals infiltrating ductal carcinoma, and a left modified radical mastectomy is performed. Pathology reports that the primary tumor is estrogen-receptor positive and that 4 of 28 lymph nodes identified are involved with tumor. Chest x-ray, bone scan, liver scan, and blood chemistries are all normal.

The most appropriate next step in the management of this case would be

(A) antiestrogen therapy (e.g., tamoxifen)
(B) appropriate combination chemotherapy
(C) postoperative radiation therapy to the left chest wall and axilla
(D) bilateral oophorectomy
(E) follow-up in 2 months

550. All the following statements concerning the immunologic abnormalities associated with Hodgkin's disease are true EXCEPT

(A) antibody production is normal in most affected persons
(B) the ability of untreated persons to respond to a battery of skin-test antigens is usually abnormal if they have stage III or stage IV disease
(C) presplenectomy pneumococcal vaccination is worthwhile
(D) the major immunologic defect in affected persons appears to reside in the T lymphocyte
(E) following successful drug or radiation therapy, affected persons regain full immunologic competence within 12 to 24 months

551. All the following are neoplasms of B-lymphocyte lineage EXCEPT

(A) chronic lymphocytic leukemia
(B) follicular lymphomas
(C) Burkitt's lymphoma
(D) mycosis fungoides
(E) small lymphocytic (well-differentiated) lymphomas

552. Regarding local therapy of operable breast cancer, which of the following statements is accurate?

(A) Axillary radiation therapy should follow modified radical mastectomy
(B) Radiation therapy administered following breast-conserving surgery has no effect on the local recurrence rate
(C) Radiation therapy administered following breast-conserving surgery has no effect on the overall survival rate
(D) All patients with a small tumor do equally well with either lumpectomy plus radiation or modified radical mastectomy
(E) Node dissection should be performed in all patients in order to reduce the chance of local spread

553. A 65-year-old woman with increasing abdominal pain is found to have a pelvic mass on physical examination. After appropriate staging studies she undergoes a laparotomy and is found to have serous carcinoma of the ovary with involvement of one ovary and several omental implants. She then undergoes a hysterectomy, bilateral salpingo-oophorectomy, liver biopsy, omentectomy, cytologic examination of abdominal washings, and extensive inspection. All evidence of disease is removed.

Assuming generally good health, an uneventful postoperative recovery, and lack of proximity to a center performing clinical trials, she should now receive

(A) no further therapy
(B) combination chemotherapy
(C) combination chemotherapy only if serum CA125 level is elevated
(D) intraperitoneal chemotherapy
(E) whole abdominal radiation therapy

554. Which of the following clinical scenarios is LEAST likely to describe a paraneoplastic syndrome resulting from small cell tumors of the lung?

(A) Weakness and fatigability, primarily of proximal muscles; electromyographic results show increasing amplitude of contraction with repetitive stimulation
(B) Cerebellar ataxia, dysarthria, deafness, pleocytosis of cerebrospinal fluid, and cerebellar atrophy on CT scan of the brain
(C) Moon facies, truncal striae, hypertension, hypokalemia, and hyperglycemia
(D) Hypercalcemia, polydipsia, polyuria, and mental status changes in the absence of bony metastases
(E) Mental status changes, muscle weakness, hyponatremia, and decreased serum osmolality with inappropriately elevated urine osmolality

555. Two years ago a 68-year-old man was found to
have a prostate nodule on routine examination. Biopsy revealed poorly differentiated prostatic adenocarcinoma;
staging studies failed to reveal any evidence of extrapros-
tatic spread. Because of a desire to maintain potency, the
patient opted for radiation therapy as primary treatment.
He did well except for requiring lower extremity revascularization for intractable claudication until recently, when
he developed pain in his right hip. Prostate specific antigen was elevated. Bone scan revealed areas of positive
uptake in the pelvis and ribs (not present on the original
staging study). The patient expresses a desire not to have
a bilateral orchiectomy, "unless it would significantly improve my quality of life or survival compared with other
therapies."

The most appropriate strategy at this point is to

(A) biopsy one of the bony lesions
(B) administer cisplatin and 5-fluorouracil
(C) administer leuprolide and flutamide
(D) administer diethylstilbestrol (DES) at low dose
(E) perform an orchiectomy

DIRECTIONS: Each question below contains five suggested responses. For **each** of the five responses listed with every question, you are to respond either YES (Y) or NO (N). In a given item **all, some, or none of the alternatives may be correct.**

556. True statements concerning the relationship between cigarette smoking and cancer include which of the following?

(A) Approximately 40 percent of all cancers are related directly or in part to cigarette smoking
(B) Bladder cancer has been associated with cigarette smoking
(C) Heavy smokers should have a yearly chest x-ray to screen for early signs of lung cancer
(D) Alcohol, asbestos, and uranium exposure act synergistically with cigarette smoking to increase the risk of cancer
(E) Women who are heavy smokers are three times as likely to develop breast cancer as are other women

557. Correct statements regarding growth factors include which of the following?

(A) Platelet-derived growth factor, produced exclusively by platelets, is primarily involved in hematopoiesis
(B) The epidermal growth factor receptor is a proto-oncogene
(C) The monocyte growth factor receptor is a molecule that catalyzes phosphorylation of certain proteins on tyrosine residues
(D) Granulocyte-macrophage colony-stimulating factor can stimulate proliferation of normal and leukemic myeloid cells
(E) Each hematopoietic growth factor acts primarily in a paracrine fashion (i.e., stimulates nearby cells)

558. True statements about doxorubicin (Adriamycin) cardiotoxicity include which of the following?

(A) Acute cardiotoxicity, which is characterized by arrhythmias and other abnormal electrocardiographic changes, is brief and rarely serious
(B) Chronic cardiotoxicity occurs in fewer than 3 percent of persons whose lifetime dose of doxorubicin is below 500 mg/m^2
(C) Weekly doxorubicin therapy is better tolerated than the same total dose given every 3 weeks
(D) Congestive heart failure frequently develops 6 months or more after the last dose of doxorubicin
(E) Previous cardiac irradiation and exposure to cyclophosphamide or anthracycline antibiotics other than doxorubicin increase the risk of cardiotoxicity

559. True statements concerning the relationship between radiation exposure and the development of neoplasia include which of the following?

(A) An unlimited linear dose-response relationship exists between radiation exposure and the development of leukemia
(B) Infants and children are at greatest risk for developing radiation-induced neoplasia
(C) Exposure to radiation below the established minimum threshold dose is considered safe
(D) The incidence of leukemia reaches a peak approximately 7 years after radiation exposure
(E) The greatest source of radiation exposure for U.S. citizens is medical diagnostic procedures

560. For a given clinical stage of Hodgkin's disease, which of the following would affect prognosis *adversely?*

(A) Presence of anergy
(B) Presence of fever
(C) Pruritus
(D) Abnormal absolute lymphocyte count
(E) Abnormal in vitro lymphocyte phytohemagglutinin response

561. Oncogenes implicated in the formation of human tumors by virtue of a chromosomal translocation include

(A) c-*myc*
(B) *Rb*-1
(C) c-*ras*^{H}
(D) c-*abl*
(E) *bcl*-2

562. Mechanisms that have been demonstrated to account for resistance of cancer cells to chemotherapy include

(A) increased level of target enzyme
(B) increased drug efflux
(C) altered target enzyme
(D) increased metabolism to inactive moiety
(E) decreased DNA repair

563. The use in combination of nitrogen mustard, vincristine (Oncovin), prednisone, and procarbazine (MOPP) in the treatment of persons who have advanced-stage Hodgkin's disease can be described by which of the following statements?

(A) Persons for whom radiotherapy has failed respond more poorly to MOPP than do previously untreated persons whose disease is of the same stage and histologic subtype

(B) Up to 80 percent of previously untreated persons achieve a complete remission with MOPP

(C) More than 75 percent of persons who achieve a complete remission with MOPP remain alive for up to 14 years

(D) Most persons who relapse do so within the first 2 years following treatment

(E) Two years of MOPP maintenance therapy, after an initial induction of remission, improves disease-free survival rate

564. Correct statements regarding the treatment of patients with non-Hodgkin's lymphoma include which of the following?

(A) Radiation therapy is curative for most patients with low-grade non-Hodgkin's lymphoma

(B) In those patients with low-grade lymphoma who require chemotherapy, only combinations of agents can change overall survival rate

(C) Over 75 percent of patients with intermediate-grade (e.g., diffuse large cell) lymphoma will achieve complete remission with combination chemotherapy

(D) Maintenance therapy (prolonged therapy after complete remission is achieved) improves survival in patients with diffuse large cell lymphoma

(E) Patients with non-Hodgkin's lymphoma who have AIDS have the same rate of response to chemotherapy as stage- and grade-matched patients without AIDS

565. True statements regarding ovarian cancer include

(A) it is second to cervical carcinoma as the leading cause of cancer death from gynecologic malignancies

(B) nulliparity is a risk factor

(C) a history of breast cancer is a risk factor

(D) stromal cell and germ cell tumors of the ovary are the most common histologic subtypes

(E) histologic grade is an important prognostic factor

566. Correct statements concerning staging laparotomy for Hodgkin's disease include which of the following?

(A) While those who have a large spleen preoperatively are virtually certain to have splenic involvement, a normal-size spleen requires assessment at laparotomy

(B) If a staging laparotomy is planned, a lymphangiogram is useful

(C) Laparotomy should nearly always be performed if positive findings would advance the stage of the disease

(D) The spleen should nearly always be removed during staging laparotomy

(E) Removal of the spleen at laparotomy is associated with better tolerance of chemotherapy

567. Which of the following factors will influence the frequency of dissemination of cutaneous malignant melanoma?

(A) Primary tumor site

(B) Dermatologic level of invasion

(C) Thickness of the primary lesion

(D) Geographic area of residence

(E) Presence of microscopic tumor satellites

568. A 22-year-old man undergoes an inguinal orchiectomy because of a left testicular mass. He was found to have an embryonal cell tumor with no lymphatic, vascular, or extratesticular extent. Abdominal-pelvic CT scan, chest x-ray, and tumor markers 3 weeks postoperatively are normal. Before the operation, his serum alphafetoprotein (AFP) had been three times normal. Which of the following would constitute reasonable approaches at this time?

(A) Chemotherapy with bleomycin, etoposide, and cisplatin

(B) Chemotherapy with vinblastine, actinomycin D, bleomycin, and cyclophosphamide

(C) Retroperitoneal lymph node dissection

(D) Radiation therapy

(E) Observation

569. Correct statements regarding carcinoma of the prostate include

(A) histologic grade is an important prognostic indicator
(B) most prostate cancers arise from the transitional cell epithelium
(C) cancer of the prostate is the second most common malignancy in men
(D) cancer of the prostate may spread hematogenously, via lymphatics, or by direct extension
(E) an elevated prostate specific antigen indicates metastatic disease

570. Characteristics of dysplastic nevi include which of the following?

(A) Dysplastic nevi serve only as markers for the risk of melanoma; melanomas arise only in apparently normal skin
(B) Dysplastic nevi tend to have a uniform appearance in a given individual
(C) Dysplastic nevi are usually more than 6 mm in diameter
(D) If two family members have melanoma, there is a 50 percent risk of developing melanoma in the patient with dysplastic nevi
(E) Patients commonly have nevi on areas not exposed to the sun

DIRECTIONS: The group of questions below consists of five lettered headings followed by a set of numbered items. For each numbered item select the **one** lettered heading with which it is **most** closely associated. Each lettered heading may be used **once, more than once, or not at all**.

Questions 571–574

Match each of the following chemotherapeutic agents to its appropriate mechanism of action.

   (A)   Inhibits DNA synthesis and reacts with DNA to cause strand scission
   (B)   Binds with DNA and causes untwisting of the double helix
   (C)   Blocks thymidylate synthetase
   (D)   Produces metaphase arrest by direct binding to tubulin
   (E)   Causes depurination and miscoding errors by its alkylating action

571. Bleomycin

572. Doxorubicin

573. Vinblastine

574. 5-Fluorouracil

Neoplasia

Answers

530. The answer is D. *(Wilson, ed 12. chap 310.)* The most common paraneoplastic syndrome is a distal sensorimotor polyneuropathy due mainly to segmental demyelination. A neuromuscular disease produced by distant cancer, Eaton-Lambert syndrome, differs from myasthenia gravis in that the ocular muscles are spared. In addition, there is an incremental response in power when an affected muscle is stimulated rapidly; the opposite effect occurs in myasthenia gravis. Eaton-Lambert syndrome is believed to be due to decreased release of acetylcholine caused by the presence of an autoantibody. The relationship between cancer and polymyositis and dermatomyositis still is controversial, but a noninflammatory myopathy has not been related to tumors. Cranial nerve palsies are usually related to carcinomatous meningitis rather than to distant effects.

531. The answer is E. *(Wilson, ed 12. chap 307.)* Basal cell carcinoma is the most common malignancy occurring in the United States. The typical appearance is that of a slowly enlarging, pearly translucent papule with rolled borders and overlying telangiectasias. As the lesion enlarges, central ulceration may occur (rodent ulcer). Sun-exposed areas are most commonly involved—about 90 percent of tumors occur on the head and neck—and fair-skinned persons are at greatest risk. Dermal nevi, which occur commonly on the faces of adults, lack the translucency seen in basal cell carcinoma. Sebaceous hyperplasia usually is smaller and has a distinct yellowish color. Diagnosis of basal cell carcinoma is easily established by punch or incisional biopsy.

532. The answer is D. *(Wilson, ed 12. chap 308.)* The characteristics distinguishing superficial spreading malignant melanoma from a normal mole include irregularity of its border and variegation of color. Instead of the homogeneous color and regular borders of a "normal" mole, the lesion shows disorderliness and irregularity. The first changes noted by persons who develop melanoma in a preexisting mole are a "darkening" in color or a change in the borders of the lesion. Irregularity of the borders in an expanding, darkening mole is melanoma until proven otherwise; biopsy should be done promptly, because early diagnosis and excision reduce the mortality rate.

533. The answer is E. *(Wilson, ed 12. chap 300.)* The value of screening mammography in reducing the mortality rate in breast cancer in those over age 40 is well-established. Current guidelines dictate a baseline mammogram between ages 35 and 40, every other year from ages 40 to 49, and annually thereafter. Mammograms should be supplemented by an annual professional breast examination and monthly breast self-examinations. Pelvic examinations and Pap smears should be done annually until three consecutive normal studies are obtained, whereupon the frequency may be reduced. To reduce the incidence of colorectal neoplasia, annual digital rectal examinations and testing for occult blood in the stool are indicated. Though sigmoidoscopic examinations are suggested every 3 to 5 years after two initial negative tests 1 year apart, colonoscopy is not presently recommended as a routine screening procedure.

534. The answer is B. *(Wilson, ed 12. chap 300.)* Certain familial and genetic syndromes are associated with an increased propensity to development of malignant neoplasms. Ataxia-telangiectasia, an autosomal recessive condition characterized by abnormal cellular immunity, conjunctival telangiectasias, and progressive spinocerebellar atrophy, is also associated with lymphoma. Carcinoma of the colon develops in almost all persons with familial polyposis coli and is found at the time of initial diagnosis of the polyps in about 40 percent of cases. Fanconi's anemia is one of a group of familial disorders associated with cytogenetic abnormalities and an increased risk of development of cancer. Neurofibromas undergo sarcomatous change in approximately 10 percent of affected patients. Chronic granulomatous disease of childhood is a disorder of oxidative metabolism in phagocytes and is not associated with neoplasia.

535. The answer is C. *(Wilson, ed 12. chaps 300, 301. Schilsky, Semin Oncol 9:75, 1982.)* Hyperuricemia occurs frequently in patients with acute leukemia, but it may also be associated with other malignant conditions. Secondary gout, however, is quite unusual, except in patients with polycythemia vera. The solubility of urate in the urine is increased at *alkaline* pH, and thus administration of bicarbonate may prevent the precipitation of urate crystals in the renal tubules and parenchyma. Cytotoxic therapy of highly drug-sensitive tumors may cause massive release of intracellular phosphate and potassium and lead to sudden alteration of blood electrolytes, which may result in fatal cardiac rhythm disturbances. Lactic acidosis occasionally occurs in untreated patients with leukemia and Burkitt's lymphoma because of the excessive production of lactate by these metabolically active tumors, and it may be reversed by appropriate chemotherapy. The treatment of choice for tumor-associated hypercalcemia is therapy of the underlying malignancy, but mithramycin is a useful ancillary agent, with toxicity that is limited if the drug is used in careful and recommended fashion.

536. The answer is A. *(Wilson, ed 12. chap 300. DeVita, ed 3. sec 1, chap 58.)* Obstruction of the superior vena cava, the SVC syndrome, is a complication of malignancies involving the mediastinum and upper lung fields, most commonly caused by carcinoma of the lung. The syndrome is characterized clinically by headache, conjunctival injection and suffusion, plethoric facies, distention of veins in the neck and upper extremities, loss of venous pulsations, and (in severe cases) convulsions. Lower extremity swelling and pulsus paradoxus suggest the presence of pericardial tamponade, another complication of chest malignancies. While the SVC syndrome is a serious medical problem, it is rarely a cause of death, and time is usually available to allow pursuit of a specific histologic diagnosis. During this interval, therapy with corticosteroids and diuretics may be useful, pending a diagnosis and the institution of more specific therapy, which should include local irradiation and systemic treatment of the tumor.

537. The answer is A. *(Wilson, ed 12. chap 302.)* Hodgkin's disease can be distinguished from non-Hodgkin's lymphomas (NHL) by a variety of characteristics. The "B" (or constitutional) symptoms described for Hodgkin's disease are less common in patients with NHL, although the presence of these symptoms is thought to influence the prognosis negatively. Involvement of Waldeyer's ring occurs more commonly in NHL than in Hodgkin's disease. Extralymphatic presentation is more frequent with NHL than with Hodgkin's disease, and NHL is more often disseminated at the time of diagnosis. Approximately 60 percent of all lymphomas are NHL.

538. The answer is B. *(Wilson, ed 12. chap 300.)* In about 85 percent of persons who have chronic myelogenous leukemia, the material comprising approximately one-half of the long arm of chromosome 22 is translocated to the end of chromosome 9. This abnormality, called the Philadelphia chromosome, involves all three hematopoietic cell lines. It is thought to represent an acquired somatic cell mutation in the bone marrow, with preferential survival and proliferation of the affected cell clone. The pathogenesis of chronic myelogenous leukemia is therefore a paradigm for all cancers that are believed to arise from a single cell that gives rise to the malignant clone.

539. The answer is C. *(Wilson, ed 12. chaps 300, 305.)* Ninety percent of persons with nonseminomatous germ cell tumors produce either α-fetoprotein (AFP) or β-HCG; in contrast, persons with pure seminomas usually produce neither. These tumor markers are present for some time after surgery—if the presurgical levels are high, 30 days or more may be required before meaningful postsurgical levels can be obtained. The half-lives of AFP and β-HCG are 6 days and 1 day, respectively. After treatment, unequal reduction of β-HCG and AFP may occur, suggesting that the two markers are synthesized by heterogeneous clones of cells within the tumor; thus, both markers should be followed. β-HCG is similar to luteinizing hormone except for its distinctive beta subunit.

540. The answer is A. *(Wilson, ed 12. chap 301.)* By following first-order kinetics, anticancer agents kill a constant fraction, rather than a constant number, of tumor cells. A course of therapy that has been shown to be capable of killing three orders of magnitude of cells (i.e., 3 logs) will do so regardless of total number of tumor cells. Because most chemotherapeutic agents have been found to reduce the number of tumor cells by only 1 to 3 logs, their effectiveness in treating cancers with a trillion cells (10^{12}) has been limited, unless the tumor burden is reduced first.

541. The answer is A. *(Wilson, ed 12. chap 301.)* The most prominent general side effects of chemotherapy relate to the effect of these drugs on dividing cells, including myelosuppression, stomatitis, and alopecia. Certain drugs, such as L-asparaginase and vincristine, can be administered during periods of low white blood cell count because they are relatively nonmyelosuppressive. Alkylating agents, such as melphalan, cyclophosphamide, and nitrogen mustard, damage bone marrow stem cells, an effect associated with the development of secondary myelodysplastic syndromes and acute leukemias. Anthracyclines are myelosuppressive, but they inhibit more committed hematopoietic cells than do the alkylating agents. Cisplatin is quite emetogenic; however, vomiting can be managed successfully with the use of a number of agents, including dexamethasone and metoclopramide. Massive losses of potassium and magnesium (in turn leading to hypocalcemia) must be anticipated with the use of cisplatin because of drug-induced renal tubular damage.

542. The answer is D. *(Wilson, ed 12. chap 302.)* There is an increased incidence of lymphoma in diseases of inherited and acquired immunodeficiency as well as in certain autoimmune diseases. Thus, children with Chédiak-Higashi syndrome, a congenital disorder of neutrophil function with associated granulomatous infections, are at risk for subsequent lymphomas as well. Ataxia telangiectasia and Wiskott-Aldrich syndromes also predispose to lymphoma. In addition to AIDS, in which the incidence of non-Hodgkin's lymphomas (especially primary lymphoma of the central nervous system) is high, patients with other acquired immunodeficiency states, including drug-induced immunosuppression, may also develop lymphoma. Sjögren's syndrome, rheumatoid arthritis, sprue, and systemic lupus are among those autoimmune diseases associated with an increased incidence of lymphoma, thereby suggesting a pathogenetic basis in immune dysregulation. Many patients receiving phenytoin will develop atypical lymphoid hyperplasia, but a few will go on to develop frank lymphoma even after the drug is stopped. Although a fatal course is possible, certain lymphoproliferative disorders associated with Epstein-Barr virus will regress if immunosuppression is discontinued.

543. The answer is C. *(Wilson, ed 12. chaps 301, 303.)* Tamoxifen is a useful antiestrogen agent in the treatment of metastatic breast cancer and usually is very well tolerated. However, it can be associated with hot flashes, nausea, mild fluid retention, and acute hypercalcemia. Virilization is uncommon with tamoxifen.

544. The answer is D. *(Wilson, ed 12. chap 303.)* The appropriate systemic therapy for postmenopausal women with estrogen-recepter–positive breast cancer metastatic to bone is either tamoxifen, 10 mg twice daily, or diethylstilbestrol. Radiation therapy can relieve bone pain and may prevent fractures if used prophylactically to treat lesions of weight-bearing bones. For lytic lesions greater than 2.5 cm in diameter in weight-bearing bones, prophylactic internal fixation followed by radiation therapy is the treatment of choice, especially if the lesions involve the cortex.

545. The answer is C. *(Wilson, ed 12. chap 305.)* Persons with disseminated teratocarcinoma treated with combination chemotherapy achieve complete remission in more than 70 percent of cases. Occasionally, residual masses remain after chemotherapy and on biopsy prove to be benign mature teratomas rather than residual malignant disease. In these cases, partial responders can be converted to complete responders—and even cured—by surgical removal of residual masses. If viable cancer is detected in the surgical specimen, then additional chemotherapy should be administered.

546. The answer is D. *(Wilson, ed 12. chaps 19, 300. DeVita, ed 3. sec 2, chap 58.)* Epidural spinal cord compression is an important complication of metastatic cancer. Local or radicular pain is the most frequent and earliest clinical symptom; subsequently, weakness and bladder and bowel dysfunction can develop. The diagnosis, which should always be considered even if neurologic examination is normal, is confirmed by demonstrating a lesion on MRI or CT scan. Lumbar spinal taps should be avoided because herniation of the cord into a decompressed region can occur after withdrawal of fluid. Surgery usually is recommended for persons with rapidly progressive neurologic signs; radiation is useful in treating persons who have slowly progressive deficits due to radiosensitive tumors. Neither systemic chemotherapy nor corticosteroids should be employed in place of surgery or radiotherapy.

547. The answer is A. *(Wilson, ed 12. chap 303. Chu, J Natl Cancer Inst 80:1125, 1988.)* The Health Insurance Plan of New York evaluated mammography as a screening tool in 62,000 persons. Their screening procedure included physical examination as well. Though an earlier report had demonstrated a benefit for screening only in those over age 50, a more recent analysis with an 18-year follow-up describes a statistically significant 24 percent reduction in mortality for all age groups. While the high frequency of physical examinations in the HIP study may have been the most important factor in reducing mortality, a Swedish trial more clearly demonstrated the benefits of screening mammograms, at least in patients over age 50.

548. The answer is E. *(Wilson, ed 12. chap 303.)* Early menarche, late menopause, nulliparity, and irregularity of the menstrual cycle all increase a woman's risk of developing breast cancer. Women who have undergone artificial menopause before the age of 35 years and women who bear their first child before the age of 18 years have a lower risk overall. These risk factors hold true throughout the woman's life.

549. The answer is B. *(Wilson, ed 12. chap 303. Early Breast Cancer Trialists' Collaborative Group, N Engl J Med 319:1681, 1988.)* For premenopausal women who have stage II carcinoma of the breast (axillary metastases only), the drug regimen combining cyclophosphamide, methotrexate, and 5-fluorouracil (CMF), when employed as an adjuvant therapy, leads to a statistically significant reduction in recurrence rate. It is the treatment of choice following mastectomy in this group of women. Mortality rate after 5 years is decreased approximately 30 percent in women treated with CMF. Median survival is prolonged by approximately 3 years with CMF treatment.

550. The answer is E. *(Wilson, ed 12. chap 302.)* While humoral immunity is well-preserved in patients with untreated Hodgkin's disease, those affected with all stages of the disease display defective cellular immunity manifested by anergy to routine skin tests. Not only are baseline immunoglobulins normal, but a normal protective response to pneumococcal vaccine will be mounted in patients about to be splenectomized prior to therapy. The anergy is associated with a decrease in the ratio of CD4+ T cells to CD8+ T cells. Abnormalities in skin testing, especially to neoantigens, persist even long after successful therapy. Though it is of no independent prognostic significance, the degree of cutaneous anergy correlates with advanced stage and the presence of systemic symptoms.

551. The answer is D. *(Wilson, ed 12. chap 302.)* Neoplasms may be classified as to their cell of origin by the use of antisera and monoclonal antibodies against certain cell surface phenotypic markers and, more recently, by the use of DNA probes for immunoglobulin genes and genes for the beta chain of the T-cell receptor. The malignant cell in chronic lymphocytic leukemia is a morphologically normal but functionally abnormal B lymphocyte. Follicular lymphomas arise from the proliferative part of the B-cell system, the lymphoid follicle, while the diffuse, small lymphocytic lymphomas are derived from the secretory compartment of the medullary cords. The Burkitt's lymphoma cell is a malignant cell of B-lymphocyte lineage; in many cases it bears a characteristic chromosomal translocation. In contrast to these B-cell neoplasms, mycosis fungoides is a peripheral T-cell lymphoma in which helper-cell function and phenotype have been identified.

552. The answer is C. *(Wilson, ed 12. chap 303.)* Other than in the performance of early local therapy rather than late local therapy based on mammographic detection, no surgical or radiotherapeutic procedure has been shown to affect survival. In other words, survival is determined by the extent and response of systemic disease. The decision between lumpectomy plus radiation therapy and modified radical mastectomy therefore rests on which modality offers the best chance for local control. Although no survival benefit can be shown, radiation therapy should be administered along with lumpectomy because at least one study has documented a higher recurrence rate in those treated with lumpectomy alone (28 percent) compared with lumpectomy plus radiotherapy (5 percent). In most cases, local control can be achieved equally well with either approach. However, certain subgroups—especially those with extensive intraductal carcinoma or with positive lumpectomy resection margins—will experience a higher local recurrence rate if breast conservation is employed. Axillary lymph node dissection is appropriate in all patients for diagnostic (in order to determine the appropriate systemic therapy), not therapeutic, purposes.

553. The answer is B. *(Wilson, ed 12. chap 304.)* The overall 5-year survival of those with disease that extends beyond the ovaries is 40 percent; however, some patients who are able to undergo complete or nearly complete initial cytoreductive surgery may be cured with combination chemotherapy. Presumably such therapy eradicates residual subclinical disease, which is invariably present despite the apparently complete resection. Although the optimal regimen has not been established, effective drugs include cisplatin, cyclophosphamide, hexamethylmelamine, and doxorubicin. Since some patients may have recurrent disease without an elevation of CA125, which is a useful antigen in monitoring response to therapy in those who have elevated levels, delaying therapy pending a rise in this level would not be prudent. No clear survival benefits have been yet shown for the fairly toxic regimen of whole abdominal radiation therapy. Intraperitoneal chemotherapy holds promise in the eradication of minimal disease, but its role remains to be defined by further clinical trials.

554. The answer is D. *(Wilson, ed 12. chaps 309, 310. Broadus, N Engl J Med 319:556, 1988.)* Small cell neoplasms of the lung are associated with a wide variety of paraneoplastic syndromes, some of which are humorally mediated, while others are of unknown pathophysiology. The Eaton-Lambert syndrome, characterized by proximal muscle weakness and the characteristic electromyographic findings, is associated almost exclusively with small cell tumors. Subacute cortical cerebellar degeneration is associated with the findings outlined in scenario B and also with small cell tumors and some cases of ovarian cancer, carcinoma of the breast, and Hodgkin's disease. Cushing's syndrome, with all the effects of hypersecretion of glucocorticoids, and the syndrome of inappropriate secretion of antidiuretic hormone are also associated with small cell lung tumors, in addition to other cancers. Hypercalcemia is infrequently associated with small cell neoplasms, but it is not an infrequent manifestation of squamous and large cell lung tumors, in which cases it may be a result of secretion of substances with parathyroid hormone-like activity or of another factor associated with the humoral hypercalcemia of malignancy.

555. The answer is C. *(Wilson, ed 12. chap 306. Crawford, N Engl J Med 321:419, 1989.)* Given the poorly differentiated histology at presentation with the associated high recurrence risk and the characteristic indicators of metastatic prostate cancer, biopsy is unnecessary. Since the patient has symptomatic disease, he should be started on androgen deprivation therapy, which is likely to cause a decrease in his pain. An equivalent response rate has been demonstrated with bilateral orchiectomy, diethylstilbestrol, and LHRH analogues such as leuprolide. Given his desire not to have an orchiectomy and his vascular disease, LHRH analogues would be the best approach. A recent study has documented a benefit to providing "total androgen blockade" with flutamide plus leuprolide compared with leuprolide alone. Prostatic carcinoma is poorly responsive to chemotherapy.

556. The answer is A-Y, B-Y, C-N, D-Y, E-N. *(Wilson, ed 12. chap 300.)* More than 15 carcinogens have been isolated from tobacco smoke. Approximately 40 percent of all cancers and one-third of all male cancer deaths have been related to cigarette smoking. The incidence not only of lung cancer but also of head and neck, esophageal, and bladder cancer is increased in smokers. In addition, use of alcohol and exposure to asbestos and uranium act synergistically to increase the risk. Yearly chest x-rays are not helpful in increasing the cure rate of lung cancer. The incidence of breast cancer does not seem to be affected by smoking.

557. The answer is A-N, B-Y, C-Y, D-Y, E-N. *(Wilson, ed 12. chap 9. Slamon, Science 244:707, 1989.)* Growth factors are believed to play a role in the pathogenesis of many diseases, both neoplastic and nonneoplastic. Platelet-derived growth factor is a 32-kDa heterodimer elaborated by a number of cells, including platelets, endothelial cells, smooth muscle–like cells, and activated macrophages. This molecule stimulates fibroblast proliferation and may aid in wound healing, but it may also be involved in atherosclerosis and in the pathogenesis of certain malignancies. Epidermal growth factor stimulates the proliferation of epithelial cells and fibroblasts. The epidermal growth factor receptor bears significant homology to the v-*erb*B viral transforming gene and to the HER-2/*neu* proto-oncogene, which is amplified in certain aggressive breast and ovarian tumors. Hematopoietic growth factors include CSF-1 (macrophage colony-stimulating factor), GM-CSF (granulocyte-macrophage colony-stimulating factor), G-CSF (granulocyte colony-stimulating factor), IL-3 (multipotent colony-stimulating factor), and erythropoietin (red blood cell–stimulating factor). Except for erythropoietin, which is made in the kidney in response to hypoxia and stimulates erythroid activity in the fashion of a classic hormone, the hematopoietic growth factors are believed to act mainly on adjacent cells (paracrine stimulation). GM-CSF and G-CSF may be helpful in augmenting recovery from chemotherapy-induced myelosuppression and other neutropenic states, but must be used with care in those with leukemia since it has been demonstrated that certain myeloid leukemias can also proliferate in response to these factors. The c-*fms* tyrosine kinase proto-oncogene codes for the transmembrane CSF-1 receptor.

558. The answer is A-Y, B-Y, C-Y, D-Y, E-Y. *(Wilson, ed 12. chap 301. DeVita, ed 3. sec 4, chap 60.)* Two types of cardiotoxicity are associated with doxorubicin (Adriamycin) therapy. Acute cardiotoxicity produces electrocardiographic abnormalities, such as arrhythmias, but rarely is serious. Chronic cardiotoxicity, which rarely develops with total doxorubicin doses less than 500 mg/m^2, leads to congestive heart failure; it occurs with increased frequency in persons who also have received cardiac irradiation, cyclophosphamide, or anthracycline compounds other than doxorubicin. Up to half of all cases of cardiotoxicity occur 6 months or more after completion of therapy. Efforts to limit cardiotoxicity and thereby enable the administration of a higher total dose of anthracycline include weekly or continuous intravenous schedules, anthracycline analogues, and cardioprotective agents that limit free-radical–induced myocardial damage.

559. The answer is A-N, B-Y, C-N, D-Y, E-N. *(Wilson, ed 12. chap 300. DeVita, ed 3. chap 9.)* A minimum acceptable safe dose of radiation does not seem to exist. Increasing doses of radiation increase the risk of developing leukemia, until a plateau is reached beyond which the chance of developing malignancy is not increased. Leukemia resulting from radiation peaks in incidence approximately 7 years after exposure. Based on research in atomic bomb survivors, infants and children are most susceptible to radiation-induced neoplasia. While 90 percent of all man-made radiation comes from medical diagnostic procedures, most radiation exposure is derived from natural sources, especially radon.

560. The answer is A-N, B-Y, C-N, D-N, E-N. *(Wilson, ed 12. chap 302.)* Within a given clinical stage of Hodgkin's disease, a recent history of fever, night sweats, or weight loss adversely influences prognosis. Persons who have these symptoms have substage "B" disease; persons who do not have these symptoms have substage "A" disease. Given modern therapeutic techniques, pruritus, anergy, absolute lymphocyte count, and in vitro lymphocyte phytohemagglutinin response all have no bearing on the outcome of Hodgkin's disease.

561. The answer is A-Y, B-N, C-N, D-Y, E-Y. *(Wilson, ed 12. chap 10. Bishop, Science 235:305, 1987.)* Proto-oncogenes, cellular homologues to viral genes capable of inducing malignant transformation, generally play a role in normal cell growth. Mutations or changed position on the genome, however, can lead to altered expression or function and concomitant malignant transformation. The translocation of chromosomes 8 and 14 in Burkitt's lymphoma brings the c-*myc* locus on chromosome 8 and the immunoglobulin heavy chain gene locus on chromosome 14 into close proximity, thereby dysregulating c-*myc* expression. The abnormal regulation of the c-*myc* nuclear-associated proto-oncogene involved in DNA synthesis may play a role in the pathogenesis of this tumor. Virtually every patient with chronic myelogenous leukemia has a translocation between chromosomes 9 and 22 (producing the Philadelphia chromosome) that brings a portion of the c-*abl* tyrosine kinase proto-oncogene next to a region called *bcr,* creating a fusion protein with similar properties to those of the v-*abl* oncogene. Low-grade follicular lymphomas frequently display a 14–18 translocation that brings an immunoglobulin gene locus adjacent to a region of unknown function, *bcl*-2, on chromosome 18. Activating point mutations in members of the *ras* gene family have been found in myeloid leukemias and in other tumors. Loss of heterozygosity (i.e., no functional copies of the normal gene remain) for the so-called antioncogene (recessive oncogene) *Rb*-1 on chromosome 13 is associated with familial retinoblastoma. Recently, recessive oncogenes, likely to play an important role in human neoplasia, have been described in association with other tumors, including colonic carcinoma, Wilms's tumor, and renal cell carcinoma.

562. The answer is A-Y, B-Y, C-Y, D-Y, E-N. *(Wilson, ed 12. chap 301.)* One of the major obstacles to curative chemotherapy is the emergence of resistance in the neoplastic population. The longer a tumor remains before eradication, the more selective pressures will increase the chances of mutations that confer drug resistance. A recently recognized, important mechanism of resistance is the expression of a 170-kDa membrane-bound glycoprotein (P170) capable of causing the efflux of a wide range of naturally occurring chemotherapeutic agents. Studies employing agents such as verapamil and quinidine, which can "block" the P170-mediated efflux, are underway. Gene amplification leading to an increased protein product level, as in the case of the dihydrofolate reductase enzyme (the target of methotrexate action), is another mechanism of resistance. Alteration of the target enzyme (topoisomerase) for etoposide action will lead to drug resistance. Increased DNA repair enzyme activity can make BCNU, an alkylating agent, a less effective molecule. Activation or increased levels of catabolic enzymes with subsequent conversion of the active drug to an inactive form (e.g., increased aldehyde dehydrogenase in the case of cyclophosphamide) is yet another mechanism whereby resistance may occur.

563. The answer is A-N, B-Y, C-N, D-Y, E-N. *(Wilson, ed 12. chap 302.)* Combination chemotherapy with nitrogen mustard, vincristine (Oncovin), prednisone, and procarbazine—MOPP—currently is the treatment of choice for most persons with advanced-stage Hodgkin's disease. Use of the MOPP regimen has led to remission in as many as 80 percent of affected persons, with about 50 percent survival at 14 years. Those persons who relapse usually do so within 2 years. Maintenance chemotherapy with MOPP has not been shown to prolong the disease-free state. Persons who did not respond to radiotherapy are no less likely than other affected persons to respond to MOPP. ABVD (Adriamycin, bleomycin, vincristine, dacarbazine) is an effective salvage regimen for those who relapse after MOPP therapy and seems to have equal efficacy when used in advanced, untreated patients. ABVD has less profound effects on germ-cell function and may be less leukemogenic than MOPP.

564. The answer is A-N, B-N, C-Y, D-N, E-N. *(Wilson, ed 12. chap 302.)* Stage (extent of disease) and tumor grade (histologic appearance) are the most important factors for determining treatment of the non-

Hodgkin's lymphomas. Since 80 to 90 percent of patients with low-grade lymphomas—small lymphocytic (diffuse, well-differentiated lymphocytic) or follicular, small cleaved cell (nodular, poorly differentiated lymphocytic)—present with disseminated disease, radiation therapy essentially can never be considered curative. On the other hand, such diseases behave in an indolent fashion and can be treated effectively in a palliative manner with single-agent alkylator therapy; the use of more aggressive combination regimens produces a higher complete response rate, but has never been conclusively shown to affect the natural history of the disease. Most patients with diffuse large cell lymphoma, the most common intermediate-grade histology, achieve complete remission and many can be cured with combination chemotherapy regimens, including cyclophosphamide, doxorubicin, vincristine, and corticosteroids (and possibly also etoposide or methotrexate, among others). Prolonged (greater than 1 year) maintenance therapy is of no value. A lymphoma presenting in a patient with AIDS has a much lower chance (less than 25 percent complete response rate) of responding to combination chemotherapy than does a lymphoma of similar histologic appearance in an immunocompetent patient.

565. The answer is A-N, B-Y, C-Y, D-N, E-Y. *(Wilson, ed 12. chap 304.)* Though the incidence of ovarian carcinoma is low, the propensity to present at an advanced stage (only 25 percent of patients have disease limited to one or both ovaries) helps to explain why this disease is the most common cause of death among all gynecologic malignancies. Only about 15 percent of ovarian cancers arise from nonepithelial elements. Epithelial tumors are most common in peri- or postmenopausal women, especially nulliparous women or those with few children. Prior breast cancer increases the risk of developing ovarian cancer by two- to fourfold. An advanced stage and a larger size of residual tumor after initial surgery carry an adverse prognosis, as do poorly differentiated ovarian carcinomas, which have a 5-year survival of well under 20 percent.

566. The answer is A-N, B-Y, C-N, D-Y, E-N. *(Wilson, ed 12. chap 302.)* Staging laparotomy for persons who have Hodgkin's disease carries a mortality rate of 1.5 percent and a complication rate of 12 percent. It should not be considered a routine procedure but should be performed if the result would change the treatment plan, not just the stage of the disease. Staging laparotomy should include careful needle and wedge biopsies of the liver lobes and edge, biopsy of retroperitoneal lymph nodes identified by preoperative lymphangiography, and biopsies of any suspicious area. The spleen should be removed for complete pathologic examination; however, splenectomy does not improve tolerance to chemotherapy. Based on clinical assessment of spleen size alone, the false-positive and false-negative rates for splenic involvement with Hodgkin's disease are 25 and 35 percent, respectively. Lymphangiograms done before laparotomy can be used to guide the surgeon to biopsy potentially involved nodes.

567. The answer is A-Y, B-Y, C-Y, D-N, E-Y. *(Wilson, ed 12. chap 308.)* Primary malignant melanoma of the skin is the leading cause of death among all diseases arising in the skin. A number of factors have been identified that correlate with increased or decreased likelihood of dissemination. The most common site for melanoma in males is the torso, and lesions occurring on the torso offer a worse prognosis than do those occurring on a lower extremity. Both dermatologic level of invasion and thickness of the primary lesion are predictive of dissemination and, hence, of survival. For example, melanomas less than 0.76 mm thick are almost always surgically cured; those that penetrate $\geq$ 3.65 mm have a 60 percent rate of distant metastases. While geographic area of residence is an important determinant of risk of development of melanoma, with incidence of disease higher in latitudes with greater sun exposure, it does not appear to affect risk of dissemination in those with diagnosed clinically localized disease. The presence of an ulcer in the primary tumor, mitotic rate, and the demonstration of tumor satellites (microscopic foci of tumor distinct from the primary tumor in the reticular dermis or subcutaneous fat) are also prognostic factors.

568. The answer is A-N, B-N, C-Y, D-N, E-Y. *(Wilson, ed 12. chap 305. Fung, J. Clin Oncol 6:734, 1988.)* This patient has stage I nonseminomatous testicular cancer by virtue of his histology, negative radiologic evaluation, and the fall to normal of AFP after surgery. His chance of cure is 97 percent. The goal is to achieve this excellent result with the minimum of long-term consequences. Routine treatment for stage I patients would involve a retroperitoneal lymph node dissection (RPLND) because of the 35 percent false-negative rate for involved nodes on CT scanning. If surgical findings were negative or if only microscopic disease was found at RPLND, the patient would probably never need further therapy. Another reasonable approach is surveillance alone, which would spare the patient surgery and the attendant morbidity, including retrograde ejaculation. In the relatively unlikely event that relapse occurs, chemotherapy can produce extremely high cure rates. In order for observation alone to be successful, the patient must be aware of the importance of careful follow-up.

569. The answer is A-Y, B-N, C-Y, D-Y, E-N. *(Wilson, ed 12. chap 306.)* Foci of prostatic carcinoma are frequently noted at autopsy, but only about one-third of such cases are clinically apparent. Nonetheless, prostatic carcinoma is the second most common cancer type in men and the third leading cause of male cancer deaths. Ninety-five percent of prostate cancers are adenocarcinomas. The grade of cellular differentiation is an extremely important prognostic variable; a higher Gleason grade (ranging from 2 to 10) indicates a biologically more aggressive tumor. Though the prostate capsule is a natural barrier to spread, dissemination may occur directly to the seminal vesicles and bladder floor, via lymphatics to the obturator, iliac, presacral, or paraaortic nodes, or hematogenously—usually to the bones, especially the pelvis and lumbar vertebrae. Staging consists of clinical examination of the prostate, pelvic CT or MRI, bone scan (with correlative x-rays for positive areas), and detection of serum markers, including acid phosphatase and the more sensitive prostate specific antigen (PSA). An elevated PSA is not pathognomonic for metastatic disease, but it is more common in those with spread to the bones. Though CT scans are helpful, the only certain way to determine local and regional lymph node spread is via surgical staging.

570. The answer is A-N, B-N, C-Y, D-Y, E-Y. *(Wilson, ed 12. chap 308. Rigel, Cancer 63:386, 1989.)* A distinctive pigmented lesion, the dysplastic nevus, occurs in families with a high incidence of melanoma. The recognition of this syndrome is important because the patient and family members can undergo intense dermatologic follow-up with early detection of malignant lesions. Patients with dysplastic nevi and two family members with melanoma have a 50 percent lifetime risk of developing melanoma. Dysplastic nevi tend to have irregular borders and be variable in color and shape on a given individual. They are usually large (minimum diameter of 6 mm) compared with benign nevi. The back is the most common site of dysplastic nevi, but they may also be seen on the scalp, buttocks, and breasts. Though dysplastic nevi do serve as markers for the development of melanoma on normal skin, they also serve as precursor lesions, which makes it vital to watch each dysplastic nevus carefully.

571–574. The answers are: 571-A, 572-B, 573-D, 574-C. *(Wilson, ed 12. chap 301.)* Bleomycin is an antibiotic complex consisting of seven structurally related polypeptides. It both inhibits DNA synthesis and reacts with DNA to cause strand scission. Indications for the use of bleomycin include lymphomas and tumors of the head and neck, skin, testes, and penis. Doxorubicin (Adriamycin), another antitumor antibiotic, inhibits DNA synthesis and DNA-dependent RNA synthesis. It acts by binding with DNA and causing untwisting of the helix, which facilitates intercalation. Doxorubicin is useful in treating a wide variety of tumors.

5-Fluorouracil, a pyrimidine analogue, blocks thymidylate synthetase, an enzyme important in the synthesis of thymidylate and DNA. Its active form is the metabolite 5-fluorodeoxyuridine monophosphate. Used topically, 5-fluorouracil is effective in treating certain neoplastic skin disorders, including superficial basal cell carcinoma. Recent studies suggest potentiation of 5-fluorouracil action by leucovorin, which induces tighter binding to thymidylate synthase.

Vinblastine and vincristine are plant alkaloids. They cause metaphase arrest in dividing cells by binding directly to tubulin; in addition, they interfere with the assembly of spindle proteins. Vinblastine is used in the treatment of persons who have Hodgkin's disease and testicular cancer.

Endocrine, Metabolic, and Genetic Disorders

DIRECTIONS: Each question below contains five suggested responses. Select the **one best** response to each question.

575. The use of repeated phlebotomy in the treatment of persons with symptomatic hemochromatosis may be expected to result in

(A) increased skin pigmentation
(B) improved cardiac function
(C) return of secondary sex characteristics
(D) protection from the development of hepatocellular carcinoma
(E) a 5-year survival rate of 50 percent

576. A 27-year-old hiker is bitten on the wrist by a coral snake. Within minutes, he notes numbness and tingling in the vicinity of the bite. He reaches an emergency room within 60 minutes of the bite, and other than minimal local swelling and fang marks on his hand, physical examination is normal. The most important measure in the treatment of this man would be to

(A) perform cutdown and suction of the bite site
(B) put ice on the bite area to neutralize the venom
(C) give coral-snake antivenom intravenously
(D) perform a wide surgical debridement of the bite site
(E) reassure him that there is no significant risk with coral-snake bites and that the numbness will soon disappear

577. All the following are features of X-linked recessive disorders EXCEPT

(A) for an affected female to be born, the father must be affected
(B) affected males transmit the disease to their sons in 50 percent of cases
(C) male offspring of female carriers have a 50 percent chance of being affected
(D) all female offspring of affected males are carriers
(E) the pedigree pattern tends to be oblique (uncles and nephews) rather than vertical (parents and children) or horizontal (siblings)

578. A 23-year-old woman with chronic sinusitis is noted to have an enlarged sella turcica on an x-ray series of the paranasal sinuses. She has no other recognized medical problems. The next step in the evaluation of this woman should be

(A) measurement of plasma prolactin
(B) CT scanning of the head
(C) measurement of plasma gonadotropins
(D) visual field testing by Goldmann perimetry
(E) repeat sella x-rays in 6 months

579. A 26-year-old diabetic man is evaluated for poor control of diabetes. He had taken 30 units of NPH insulin each morning for several years and had consistently negative or trace urine sugars before meals. However, during the last few weeks he increased the dosage to 38 units each morning because of increasing glycosuria, detected in the bedtime urine sample. He has gained 2.2 kg (5 lb) during the last month. He has noted increasingly severe hunger pangs and headaches before dinner for the last week, but bedtime urine sugars have not diminished.

The most appropriate management at this point would be to

(A) begin the man on regular insulin at 5 P.M., according to the plasma glucose level at bedtime
(B) increase the dosage of NPH insulin, according to the plasma glucose level at bedtime
(C) decrease the dosage of NPH insulin gradually (initially by 10 percent)
(D) continue the same dosage of insulin but decrease the caloric intake at dinner
(E) switch from ordinary NPH to pork NPH insulin

580. Evidence of continuing ovarian estrogen production in a 29-year-old woman being evaluated for secondary amenorrhea is

(A) normal plasma estrone and luteinizing hormone (LH) levels
(B) normal plasma prolactin level
(C) an increase in plasma estradiol level following administration of human chorionic gonadotropin (hCG)
(D) appearance of menses following a short course of progestogen therapy
(E) normal bone density

581. A 7-year-old girl is referred for evaluation of vaginal bleeding for 2 months. The mother says that she has not been exposed to exogenous estrogens. Physical examination reveals height at the 98th percentile, Tanner stage III breast development, and no axillary or pubic hair. No abdominal or pelvic masses are palpated. Neurologic examination is normal. Radiographic and laboratory evaluations reveal the following:

> Skull films: normal sella; no intracerebral calcifications
> Bone age: 10 years
> Urinary 17-ketosteroids: 1.7 μmol (0.5 mg)/g creatinine/24 h
> Urinary gonadotropins: undetectable

The appropriate next step in the management of this girl would be

(A) exploratory laparotomy
(B) treatment with medroxyprogesterone acetate
(C) measurement of plasma androstenedione level
(D) abdominal CT scanning and pelvic sonography
(E) karyotype analysis

582. Which of the following pairs of chromosomal trisomies is most likely to allow survival of a patient into adult life?

(A) 47,XXY and trisomy 18
(B) Trisomies 21 and 13
(C) Any two autosomal trisomies
(D) 47,XXX and trisomy 21
(E) Trisomies 16 and 13

583. A 42-year-old man (indicated by the star in the family history below) has renal failure due to Alport's syndrome, which is nephritis associated with sensorineural deafness and is inherited as an autosomal dominant defect. He is being evaluated for a renal transplant from a living related donor. The best candidate for evaluation as a potential kidney donor for this man would be

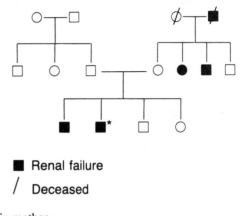

■ Renal failure
/ Deceased

(A) his mother
(B) his father
(C) his unaffected brother
(D) his sister
(E) none of the above

584. Peripheral blood cells are obtained from members of a family; the DNA is extracted, treated with restriction endonuclease E, run on an agarose gel, transferred to nitrocellulose paper, probed with a 4-kilobase (kb) radiolabeled segment of DNA, and exposed to x-ray film. In the following pattern, solid blocks indicate segments of DNA hybridizing to the probe, and numbers indicate DNA length in kilobases.

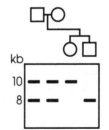

What most likely accounts for the fact that only one band appears in the son and only one (different) band appears in the daughter?

(A) A gene deletion in each child
(B) Chromosome segregation in the offspring
(C) Linkage disequilibrium in the offspring
(D) Parents who are heterozygotes for restriction fragment length polymorphism
(E) Loss of restriction site for endonuclease E in both the children

585. A 42-year-old alcoholic man has eaten poorly for the last 10 days but has continued to drink. His family brings him to the emergency room. On neurologic examination he is confused but otherwise normal. Blood glucose concentration is 2.8 mmol/L (50 mg/dL). Intravenous infusion of a bolus of 50% glucose solution is given. His confusion worsens, and he develops horizontal nystagmus, ataxia, and a heart rate of 130 beats per minute.

At this point, the man's physician should

(A) order an immediate CT scan of the head
(B) perform a lumbar puncture
(C) administer another bolus of 50% glucose solution
(D) administer intravenous folic acid, 5 mg
(E) administer intramuscular thiamine, 50 mg

586. A 32-year-old alcoholic man is admitted to the hospital because of acute abdominal pain. Hemorrhagic necrosis of the pancreas is found during emergency laparotomy. Postoperatively, he becomes septic and hyperglycemic. Mechanical ventilation for respiratory failure is required, and attempts to wean him from the ventilator are begun 3 days later. Which of the following daily regimens would provide the most appropriate form of nutrition for this man (assuming that each regimen would include the required amounts of calories, vitamins, and minerals and that the hyperglycemia can be controlled with insulin)?

(A) A defined-formula liquid diet given through a small-bore nasogastric tube
(B) Peripheral intravenous infusion of 3 L of a 25% dextrose solution containing 2% amino acids
(C) Central intravenous infusion of 3 L of a 25% dextrose solution containing 2% amino acids
(D) Peripheral intravenous infusion of 1.5 L of a 25% dextrose solution containing 4% amino acids and mixed with 1 L of a 10% lipid solution
(E) Peripheral intravenous infusion of 1 L of a 12% dextrose solution containing 6% amino acids and mixed with 2 L of a 10% lipid solution

587. After apical scars are found on chest x-ray in a 48-year-old postmenopausal woman, chemoprophylaxis with isoniazid is begun. Two months later the woman complains of weakness, nausea, and tingling in the feet. Physical examination is unremarkable, and routine blood and urine tests are normal. Four weeks later she has a grand-mal seizure and is admitted to the hospital. Findings on the admission physical include seborrheic dermatitis, glossitis, and absent ankle and knee tendon reflexes; hematologic testing reveals microcytic anemia.

At this point, the woman's physician should

(A) order immediate electroencephalography
(B) order CT scan of the brain
(C) discontinue isoniazid and begin treatment with rifampin
(D) administer intramuscular pyridoxine, 100 mg, then give 50 mg orally daily
(E) administer intramuscular cyanocobalamin, 100 μg, then give 100 μg daily for 1 week

588. A 78-year-old man who lives alone and prepares his own food is found to have numerous ecchymotic areas on the posterior aspect of his lower extremities. On closer examination of the skin, he has hemorrhagic areas around hair follicles; the hairs are fragmented. Splinter hemorrhages are present in the nail beds, and several hematomas are present in the muscles of the arms and legs. Except for the absence of teeth, the rest of the physical examination is unremarkable. Laboratory examination reveals a normal PT, PTT, and CBC, except for a hematocrit of 28 percent (red blood cell indices are normal).

This clinical syndrome is most likely due to a deficiency of

(A) vitamin A
(B) vitamin C
(C) folate
(D) vitamin K
(E) pyridoxine

589. A 25-year-old man with a renal allograft and history of an intracerebral abscess is evaluated for profound polyuria. He is admitted to the hospital for a water deprivation test. No fluids are given after 12 midnight. By 11 A.M. he has lost 1 kg, and urine osmolality has been 120 mosm/kg for the last 3 h. Plasma osmolality is 320 mosm/kg (serum sodium is 155 mmol/L). At 11 A.M. 1 μg desmopressin is given by subcutaneous injection; 45 min later the urine osmolality is measured at 121 mosm/kg. The patient is then allowed to drink.

Treatment of this patient should include

(A) vasopressin tannate in oil
(B) hydrochlorothiazide
(C) desmopressin
(D) chlorpropamide
(E) none of the above

590. A person with hypercalcemia due to sarcoidosis would likely have all but which one of the following?

(A) An abnormal chest x-ray
(B) Increased absorption of calcium from the gastrointestinal tract
(C) Hypercalciuria
(D) Increased serum parathyroid hormone level
(E) Hypergammaglobulinemia

591. A 67-year-old man with chronic arthritis is found to have passed a uric acid stone after an episode of renal colic. On workup he is found to have multiple radiolucent stones in the left renal pelvis, uric acid excretion of 5.4 mmol/d (900 mg/d), a serum uric acid concentration of 580 μmol/L (9.8 mg/dL), a serum creatinine concentration of 160 μmol/L (1.8 mg/dL), and monosodium urate crystals in an effusion in the left knee. The drug of choice for long-term therapy in this patient is

(A) probenecid alone
(B) probenecid and sodium bicarbonate
(C) allopurinol
(D) colchicine
(E) sulfinpyrazone

592. A patient has a serum triglyceride concentration of 45 mmol/L (4000 mg/dL), a serum cholesterol concentration of 15.5 mmol/L (600 mg/dL), eruptive xanthomas, and lipemia retinalis. The serum shows a creamy upper layer with a turbid infranatant after overnight refrigeration. These findings are most consistent with which of the following plasma lipoprotein patterns?

(A) Type 1
(B) Type 2
(C) Type 3
(D) Type 4
(E) Type 5

593. An obese woman has hypertriglyceridemia without hypercholesterolemia. The most appropriate first step in the treatment of this woman would be

(A) abstinence from alcohol
(B) weight reduction
(C) avoidance of oral contraceptives
(D) clofibrate therapy
(E) bile acid-binding resin therapy

594. In designing a hormone replacement program for patients with coexistent thyroid and adrenal failure,

(A) the dose of glucocorticoid must be increased slowly once thyroid replacement has been initiated
(B) the dose of thyroid hormone must be increased slowly once glucocorticoid replacement has been initiated
(C) mineralocorticoid replacement must also be included if combined therapy is required
(D) thyroid replacement must not be initiated until treatment with glucocorticoid has been instituted
(E) growth hormone replacement must also be included if combined therapy is required

595. A 35-year-old clinically euthyroid woman is seen because of a neck mass. She has no history of prior neck irradiation. A 2-cm, firm nodule is palpated in the left lobe of an otherwise normal gland. Fine needle aspiration of this lesion reveals sheets of follicular cells. The next appropriate procedure is

(A) subtotal thyroidectomy
(B) levothyroxine suppressive therapy
(C) repeat fine needle aspiration
(D) follow-up examination in 6 months
(E) radionuclide scan

596. Cholestyramine and colestipol are binding resins that are used to treat patients with hypercholesterolemia. Their serum-cholesterol-lowering effects are thought to be mediated by

(A) causing mild diarrhea and a mild degree of fat malabsorption
(B) binding of intestinal cholesterol, thus decreasing its net absorption
(C) decreasing the intestinal synthesis of very low density lipoproteins
(D) interrupting the enterohepatic circulation of cholesterol by sequestering bile acids in the intestine
(E) none of the above

597. A 28-year-old woman who is 15 kg (33 lb) over ideal body weight wants to begin dieting. The best initial regimen for weight loss would be

(A) a low-calorie balanced diet
(B) a low-calorie, liquid protein diet ("protein-sparing modified fast")
(C) total starvation
(D) use of amphetamines to curb appetite
(E) an increase in exercise but no dietary changes

598. Obese persons are at an increased risk for all the following disorders EXCEPT

(A) hypothyroidism
(B) cholelithiasis
(C) diabetes mellitus
(D) hypertension
(E) hypertriglyceridemia

599. A 45-year-old woman is seen because of headaches, fatigue, and weakness. She takes no medicines. Except for a blood pressure of 150/95, the physical examination is normal. Electrocardiogram discloses prominent QRS voltage consistent with left ventricular hypertrophy and U waves. Serum electrolytes reveal the following: sodium, 148 mmol/L; potassium, 2.9 mmol/L; chloride, 110 mmol/L; and bicarbonate, 35 mmol/L.

Which of the following measurements would be the most helpful in establishing a diagnosis of primary mineralocorticoid excess?

(A) Urinary 17-ketosteroids
(B) Plasma renin activity
(C) Plasma renin following administration of 20 mg furosemide
(D) Plasma aldosterone following saline loading
(E) Abdominal CT scan

600. Which of the following regimens is best for the preoperative management of a patient with a known pheochromocytoma?

(A) Propranolol alone
(B) Propranolol followed by phenoxybenzamine
(C) Phenoxybenzamine followed by propranolol
(D) Prazosin alone
(E) Propranolol followed by prazosin

601. A person with Cushing's disease undergoes transsphenoidal removal of an ACTH-secreting microadenoma. Routine endocrinologic management after recovery from surgery should include administration of

(A) hydrocortisone, 30 mg/d
(B) hydrocortisone, 100 mg/d
(C) hydrocortisone, 30 mg/d, and levothyroxine, 0.1 mg/d
(D) hydrocortisone, 100 mg/d, and desmopressin, 0.2 μg/d
(E) none of the above

602. Which of the following statements is true regarding Cushing's disease caused by bilateral adrenal hyperplasia?

(A) Cortisol production may increase during administration of metyrapone
(B) Urinary 17-ketosteroid excretion is usually normal
(C) Plasma cortisol concentration may be maintained at a level less than 550 nmol/L (20 μg/dL)
(D) Administration of dexamethasone, 8 mg/d for 2 days, reduces cortisol production only minimally
(E) Administration of dexamethasone, 2 mg/d for 2 days, is not followed by a reduction in urinary free cortisol excretion

603. All the following statements concerning Wilson's disease are true EXCEPT

(A) hepatic involvement is present in half the patients
(B) the absence of Kayser-Fleischer corneal rings excludes the diagnosis of neuropsychiatric Wilson's disease
(C) a low serum ceruloplasmin value is consistent with the diagnosis
(D) administration of penicillamine is the treatment of choice
(E) treatment should be interrupted routinely to minimize side effects

604. Each of the following may be a direct consequence of severe magnesium deficiency EXCEPT

(A) digitalis-induced arrhythmias
(B) hypocalcemia
(C) hypokalemia
(D) hyponatremia
(E) confusion

605. A 42-year-old woman has obesity, weakness, and mild hypertension. She complains of menstrual irregularity for the last few months. Physical examination discloses some pink abdominal striae. Fasting blood glucose level is 10 mmol/L (189 mg/dL). The most appropriate means to rule out Cushing's syndrome in this woman would be

(A) CT of the pituitary gland
(B) measurement of 24-h urinary free cortisol excretion
(C) 2-day dexamethasone suppression test (8 mg/d)
(D) overnight dexamethasone suppression test
(E) measurement of the morning plasma ACTH level

606. A 28-year-old woman is referred because of failure to menstruate during the 7 months since the delivery of an infant. She is still nursing the baby. Measurement of a random serum prolactin level obtained elsewhere was 310 μg/L. After obtaining a pertinent history and physical examination, your next step in the evaluation of this patient's condition would be which of the following?

(A) Trial of low-dose bromocriptine to assess suppressibility of the hyperprolactinemic state
(B) Computed tomography of the head and pituitary gland with contrast
(C) Goldmann visual field assessment
(D) Measurement of serum prolactin levels before and after nursing
(E) Delay in any further evaluation until she stops nursing

607. In the assessment of a 10-year-old girl with short stature and an abnormal growth rate, all the following studies are of value in the initial workup EXCEPT

(A) serum thyroxine concentration
(B) measurement of random insulin-like growth factor I/somatomedin C (IGF-I/SM-C) concentration
(C) measurement of random plasma growth hormone concentration
(D) radiographic assessment of bone age
(E) chromosomal karyotype

608. A 64-year-old man seeks medical attention because of an annoying cough. Physical examination is remarkable only for supraclavicular lymphadenopathy. Chest x-ray shows a parahilar mass and paratracheal lymph node enlargement. Serum and urine chemistries are as follows:

Sodium: 120 mmol/L
Potassium: 4 mmol/L
Bicarbonate: 23 mmol/L
Serum osmolality: 250 mosmol/kg H_2O
Urine osmolality: 600 mosmol/kg H_2O
Urine sodium: 80 mmol/L

The most likely pathophysiologic basis for this man's hyponatremia is

(A) production of a vasopressin-like molecule by tumor tissue
(B) production of authentic vasopressin by tumor tissue
(C) potentiation of vasopressin action on the renal tubule by a tumor product
(D) stimulation of neurohypophyseal vasopressin secretion by a tumor product
(E) central nervous system metastases resulting in loss of vasopressin regulation

609. In a person who has chronic inappropriate AVP (vasopressin) secretion due to bronchogenic carcinoma, the agent most likely to be effective in supplementing the benefit of a water restriction regimen would be

(A) ethanol
(B) phenytoin
(C) lithium
(D) desmopressin
(E) demeclocycline

610. Impaired peripheral conversion of thyroxine (T_4) to triiodothyronine (T_3) is associated with the administration of all the following agents EXCEPT

(A) propylthiouracil
(B) dexamethasone
(C) methimazole
(D) propranolol
(E) oral cholecystography dye

611. Eight years after surgical resection of a benign nodule in the left lobe of her thyroid gland, a 35-year-old woman presents with a right-sided neck mass. Her thyroid scan is shown below. She is asymptomatic and takes no medication. Which of the following should her physician advise?

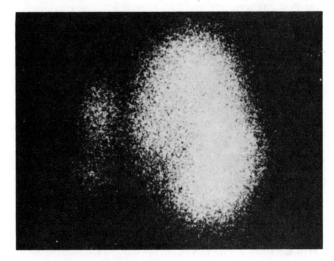

(A) Diagnostic ultrasonography
(B) Surgical exploration of the right side of the neck
(C) Measurement of plasma calcitonin concentration
(D) Reevaluation in 1 year
(E) Exogenous thyroid hormone therapy

612. A 26-year-old pregnant woman has a goiter but is clinically euthyroid. Thyroid function tests reveal a free thyroxine index that is slightly elevated. An ultrasensitive TSH test reveals a level of 0.3 mU/L. The test that would be most appropriate in determining whether the woman is euthyroid or hyperthyroid is

(A) radioactive iodine uptake
(B) technetium thyroid scan
(C) T_3 suppression test
(D) thyrotropin-releasing hormone (TRH) stimulation test
(E) serum T_3 by radioimmunoassay

613. A 24-year-old woman develops Graves' disease during the third trimester of pregnancy. The most appropriate treatment would be

(A) subtotal thyroidectomy
(B) propylthiouracil
(C) propylthiouracil and levothyroxine
(D) radioactive iodine
(E) propranolol

614. In a 44-year-old woman with a subnormal serum thyroxine level and a history of treatment at the age of 29 years with radioactive iodine for Graves' disease, the best confirmatory test for suspected primary hypothyroidism is measurement of which of the following?

(A) Serum triiodothyronine (T_3) concentration
(B) Serum reverse triiodothyronine (rT_3) concentration
(C) Serum thyroid-stimulating hormone (TSH) concentration
(D) 24-h radioactive iodine uptake
(E) Thyrotropin-releasing hormone (TRH) stimulation test to measure TSH reserve

615. A 20-year-old man who has been treated with high-dose daily steroids for 3 weeks during an exacerbation of asthma is switched to alternate-day prednisone therapy. Four days later, he complains of muscle weakness, arthralgias, and fatigue; in addition, his temperature is 37.8°C (100°F). His physician should

(A) order a blood sample for antinuclear antibody determination
(B) order a blood sample for creatine phosphokinase determination
(C) search for an occult infection
(D) immediately switch back to daily steroid administration
(E) reassure the man that this problem is common and self-limited

616. In persons with congenital adrenal hyperplasia due to inherited defects of adrenal steroid C-21 hydroxylase, excessive androgen production is the result of

(A) autonomous adrenal production of steroids
(B) autonomous pituitary production of ACTH
(C) extraglandular formation from large amounts of nonandrogenic adrenal steroids
(D) failure of production of an adrenal product necessary for negative feedback on pituitary ACTH secretion
(E) positive feedback on pituitary ACTH secretion by abnormal adrenal products

617. A 38-year-old woman with obesity, dermal striae, and hypertension is referred for endocrinologic evaluation of possible cortisol excess. The woman receives a midnight dose of 1 mg of dexamethasone; a plasma cortisol level drawn at 8 A.M. the next day is 386 nmol/L (14 μg/dL). At this point in the evaluation, the most appropriate diagnostic maneuver would be

(A) CT scanning of the pituitary gland
(B) abdominal CT scanning
(C) measurement of 24-h 17-hydroxycorticosteroid excretion in urine
(D) 2-day low-dose dexamethasone suppression test (0.5 mg every 6 h for 48 h)
(E) 2-day high-dose dexamethasone suppression test (2.0 mg every 6 h for 48 h)

618. In a 36-year-old woman who has had insulin-dependent diabetes mellitus since the age of 14, hyperkalemia is being evaluated. On physical examination her blood pressure is 146/96 mmHg. Laboratory evaluation discloses the following:

Fasting plasma glucose: 6 mmol/L (110 mg/dL)
Serum creatinine: 194 μmol/L (2.2 mg/dL)
Serum sodium: 135 mmol/L
Serum potassium: 6.2 mmol/L
Serum chloride: 116 mmol/L
Serum bicarbonate: 14 mmol/L

After a short ACTH infusion test, the plasma cortisol concentration increases from 386 to 717 nmol/L (14 to 26 μg/dL). After administration of 80 mg of furosemide and 3 h of upright posture, the plasma renin activity and aldosterone concentration are unchanged from baseline values.

The most appropriate therapeutic regimen to correct the electrolyte imbalance would be

(A) administration of fludrocortisone
(B) administration of furosemide
(C) administration of hydrocortisone and furosemide
(D) hemodialysis
(E) administration of potassium-binding anion-exchange resins

619. The best indicator of how well a person's diabetes mellitus has been controlled over an extended length of time (months) is

(A) hemoglobin A_{1c} concentration
(B) glycosylated albumin concentration
(C) plasma C-peptide concentration
(D) mean of the blood sugar levels measured through the day
(E) 24-h urine glucose excretion

620. A 22-year-old woman who has had diabetes mellitus for 6 years now wishes to become pregnant. She takes 32 units of NPH insulin each morning, and her urine glucose values (done twice daily) are "usually trace or 1+." Her hemoglobin A_{1c} level is 9.8 percent (normal: 5 to 8 percent). She takes oral contraceptive pills. Her physician should advise her that

(A) home glucose monitoring and a daily regimen of multiple subcutaneous injections of regular insulin are necessary now
(B) oral contraceptive agents can falsely elevate HbA_{1c} levels
(C) attempts to achieve better diabetic control can wait until she has become pregnant
(D) the current insulin regimen probably will be adequate until the last trimester of pregnancy
(E) hospitalization will probably be necessary for most of her pregnancy to ensure normal delivery and perinatal survival

621. A 24-year-old man with diabetes since the age of 9 years sees his physician for a routine checkup. He has no complaints and is taking 40 units NPH and 5 units regular insulin each morning as prescribed. Funduscopic examination reveals the findings in Color Plate I. Based on these findings, his physician should recommend

(A) vitrectomy
(B) photocoagulation
(C) hypophysectomy
(D) more vigorous control of the blood sugar level
(E) followup examination in 3 months

622. A middle-aged diabetic man who has been taking chlorpropamide, 0.5 g daily, becomes confused and lethargic at home. He is brought to the emergency room, where examination is otherwise negative. Blood glucose concentration is 1.3 mmol/L (24 mg/dL). He is given 50 mL of a 50% intravenous glucose solution and becomes more responsive. His physician should now

(A) send the man home with instructions to decrease the dosage of chlorpropamide to 0.25 g daily
(B) send the man home with instructions to switch to tolbutamide, 0.5 g three times daily
(C) observe the man for several more hours and send him home if no further problems develop
(D) have the man eat a meal, then administer a 5% glucose solution intravenously for 12 h and send him home if no further problems develop
(E) have the man eat a meal, then admit him to the hospital for further observation and treatment

623. An 18-year-old woman fasts for 24 h. The metabolic changes that would be expected at the end of the fasting period include all the following EXCEPT

(A) dependence by the brain on ketone metabolism
(B) breakdown of triglycerides in adipose tissue
(C) utilization of lactate, glycerol, and amino acids for hepatic gluconeogenesis
(D) a decrease in liver glycogen
(E) a fall in plasma insulin concentration and a rise in release of glucagon, cortisol, growth hormone, and epinephrine

624. In a 40-year-old man with long-standing hypogonadism resulting from total surgical castration for bilateral seminomas at the age of 17 years, the effectiveness of testosterone cypionate therapy can best be monitored by the assessment of

(A) plasma testosterone level
(B) plasma luteinizing hormone (LH) level
(C) plasma testosterone cypionate level
(D) change in muscle mass
(E) frequency of nocturnal erections

625. A 20-year-old competitive swimmer is examined because of primary amenorrhea. Her height is 170 cm (67 in) and she weighs 50 kg (110 lb). Her breasts are well developed. Findings on pelvic examination are normal, and the pelvic hair appears to be normal. Cervical mucus is abundant and demonstrates ferning upon drying. Urine spot and blood tests for pregnancy are negative. She is given 10 mg of medroxyprogesterone acetate twice a day for 5 days, and 3 days later she experiences menstrual bleeding for the first time. The most likely cause of the amenorrhea is

(A) functional hypothalamic amenorrhea
(B) 45,X gonadal dysgenesis
(C) polycystic ovarian disease
(D) chromaphobe adenoma of the pituitary
(E) prolactinoma of the pituitary

626. A 21-year-old woman is examined because of secondary amenorrhea. Cyclic menses had commenced at the age of 14 years. When she was 19 years old she became pregnant and was hospitalized during the sixth month of that pregnancy because of bleeding and hypotension that proved to be the result of a spontaneous abortion with retained placental fragments; she received ten units of blood, and a dilation and curettage was performed. No menses have occurred during the 2 years since the hospitalization. She now wishes to become pregnant.

Findings on physical examination, including rectopelvic examination, are normal. Results on complete blood counts, SMA-12, and chest x-ray are within normal limits. Serum thyroxine (T$_4$) concentration is 90 nmol/L (7 μg/dL) and an 8 A.M. plasma cortisol measurement is 470 nmol/L (17 μg/dL). No menstrual bleeding occurs after administration of 10 mg medroxyprogesterone acetate per day for 10 days or cyclic estrogen and progestogen (1.25 mg conjugated estrogens by mouth each day for 3 weeks with 10 mg medroxyprogesterone acetate per day for the last 7 days).

At this point the most appropriate diagnostic study would be

(A) CT scan of the pituitary with contrast
(B) hysterosalpingogram
(C) CT scan of the abdomen followed by wedge resection of the ovaries
(D) metyrapone test
(E) chromosomal analysis

627. A 36-year-old woman has noticed the absence of menses for the last 4 months. A pregnancy test is negative. Serum levels of luteinizing hormone and follicle-stimulating hormone are elevated, and the serum estradiol level is low. These findings suggest

(A) bilateral tubal obstruction
(B) panhypopituitarism
(C) polycystic ovarian disease
(D) premature menopause
(E) exogenous estrogen administration

628. A newborn infant with ambiguous genitalia develops vomiting and profound volume depletion. A diagnosis of congenital adrenal hyperplasia due to C-21 hydroxylase deficiency would be supported by all the following findings EXCEPT

(A) elevated urinary 17-ketosteroid concentration
(B) elevated plasma 11-deoxycortisol concentration
(C) elevated plasma 17-hydroxyprogesterone concentration
(D) elevated plasma androstenedione concentration
(E) elevated urinary pregnanediol and pregnanetriol concentrations

629. In women with gonadal dysgenesis, development of malignancy in the streak gonads is most likely when the karyotype is

(A) 46XX$_i$ (isochrome X)
(B) 46,XX
(C) 45,X
(D) 45,X/46,XY mosaicism
(E) 45X,46XX mosaicism

630. The most common presentation of primary hyperparathyroidism is

(A) peptic ulcer
(B) proximal muscle weakness
(C) osteitis fibrosa cystica
(D) calcium kidney stones
(E) asymptomatic hypercalcemia

631. The diagnosis of primary hyperparathyroidism is made in an elderly woman who has osteitis fibrosa cystica and elevated serum levels of calcium (3 mmol/L [12.0 mg/dL]) and creatinine (309 μmol/L [3.5 mg/dL]). The woman is not considered a surgical candidate because of pulmonary disease. The best medical treatment for hyperparathyroidism in this woman would be

(A) plicamycin
(B) estrogen
(C) phosphate
(D) diphosphonate
(E) thiazide

632. Prolonged immobilization has been associated with all the following consequences EXCEPT

(A) hypercalcemia
(B) hypercalciuria and nephrolithiasis
(C) osteoporosis
(D) soft-tissue calcifications
(E) elevation of serum parathyroid hormone levels

633. A 54-year-old man with peptic ulcer disease has been using aluminum hydroxide–containing antacids for the past several years to treat his symptoms. He complains of diffuse bone pain and progressive muscular weakness. These symptoms are most likely a result of

(A) malnutrition associated with his ulcer symptoms
(B) occult gastric malignancy
(C) aluminum-induced osteomalacia
(D) chronic phosphorus depletion
(E) aluminum intoxication

634. A 34-year-old woman has had three hospital admissions during the last year because of nephrolithiasis. The rate of 24-h urinary calcium excretion has been above the normal range on all three occasions and serum calcium concentrations were between 2.5 and 2.8 mmol/L (10.2 and 11.5 mg/dL). The serum phosphorus concentration was 0.77 mmol/L (2.4 mg/dL) and the parathyroid hormone level was 229 nL eq/mL (normal less than 150 nL eq/mL).

The most appropriate management at this time would be

(A) to begin administration of prednisone, 40 mg daily, and taper the dose over a period of 4 weeks
(B) to administer thiazide diuretics to decrease calcium excretion
(C) symptomatic treatment of renal lithiasis only
(D) calcium supplementation to prevent progressive bone loss
(E) surgical exploration of the neck

635. Each of the following conditions is characteristic of the presentation of osteomalacia in adults EXCEPT which one?

(A) Bowing of the tibia
(B) Pseudofractures
(C) Long-bone pain
(D) Proximal muscle weakness
(E) Hypophosphatemia

636. During a routine checkup, a 67-year-old man is found to have a level of serum alkaline phosphatase three times the upper limit of normal. Serum calcium and phosphorus concentrations and liver function test results are normal. He is asymptomatic. The most likely diagnosis is

(A) metastatic bone disease
(B) primary hyperparathyroidism
(C) occult plasmacytoma
(D) Paget's disease of bone
(E) osteomalacia

637. The vitamin D metabolite that regulates absorption of calcium from the gastrointestinal tract is

(A) dihydrotachysterol
(B) cholecalciferol
(C) $24,25(OH)_2D$
(D) $1,25(OH)_2D$
(E) 25OH vitamin D

638. A 61-year-old woman noticed severe sharp pain in her back after lifting a suitcase. A compression fracture of the T11 vertebral body is identified on x-ray examination. Routine laboratory evaluation discloses a serum calcium concentration of 2 mmol/L (8.0 mg/dL), a serum phosphorus concentration of 0.77 mmol/L (2.4 mg/dL), and increased serum alkaline phosphatase activity. The serum parathyroid hormone level was subsequently found to be elevated as well. The most likely diagnosis is

(A) Paget's disease of bone
(B) ectopic parathyroid hormone secretion
(C) primary hyperparathyroidism
(D) postmenopausal osteoporosis
(E) vitamin D deficiency

639. Which of the following conditions is associated with hypocalcemia but NOT with an increased serum level of parathyroid hormone?

(A) Severe hypomagnesemia
(B) Osteomalacia secondary to vitamin D deficiency
(C) Osteomalacia secondary to vitamin D resistance
(D) Renal failure
(E) Pseudohypoparathyroidism

640. The most important regulator of serum $1,25(OH)_2$ vitamin D concentration is

(A) serum calcium
(B) serum magnesium
(C) serum 25OH vitamin D
(D) parathyroid hormone
(E) prolactin

DIRECTIONS: Each question below contains five suggested responses. For **each** of the five responses listed with every question, you are to respond either YES (Y) or NO (N). In a given item **all, some, or none of the alternatives may be correct.**

641. Anovulatory cycles are characterized by

(A) elevated levels of plasma progesterone
(B) dysmenorrhea
(C) an absent luteal phase
(D) lack of a normal LH and FSH surge
(E) irregular uterine bleeding

642. True statements regarding the pedigree analysis of an autosomally transmitted dominant disorder include which of the following?

(A) Males and females are affected in equal proportions
(B) On average, half the siblings of an affected patient will be affected with the disorder
(C) Persons of each gender are likely to transmit the condition to male and female offspring
(D) Normal children of an affected parent will have only normal offspring
(E) Consanguinity is common among the parents of affected offspring

643. A 15-year-old boy has had hypothyroidism since early childhood. For several years, he has noticed frequent episodes of numbness and tingling of his hands, occasionally accompanied by muscle spasms. Physical examination reveals a positive Chvostek sign, short stature, and short left fourth metacarpals (absent knuckles). The boy's mother is also short and has absent knuckles. Serum calcium concentration is 1.9 mmol/L (7.5 mg/dL).

Further investigation of the boy's disorder would be expected to reveal

(A) antibodies to parathyroid and thyroid tissue
(B) elevated parathyroid hormone concentration
(C) diminished increase in urinary cyclic AMP in response to administration of parathyroid hormone
(D) calcification of the basal ganglia
(E) moniliasis

644. Diseases inherited in a multifactorial genetic fashion (i.e., not autosomal dominant, autosomal recessive, or X-linked) and seen more frequently in persons bearing certain histocompatibility antigens include

(A) gluten-sensitive enteropathy
(B) neurofibromatosis
(C) adult polycystic kidney disease
(D) Wilson's disease
(E) diabetes mellitus

645. Erectile impotence may be caused by

(A) elevated serum prolactin
(B) nifedipine
(C) cimetidine
(D) Peyronie's disease
(E) amitriptyline

646. Protein malnutrition commonly occurs in association with energy-deficient diets because

(A) diets low in carbohydrate and fat cause acute protein malabsorption
(B) amino acids are diverted from protein synthesis into oxidative metabolism
(C) normal protein synthesis requires an adequate energy supply
(D) normal protein metabolism occurs only if fat in the diet is adquate
(E) it is common for diets to be deficient in both protein and energy

647. A 34-year-old man with alcoholic cirrhosis is admitted to the hospital for evaluation of abdominal swelling, which has become progressively worse over the last 2 weeks. On physical examination, he is noted to be cachectic; the liver is enlarged, ascites and edema are present, and stool is heme-positive. Measurement of which of the following parameters would be useful in determining the extent of the man's *protein* malnutrition?

(A) Blood ammonia concentration
(B) Serum albumin and transferrin levels
(C) Present body weight as a percentage of ideal body weight
(D) Midarm circumference and triceps skin-fold thickness
(E) Ratio of 24-h creatinine excretion to height

648. Alterations characteristic of combined protein-calorie starvation include

(A) decreased serum T_4 and serum T_3 and increased serum reverse T_3 (rT_3) levels
(B) decreased serum insulin, glucagon, and cortisol levels
(C) impaired cell-mediated immunity
(D) decreased serum immunoglobulin levels and impaired humoral response to antigens
(E) increased plasma free fatty acid and ketone levels

649. In a person with severe protein starvation, which of the following conditions would increase the amount of protein needed to achieve positive nitrogen balance?

(A) Renal failure
(B) Gastrointestinal fistula
(C) Sepsis
(D) Simultaneous caloric malnutrition
(E) Thyrotoxicosis

650. In which of the following situations is total parenteral nutrition (TPN) indicated as the *first* choice to provide partial or complete nourishment?

(A) A 34-year-old man has an acute exacerbation of Crohn's disease and develops an ileocolic fistula
(B) A 70-year-old woman has chest and limb injuries and extensive burns following an airplane crash
(C) A 26-year-old woman has extensive small-bowel resection for life-threatening regional enteritis
(D) A 53-year-old man scheduled to undergo elective surgery for gallstones will be unable to eat or drink for 5 days
(E) A 26-year-old woman is unable to swallow because of a relapse of myasthenia gravis

651. Appropriate dietary restrictions have been successful in treating patients who have which of the following inherited metabolic disorders?

(A) Phenylketonuria
(B) Familial lipoprotein lipase deficiency
(C) Hyperprolinemia
(D) Tay-Sachs disease
(E) Galactosemia

652. In a patient with hypercholesterolemia, which of the following may be an appropriate treatment to lower serum cholesterol concentration?

(A) Cholestyramine
(B) Nicotinic acid
(C) Lovastatin
(D) Probucol
(E) Low-cholesterol diet

653. Disorders associated with premature coronary heart disease include familial

(A) hypercholesterolemia
(B) hyperalphalipoproteinemia
(C) hypertriglyceridemia
(D) combined hyperlipidemia
(E) lipoprotein lipase deficiency

654. Hypertriglyceridemia is frequently encountered in patients with diabetes mellitus. True statements regarding this association include which of the following?

(A) Predisposition to both diseases may be independently inherited
(B) Insulin deficiency is a major factor contributing to the hypertriglyceridemia
(C) Some patients eventually need specific pharmacologic treatment for the hypertriglyceridemia
(D) Acute pancreatitis may occur with uncontrolled diabetes mellitus and elevation of the triglyceride levels
(E) Hypertriglyceridemia may resolve with adequate control of the diabetes

655. A 29-year-old obese man is referred because of hyperlipidemia. He consulted a dermatologist because of tuberous xanthomas in both elbows and yellowish discoloration of the palmar and digital creases. Serum cholesterol and triglyceride levels were 8.4 mmol/L (328 mg/dL) and 3.9 mmol/L (345 mg/dL), respectively. True statements regarding this patient include

(A) he has lipoprotein lipase deficiency
(B) weight loss is an important feature of management to reduce his lipid levels
(C) hypothyroidism or diabetes mellitus, or both, must be excluded by appropriate testing
(D) he is homozygous for a genetic defect of lipid metabolism
(E) clofibrate may be useful in the management of his hyperlipidemia

656. Potential long-term complications of gastric bypass surgery in a 39-year-old, 160-kg (352-lb) man include

(A) polyarthritis
(B) progressive hepatic disease
(C) early satiety
(D) diarrhea
(E) nephrolithiasis

657. Insulin resistance in obese persons results from which of the following phenomena?

(A) A decrease in the number of cell-surface insulin receptors
(B) Abnormal processing of proinsulin by pancreatic beta cells
(C) Circulating insulin antagonists
(D) Accelerated insulin degradation by the liver
(E) Postreceptor, intracellular defects in glucose metabolism

658. A 24-year-old woman presents because she is concerned that she has too much facial hair. She has irregular menstrual periods but takes no drugs, has no other complaints, and feels well. On examination she is slightly overweight and has a deep voice. There is mild facial cystic acne. There is increased hair on the upper lip and eyebrows, but no other facial hair. Chest hair and pubic hair are normal. The hair on the upper lip is not coarse and there is no frontal balding. Plasma testosterone is 1.7 nmol/L (50 ng/dL); plasma dehydroepiandrosterone sulfate is 17 nmol/L (600 ng/dL).

Which of the following disorders could the patient have?

(A) Adrenocortical carcinoma
(B) Polycystic ovaries
(C) Congenital adrenal hyperplasia
(D) Idiopathic hirsuitism
(E) Arrhenoblastoma

659. Which of the following abnormalities may be seen in patients with anorexia nervosa?

(A) Episodic LH release
(B) Elevated serum prolactin
(C) Depressed growth hormone levels
(D) Elevated plasma cortisol
(E) Increased reverse triiodothyronine (rT_3) levels

660. True statements regarding human obesity include which of the following?

(A) The resting metabolic rate is lower than normal in obese persons
(B) Endocrine diseases such as hypothyroidism and Cushing's syndrome are a frequent cause of obesity
(C) The energy expenditure of exercise is decreased in obese persons
(D) Genetic predisposition may be the single most important factor in obesity
(E) Decreased activity of lipoprotein lipase is the cause of obesity in some persons

661. Characteristic manifestations of Nelson's syndrome (pituitary tumor arising after bilateral adrenalectomy) include

(A) hyperpigmentation
(B) erosion of the sella turcica
(C) increased urinary 17-ketosteroid excretion
(D) failure of high doses of dexamethasone to suppress plasma cortisol levels
(E) elevated plasma ACTH levels

662. Growth hormone secretion is increased in normal persons in a number of situations, including

(A) exercise
(B) hyperglycemia
(C) infusion of levodopa
(D) infusion of arginine
(E) administration of thyrotropin-releasing hormone

663. A 45-year-old man who has noted decreased libido and sexual potency for the last 8 months is found to have a serum prolactin level of 70 μg/L. Computed tomography of the head reveals a pituitary tumor with suprasellar extension. Appropriate management of this patient would include

(A) formal visual field testing
(B) initiation of treatment with bromocriptine, 2.5 mg daily
(C) reassurance about the return of sexual function as soon as prolactin levels return to normal
(D) initiation of prophylactic treatment with desmopressin
(E) determination of serum gonadotropin and testosterone levels

664. Low thyroidal radioactive iodine uptake (RAIU) in persons exhibiting weight loss and elevated free thyroxine index can be caused by

(A) subacute thyroiditis
(B) struma ovarii
(C) choriocarcinoma
(D) ingestion of exogenous levothyroxine
(E) recent intravenous pyelography

665. True statements concerning the "sick euthyroid" syndrome include which of the following?

(A) Thyroid hormone production is usually normal
(B) Values for free thyroxine (T_4) index may be decreased, normal, or increased
(C) Serum total T_4 concentrations are usually normal or decreased
(D) Decreased production of triiodothyronine (T_3) is a consistent feature of the disorder
(E) Although serum levels of thyroid-binding globulin and thyroid-binding prealbumin may be decreased, decreased protein binding of thyroid hormones is caused principally by a circulating inhibitor of binding

666. In a 33-year-old woman who recently had an upper respiratory tract infection, symptoms of thyrotoxicosis develop. Her thyroid gland is exquisitely tender and nodular. The 24-h uptake of radioactive iodine is 2 percent. Appropriate treatment for this woman might include

(A) subtotal thyroidectomy
(B) administration of radioactive iodine
(C) administration of glucocorticoids
(D) administration of propranolol
(E) administration of aspirin

667. In a person who has Cushing's syndrome, the diagnosis of functioning adrenal carcinoma would be suggested by

(A) a palpable abdominal mass
(B) markedly increased urinary excretion of 17-ketosteroids
(C) high plasma levels of ACTH
(D) failure to suppress 17-hydroxycorticosteroid secretion with high-dose dexamethasone
(E) a doubling of urinary 17-hydroxycorticosteroid excretion after administration of metyrapone

668. A 52-year-old woman with systemic lupus erythematosus is about to be started on a long-term course of therapy with pharmacologic doses of glucocorticoids. Pretreatment evaluation should include

(A) chest x-ray and tuberculin skin test
(B) ACTH infusion test
(C) thoracic and lumbar spine films
(D) stool test for occult blood
(E) metyrapone test

669. The syndromes of congenital adrenal hyperplasia may result in which of the following disorders?

(A) Virilization
(B) Isosexual precocious puberty
(C) Male pseudohermaphroditism
(D) Hypertension
(E) Hypotension

670. Urinary 17-ketosteroid determination can be described by which of the following statements?

(A) It is a useful measurement to assess gonadal function
(B) It assesses the production of both adrenal and gonadal androgens
(C) It is a measurement primarily of androsterone and etiocholanolone excretion
(D) It usually is elevated in persons with untreated congenital adrenal hyperplasia due to C-21 hydroxylase deficiency
(E) Testosterone production usually contributes only about 40 percent of the value in men

671. Conditions that contribute to the enhanced rate of hepatic ketogenesis common to starvation and diabetic ketoacidosis include

(A) a decline in the circulating insulin/glucagon ratio
(B) decreased hepatic malonyl CoA concentration
(C) increased levels of plasma free fatty acids
(D) increased hepatic carnitine content
(E) increased activity of hepatic carnitine palmitoyl-transferase I

672. True statements concerning type 1 diabetes mellitus include which of the following?

(A) Direct vertical transmission has been shown by pedigree analysis to occur with a high prevalence
(B) The concordance rate for monozygotic twins less than 40 years of age is over 80 percent
(C) The risk of type 1 diabetes is increased in persons carrying HLA antigens B8, B15, DR3, or DR4
(D) Circulating islet-cell antibodies are usually present in patients with juvenile-onset type 1 diabetes studied either soon before or soon after the onset of symptoms
(E) Mumps virus and Coxsackie virus have been identified as possible causative agents in juvenile-onset type 1 diabetes

673. Characteristics of hyperosmolar coma include

(A) blood glucose concentration of 55 mmol/L (975 mg/dL)
(B) marked elevation of serum free fatty acids
(C) association with thrombosis and bleeding from disseminated intravascular coagulation
(D) occurrence in elderly persons with maturity-onset diabetes
(E) best initial therapeutic response with large volumes of free water and large doses of insulin

674. The diagnosis of diabetes mellitus is certain in which of the following situations?

(A) Abnormal oral glucose tolerance in a 24-year-old woman who has been dieting
(B) Successive fasting plasma glucose concentrations of 8, 9, and 8.5 mmol/L (147, 165, and 152 mg/dL) in an asymptomatic, otherwise healthy business-women
(C) Hyperglycemic ketoacidosis that developed in an 18-year-old man after surgical reduction of a fractured leg
(D) Persistent asymptomatic glycosuria in a 30-year-old woman
(E) Hyperglycemic hyperosmolar coma that developed in a 73-year-old man after a stroke

675. A 45-year-old woman has had diabetes for the last 8 years and has been treated with either oral hypoglycemic agents or insulin. She has been doing well on human NPH insulin for the last several months. However, in the last week she has developed symptoms of hyperglycemia. Doubling her insulin dosage does not help, and she is admitted to the hospital. Physical examination of this nonobese woman shows no sign of infection, ketoacisosis, or Cushing's syndrome. Following admission, insulin dosage is increased progressively to 240 units daily, but blood glucose concentration never falls below 19 mmol/L (350 mg/dL).

True statements regarding this woman's condition include which of the following?

(A) IgG anti-insulin antibodies are likely to be present in high titer
(B) Cell-surface insulin receptors are likely to be decreased in number
(C) Anti-insulin-receptor antibodies, increased erythrocyte sedimentation rate, and other signs of autoimmune disease are likely to be present
(D) Insulin desensitization procedures should be instituted
(E) Treatment should include high-dose prednisone

676. Which of the following would be associated with a poor prognosis for development of (or progression of) symptomatic renal failure in a 29-year-old woman who has had type 1 diabetes mellitus since the age of 14 years?

(A) Urine albumin excretion of 0.12 to 0.17 g/d on three separate occasions
(B) Urine albumin excretion of 0.55 to 0.62 g/d on three separate occasions
(C) Diastolic blood pressure of 110 to 123 mmHg
(D) Nocturia, 3 times per night
(E) Insulin requirement greater than 120 units per day

677. A 40-year-old physician's assistant has had episodic confusion, diaphoresis, and palpitations for the past 4 weeks. She has had several nightmares and three syncopal episodes. Fasting hypoglycemia with inappropriately elevated plasma insulin concentration is documented in the hospital. Plasma C-peptide concentration also is increased. Her physician should

(A) measure plasma insulin antibody levels
(B) measure plasma proinsulin levels
(C) measure plasma or urine sulfonylurea levels
(D) perform abdominal CT scan
(E) consult a surgeon for pancreatic surgery

678. Causes of fasting hypoglycemia due primarily to overutilization of glucose include

(A) carnitine deficiency
(B) hepatoma
(C) insulinoma
(D) congestive heart failure from cor pulmonale
(E) hypopituitarism

679. Testosterone replacement in a patient with Klinefelter syndrome (47,XXY) would be indicated in order to

(A) maintain spermatogenesis
(B) prevent antisocial behavior
(C) maintain sexual potency
(D) cause disappearance of gynecomastia
(E) promote virilization

680. Correctly matched deficiencies of specific trace elements and their recognized features include

(A) zinc deficiency: hyperkeratosis and alopecia
(B) zinc deficiency: gonadal atrophy
(C) copper deficiency: fever
(D) cobalt deficiency: anemia
(E) selenium deficiency: heart failure

681. Correct statements concerning hormones and their receptors include which of the following?

(A) Intracellular receptors transport hormones to the nucleus where the complex enhances transcription of certain species of mRNA
(B) The steroid hormone receptor bears homology to the *src* family of tyrosine kinase oncogenes
(C) The insulin receptor is homologous to the viral oncogene *erbA*
(D) The growth hormone and prolactin receptors are homologous
(E) Luteinizing hormone (LH) binding to its receptor allows GTP (G proteins) to bind to the receptor protein

682. Increased gonadal production of estrogen is characteristic of

(A) testicular feminization
(B) polycystic ovarian disease
(C) persistent follicle cyst
(D) third trimester of pregnancy
(E) arrhenoblastoma

683. Hot flashes (menopausal flushing) characteristically are associated with which of the following?

(A) Removal of testes in a 23-year-old 46,XY woman with the syndrome of complete testicular feminization
(B) Removal of the ovaries in a 26-year-old 46,XX woman with extensive pelvic inflammatory disease
(C) Removal of the streak gonads in a woman with the 46,XY form of pure gonadal dysgenesis
(D) Premature menopause
(E) Removal of the ovaries in a 23-year-old woman with bilateral dysgerminoma of the ovaries

684. A 38-year-old woman had a bilateral oophorectomy, and 2 months later she complains of hot flashes twice a day. The indications for estrogen replacement in this patient include

(A) suppression of hot flashes
(B) prevention of atrophic vaginitis
(C) prevention of accelerated loss of bone mass
(D) avoidance of the development of hirsutism
(E) prevention of breast atrophy

685. A 30-year-old man, father of three children, has had progressive breast enlargement during the last 6 months. He does not use any drugs. Physical examination is remarkable only for bilateral gynecomastia: testicular size is normal. Evaluation at this time should include

(A) blood sampling for SGOT and serum alkaline phosphatase and bilirubin levels
(B) blood sampling for plasma estradiol, testosterone, and LH levels
(C) a 24-h urine collection for measurement of 17-ketosteroids
(D) chromosomal karyotype
(E) breast biopsy

686. Known causes of ambiguous genitalia include

(A) the sex-chromosome pattern XYY
(B) the mosaic sex-chromosome pattern 45,X/46,XY
(C) single gene mutations that impair androgen action
(D) hypogonadotropic hypogonadism
(E) maternal ingestion of a virilizing drug during pregnancy

687. True statements describing persons who have Klinefelter syndrome include which of the following?

(A) They are 20 times as likely as normal men to develop breast cancer
(B) They may have a normal peripheral-blood karyotype and testes of average size
(C) They have an increased incidence of hypospadias
(D) They almost always are mentally deficient and socially maladjusted
(E) Diagnosis usually is not made until after puberty

688. A 40-year-old woman with known alcoholism is hospitalized because of dizziness and muscle aches. Serum phosphorus concentration is 0.3 mmol/L (0.9 mg/dL) several days after admission. Clinical signs and symptoms associated with hypophosphatemia include

(A) waddling gait
(B) irritability and apprehension
(C) elevated serum creatine phosphokinase concentration
(D) bacterial infection
(E) congestive cardiomyopathy

689. Hypophosphatemia is associated with which of the following?

(A) Acute renal failure
(B) Hyperventilation
(C) Use of nonabsorbable antacids
(D) Use of insulin
(E) Junk-food diet

690. Serum concentration of 25OH vitamin D may be reduced in association with which of the following conditions?

(A) Dietary deficiency of vitamin D
(B) Chronic severe cholestatic liver disease
(C) Chronic renal failure
(D) Anticonvulsant therapy with phenobarbital or phenytoin
(E) High-dose glucocorticoid therapy

691. Correct statements concerning hypervitaminosis D include which of the following?

(A) It may result from prolonged sun exposure
(B) It usually results from a single excessive dose of vitamin D_2 or D_3
(C) Consequences include hypercalcemia, hypercalciuria, and renal impairment
(D) Anephric patients can develop vitamin D toxicity
(E) Serum 1,25(OH) vitamin D levels are elevated

692. A 60-year-old woman has low-back pain. Radiographic examination reveals diffuse demineralization and a compression fracture of the fourth lumbar vertebra. Serum calcium concentration is 2.8 mmol/L (11.5 mg/dL). This clinical picture is compatible with the presence of which of the following conditions?

(A) Postmenopausal osteoporosis
(B) Paget's disease
(C) Primary hyperparathyroidism
(D) Multiple myeloma
(E) Osteomalacia

693. A 25-year-old woman presents to her internist complaining of fatigue. Though she does not seem to be depressed, she admits to a diminished appetite and loss of interest in sex. She is also intolerant of the cold and notes that her hair is falling out. She has trouble caring for her 1½ year old and recounts a very difficult parturition with a great deal of blood loss. She is on no medicines, has been amenorrheic since the birth of the child, and did not nurse the infant.

Which of the following tests would help to diagnose her problem?

(A) Measurement of growth hormone 1 h after insulin administration
(B) Measurement of plasma cortisol 1 h after insulin administration
(C) Measurement of urinary free cortisol
(D) Thyroid function tests and TSH
(E) ACTH stimulation test

694. Manifestations of hypothyroidism include

(A) diminished QRS voltage on ECG
(B) depressed serum cholesterol
(C) microcytic anemia
(D) increased serum creatine phosphokinase
(E) increased serum lactic dehydrogenase

695. A 25-year-old man presents with a several-month history of fatigue, weakness, anorexia, and nausea. Physical examination reveals a slightly emaciated, thin, tanned man whose baseline blood pressure is 90/60. He complains of extreme lightheadedness during the assessment of orthostatic vital signs. Laboratory evaluation reveals hyponatremia and hyperkalemia. Plasma cortisol level fails to rise significantly 60 min after intramuscular administration of 250 μg cosyntropin.

Which of the following conditions could have caused this clinical picture?

(A) Withdrawal from prolonged (> 1 year) administration of steroids for asthma
(B) Disseminated tuberculosis
(C) Craniopharyngioma
(D) Disseminated cytomegalovirus infection
(E) Esophageal candidiasis requiring long-term high-dose ketoconazole therapy

696. Which of the following would be appropriate in the initial management of patients with diabetic ketoacidosis?

(A) Administer 50 units/h of insulin intravenously until the acidosis is reversed
(B) Discontinue insulin therapy when plasma glucose levels approach normal
(C) Increase insulin dosage when plasma ketones rise
(D) Administer 5% glucose solution when the plasma glucose falls below 17 mmol/L (300 mg/dL)
(E) Infuse potassium chloride if the presenting serum potassium level is normal

697. Established complications of oral contraceptive use include

(A) deep venous thrombosis
(B) thromboembolic stroke
(C) hypertension
(D) endometrial cancer
(E) breast cancer

698. In which of the following disorders of incomplete sexual development in the male would testosterone production be normal or high?

(A) Deficiency of 17β-hydroxysteroid dehydrogenase
(B) Testicular feminization
(C) Deficiency of 5α-reductase
(D) Deficiency of 17,20-desmolase
(E) Reifenstein syndrome

699. In which of the following porphyria syndromes may the diagnosis be made on the basis of a positive Watson-Schwartz reaction in the urine (detection of porphobilinogen)?

(A) Intermittent acute porphyria
(B) Congenital erythropoietic porphyria
(C) Protoporphyria
(D) Porphyria cutanea tarda
(E) Variegate porphyria

700. Correct statements concerning inherited defects of metabolism include which of the following?

(A) Niemann-Pick disease is caused by a deficiency of glucosylceramidase and is associated with a characteristic bone marrow storage cell
(B) The incidence of disease due to hexosaminidase deficiency has been reduced in North America by heterozygote detection programs
(C) Errors in glycogen elongation or branching are incompatible with a normal life expectancy
(D) Early diagnosis of phenylketonuria is possible, but of little therapeutic benefit
(E) Cystinuria, the most common inborn error of amino acid transport, is associated with increased urinary excretion of all dibasic amino acids

Endocrine, Metabolic, and Genetic Disorders

Answers

575. The answer is B. *(Wilson, ed 12. chap 327.)* In persons with symptomatic hemochromatosis, repeated phlebotomy, by removing excessive iron stores, results in marked clinical improvement. Specifically, the liver and spleen decrease in size, liver function improves, cardiac failure is reversed, and skin pigmentation ("bronzing") diminishes. Carbohydrate intolerance may abate in up to half of all affected persons. For unknown reasons there is no improvement in the arthropathy or the hypogonadism (due to pituitary deposition of iron) associated with hemochromatosis. Five-year survival rate is increased from 33 to 90 percent with treatment; prolonged survival may actually increase the risk of hepatocellular carcinoma, which affects one-third of persons treated for hemochromatosis.

576. The answer is C. *(Wilson, ed 12. chap 376. Kitchens, JAMA 258:1615, 1987.)* Coral snakes rarely bite humans, but when they do the potent neurotoxin can cause death. If it is suspected that a person has been envenomed, antivenom should be given without waiting for systemic manifestations to develop. The bite of a coral snake, though it causes little pain and swelling, produces local numbness and weakness in the region of the bite; ataxia, ptosis, palatal and pharyngeal paralysis, and other neurologic symptoms may follow. If the extremity is not promptly immobilized with a proximal constrictive band after a bite, a significant amount of toxin may be absorbed. Ice, no longer a recommended treatment for snake bite, does not neutralize the toxin. Wide surgical debridement would be unnecessary.

577. The answer is B. *(Wilson, ed 12. chap 5.)* The genes responsible for X-linked recessive disorders, such as hemophilia A, nephrogenic diabetes insipidus, Duchenne's muscular dystrophy, and testicular feminization, are on the X chromosome. Males, who are XY, will demonstrate the full syndrome whenever they inherit the altered gene from a mother who is heterozygous (or rarely homozygous). Homozygously affected females can only arise from the union of an affected male and a carrier (or homozygous) female. Thus, the disease tends to be seen in uncles and nephews rather than fathers and sons. In fact, an affected father cannot give rise to affected males, since they will inherit his Y chromosome. Assuming marriage to a normal female, all the affected male's female offspring will be carriers, since they will all get the single abnormal gene from their father. A female carrier (having one of her two X chromosomes carrying the mutant allele) will have sons with a 50 percent chance of being affected and daughters with a 50 percent chance of being carriers.

578. The answer is B. *(Wilson, ed 12. chap 313. Jordon, Am J Med 62:569, 1977.)* The first step in evaluating a person found to have an enlarged sella turcica but no symptoms that can be related to a pituitary tumor is to rule out the possibility of an empty sella. A CT scan of the head is now the procedure of choice in examining for an empty sella. If an empty sella is documented by a CT scan in an asymptomatic person, no specific endocrinologic evaluation is necessary.

579. The answer is C. *(Wilson, ed 12. chap 319. Cryer, Diabetes 38:1183, 1983.)* Hypoglycemia is common in patients with type 1 diabetes mellitus, particularly when aggressive efforts are made to bring the fasting glucose concentrations into the normal range and to control postprandial hyperglycemia. Hypoglycemia can worsen diabetic control, in large part by triggering the release of counterregulatory hormones, such as glucagon. This phenomenon of "hypoglycemic hyperglycemia," called the Somogyi effect, should be suspected when wide swings in blood or urine sugar levels occur over a short period of time. Other clues suggesting a Somogyi effect are worsening of diabetic control as insulin dosage is increased and increased hunger and weight gain despite worsening hyperglycemia or glycosuria. By contrast, poor control due to underdosage of insulin usually causes weight loss from caloric wastage in the urine (ketonuria and glycosuria). The correct therapy for the man described in this question is to decrease the morning dose of NPH insulin rather than to administer more or different insulin, to treat the rebound hyperglycemia, or to decrease food intake at supper.

580. The answer is D. *(Wilson, ed 12. chaps 53, 322.)* Progestogen therapy results in secretory differentiation of an estrogen-primed proliferative endometrium, and the endometrium is sloughed following progestogen withdrawal only if it has been stimulated first by estrogen. Thus, in a woman being evaluated for secondary amenorrhea, the appearance of menses following a short course of progestogen is indicative of an estrogen-primed endometrium and is good evidence of ovarian estrogen secretion. Estrone levels do not reflect direct ovarian estrogen secretion, because estrone is derived principally from the peripheral conversion of androstenedione, which is secreted from the adrenal glands and the ovaries. A woman with amenorrhea caused by hypogonadotropic hypogonadism has deficient ovarian estrogen secretion but may demonstrate an increase in plasma estradiol following human chorionic gonadotropin (hCG) administration. Prolactin secretion is increased by estrogen stimulation, accounting for a slightly higher mean prolactin level in women compared with that in men. However, a normal prolactin level is not evidence of persistent estrogen secretion.

581. The answer is D. *(Wilson, ed 12. chaps 53, 322.)* In a 7-year-old girl, isosexual precocity that is associated with undetectable levels of gonadotropins and urinary 17-ketosteroid levels appropriate for her chronologic age is most likely due to an estrogen-secreting tumor. Tumor localization procedures, such as abdominal CT scanning and pelvic sonography, should be performed before laparotomy. Plasma androstenedione measurement is unlikely to be helpful if urinary 17-ketosteroid excretion is low or normal. In idiopathic precocious puberty, a diagnosis of exclusion, urinary gonadotropins are either normal for chronologic age or elevated; in addition, if plasma gonadotropins are measured frequently during a 24-h period, the characteristic pubertal nocturnal surge should be seen in patients with idiopathic precocious puberty.

582. The answer is D. *(Wilson, ed 12. chap 7.)* Most autosomal chromosomal trisomies cause death in utero. Among live-born infants with trisomies (21, 18, and 13), trisomies 18 and 13 cause death in infancy. Patients with trisomy 21 (Down's syndrome) may reach adulthood, although with a shortened life expectancy because of an increased incidence of severe infections and complications from associated malformations. On the other hand, sex chromosome trisomies are compatible with intrauterine survival and are usually associated with a normal life expectancy.

583. The answer is B. *(Wilson, ed 12. chaps 5, 228.)* Many autosomal dominant disorders vary in the time of onset and severity of expression. Therefore, persons such as the two apparently unaffected siblings who are at risk for development of hereditary nephritis, even in the absence of overt evidence of renal impairment, are poor candidates as donors for a kidney. In addition, the mother is clearly a carrier and a poor candidate. The father is the best close relative to evaluate as a potential donor.

584. The answer is D. *(Wilson, ed 12. chap 6.)* One of the most important techniques for identifying genomic sites responsible for inherited diseases and for prenatal diagnosis is the identification of restriction fragment length polymorphisms (RFLPs). Such RFLP sites are the consequences of variable sequences that may or may not allow a specific restriction endonuclease (an enzyme recognizing a specific, usually four-to-seven-base DNA sequence) to cut at that site. In the Southern blots of the depicted family, the parents are heterozygous for a restriction site that is 2 kb away from one nonpolymorphic site and 8 kb away from another nonpolymorphic site in the other direction (which is the section the probe recognizes). In one of each of the parents' chromosomes the polymorphic site is present; in the other chromosome it is not. Thus, upon digestion of the parents' DNA, both a 10-kb fragment, representing the chromosome that lacks the polymorphic site, and an 8-kb fragment, representing the chromosome that has this site, exist. The son has inherited the chromosome with the site present from both his father and his mother, while the daughter has inherited the chromosome without the sequence that does not allow the extra cut from both parents. If the polymorphic sequence that allows cutting were associated with an autosomal recessive disease (by virtue of its being proximate on the genome), then such a marker could be used to predict the presence of the disease in the son or a fetus with a similar pattern on Southern blotting of DNA.

585. The answer is E. *(Wilson, ed 12. chaps 76, 357.)* Causes of thiamine deficiency in alcoholic persons include poor dietary intake, impaired absorption and storage, and accelerated destruction of thiamine diphosphate. Both the cardiovascular and the neurologic signs of thiamine deficiency (beriberi) can become abruptly evident following the administration of glucose to thiamine-depleted, asymptomatic persons. Nystagmus, ataxia, and confusion, often accompanied by ophthalmoplegia, are strongly suggestive of Wernicke's encephalopathy; cardiovascular involvement may be signaled by tachycardia as an early manifestation of peripheral vasodilation. Thiamine should be administered promptly—and preferably before glucose is given—to any person in whom subclinical thiamine deficiency is suspected.

586. The answer is E. *(Wilson, ed 12. chap 75.)* The first decision regarding the administration of a dietary formula is the choice of route. In the case presented, the underlying disorder (hemorrhagic pancreatitis) and recent abdominal surgery are contraindications to enteral therapy. Both lipids and carbohydrates may be infused with amino acids to meet metabolic needs, but several considerations should be taken into account in choosing which mixture to use. First is osmolality—concentrated glucose solutions are hypertonic and cause peripheral vein thrombosis. Another factor is the metabolic state of the patient; both pancreatic insufficiency and hyperglycemia are relative contraindications to using hypertonic glucose solutions. Second, carbohydrate as the sole source of calories raises the metabolic rate and thus the production of carbon dioxide; in a patient being weaned from ventilatory assistance, giving more nonprotein calories as fat reduces CO_2 excretion. Third, lipid infusions provide essential fatty-acid requirements, and because lipids do not raise insulin levels or require insulin for metabolism, they may be discontinued abruptly (e.g., if emergency surgery is needed) without risk of hypoglycemia. In summary, a regimen providing 85 percent of nonprotein calories as lipid and 15 percent as glucose is near isotonic and probably optimal in the case described.

587. The answer is D. *(Wilson, ed 12. chap 76.)* The combination of peripheral neuritis, dermatitis, glossitis, microcytic anemia, and convulsions suggests the presence of pyridoxine deficiency. Naturally occurring pyridoxine deficiency is rare, owing to the widespread distribution of the vitamin in food. It is therefore paradoxical that clinical deficiency is frequent, because many commonly used drugs act as pyridoxine antagonists. Pyridoxal phosphate is the active cofactor for numerous enzymatic reactions in amino acid metabolism and in heme synthesis; it is also important for normal neuronal excitability. Estrogens inhibit the role of pyridoxine in tryptophan metabolism, and hydrazines such as isoniazid can inhibit various enzymes that use pyridoxine as a cofactor and thereby induce convulsions. Cycloserine and penicillamine act similarly. The appropriate management for persons receiving drugs capable of causing pyridoxine deficiency is dietary supplementation (at least 30 mg of pyridoxine daily); overt deficiency, when present, requires immediate parenteral therapy.

588. The answer is B. *(Wilson, ed 12. chap 76. Revler, JAMA 253:805, 1985.)* Humans, unlike many animals capable of synthesizing ascorbic acid from D-glucose, require exogenous vitamin C. Ascorbic acid functions as a redox agent, and its most important role is in the synthesis of appropriately hydroxylated collagen. Features of scurvy result from defective collagen synthesis and include capillary fragility resulting in ecchymoses (due to impaired collagen formation in blood vessels), poor wound healing, and abnormal hair development. This syndrome is common in edentulous, elderly men who reside alone and ingest a diet deficient in milk, fruits, and vegetables. Resolution of bleeding occurs rapidly after administration of oral ascorbic acid. Vitamin A deficiency tends to produce night blindness and xerophthalmia. Bleeding is seen in vitamin K deficiency but should be accompanied by an elevated prothrombin time caused by impaired synthesis of clotting factors. The anemia of folate deficiency, often seen in concert with scurvy, is macrocytic. Patients with insufficient quantities of available pyridoxine can develop seizures.

589. The answer is B. *(Wilson, ed 12. chap 315.)* The evaluation of polyuric syndromes should include simultaneous measurements of urine and plasma osmolality. Ideally, the plasma osmolality should be elevated so that determination of an inappropriately dilute urine is possible. Such an effort may require an overnight water deprivation test. This test must be carried out carefully to insure that a dangerous level of dehydration does not occur. Once 1 kg of body weight is lost and the plasma osmolality is elevated, the finding of a urine osmolality stable for 3 h at a low level confirms the diagnosis of diabetes insipidus. At that point vasopressin is administered, and the urine osmolality is checked between 30 and 60 min thereafter. In cases of central diabetes insipidus, the rise in urine osmolality exceeds 9 percent, whereas in nephrogenic diabetes insipidus, frequently due to renal dysfunction as in the case presented, there is little, if any, increment. The treatment for nephrogenic diabetes insipidus consists of the administration of diuretics to cause a fall in glomerular filtration rate and a concomitant increase in proximal tubular fluid resorption, decreased distal fluid delivery, and diminished production of dilute urine. This therapeutic strategy should be accompanied by sodium restriction.

590. The answer is D. *(Wilson, ed 12. chaps 339, 340.)* The hypercalcemia of sarcoidosis is usually associated with disseminated disease. Therefore, almost all persons with sarcoidosis who have hypercalcemia also have an abnormal chest x-ray (diffuse fibronodular infiltration or marked enlargement of hilar nodes, or both). This is an important point in the differential diagnosis of hypercalcemia—sarcoidosis is unlikely as a cause of hypercalcemia if the chest x-ray is normal. Hypergammaglobulinemia is another helpful clue to the presence of sarcoidosis. The hypercalcemia of sarcoidosis is thought to be the consequence of increased synthesis of $1,25(OH)_2$ vitamin D_3 and the subsequent increased intestinal absorption of calcium. Elevated serum calcium concentration in sarcoidosis causes a decreased level of serum parathyroid hormone, resulting in marked hypercalciuria.

591. The answer is C. *(Wilson, ed 12. chap 329.)* Colchicine is useful in the treatment of acute gouty arthritis but not chronic tophaceous gout. However, it can be a useful ancillary drug in treatment of chronic gout at the start of allopurinol therapy to prevent the precipitation of acute gouty arthritis. Chronic gout can be treated either with uricosuric agents (probenecid or sulfinpyrazone) or with an inhibitor of uric acid synthesis (allopurinol). The ideal candidate for uricosuric agents is a patient under the age of 60 years who has normal renal function, a uric acid excretion of less than 700 mg per day, and no history of renal stones. Specific indications for choosing allopurinol over a uricosuric agent include the presence of uric acid nephrolithiasis, high uric acid excretion, and impairment of renal function; hence, allopurinol is the appropriate initial drug in this patient. Combinations of allopurinol and uricosuric agents may be employed when uric acid levels cannot be controlled with either drug alone.

592. The answer is E. *(Wilson, ed 12. chap 326.)* The patient described in the question has type 5 hyperlipoproteinemia. This usually familial disorder, a variant of familial hypertriglyceridemia, is characterized by elevated levels of chylomicrons and VLDL. (The fact that VLDL levels are increased in the patient described is shown by the high triglyceride-to-cholesterol ratio and by the turbid infranatant layer; high levels of chylomicrons are indicated by the presence of the creamy upper layer in standing plasma.) Diabetes, pancreatitis, and hyperuricemia are common in persons with the disorder. Hypertriglyceridemia may be exacerbated by obesity, dietary factors, and alcoholism. Type 5 hyperlipoproteinemia can also be seen in the rare autosomal recessive disorder familial apoprotein CII deficiency. In this disorder lipoprotein lipase is not activated, so the two substrate lipoproteins, chylomicrons and VLDL, accumulate in the blood.

593. The answer is B. *(Wilson, ed 12. chap 326.)* Whether hypertriglyceridemia in an overweight person is due to familial hypertriglyceridemia, multiple lipoprotein-type hyperlipemia, or sporadic hypertriglyceridemia, the primary mode of therapy should be weight reduction. Dietary saturated-fat content should be restricted as part of the weight reduction regimen. Hypothyroidism and diabetes mellitus, if present, should be treated, and use of alcohol and oral contraceptives should be avoided. If these measures are inadequate, drug therapy with clofibrate should be tried. Bile acid–binding resins, such as cholestyramine or colestipol, are used in the treatment of hypercholesterolemia but are not useful for treating hypertriglyceridemia.

594. The answer is D. *(Wilson, ed 12. chap 316.)* In most instances of hypothyroidism in adults, replacement therapy should be initiated with gradually increasing doses of thyroid hormone. However in cases of neonatal, infantile, and juvenile hypothyroidism full replacement should be begun immediately to increase the chances of normal intellectual and anatomic development. In patients with secondary hypothyroidism or when coexistent adrenal insufficiency is suspected, it is important that thyroid replacement not be initiated until treatment with glucocorticoid has begun. Adrenocortical insufficiency can be precipitated by an increase in the clearance rate of glucocorticoids engendered by correction of the hypothyroid state.

595. The answer is E. *(Wilson, ed 12. chap 316. Rojeski, N Engl J Med 313:428, 1985.)* The finding of a solitary thyroid nodule should raise the suspicion of thyroid carcinoma. However, surgery should be reserved for those patients in whom the diagnosis of thyroid cancer is definite or at least highly probable. Fine needle aspiration is almost always the procedure of first choice in the evaluation of such solitary nodules. Surgery is indicated in the case of definite lymphoma or carcinoma (papillary, medullary, poorly differentiated, or follicular). If small groups of uniform, colloid-poor cells are seen, these inconclusive results should be met by repeating the fine needle aspiration. If repeat results are similar, then a trial of levothyroxine suppression should be initiated and follow-up in 6 months planned. If there are sheets of follicular cells reported on pathology from the initial fine needle aspiration, then the nodule could represent either follicular carcinoma or adenoma. In this situation, a radionuclide scan demonstrating a functioning nodule would be reassuring and merely mandate an evaluation for hyperthyroidism; a "cold" nodule would require subtotal thyroidectomy.

596. The answer is D. *(Wilson, ed 12. chap 326. Schaefer, N Engl J Med 312:1300, 1985.)* Cholestyramine and colestipol are bile acid–binding resins that decrease the reabsorption of bile acids from the intestine, thus secondarily decreasing the enterohepatic circulation of cholesterol. The liver responds to the acid depletion by increasing the synthesis of bile acids. The additional cholesterol required for bile acid synthesis is obtained by the liver by increasing the number of low density lipoprotein (LDL) receptors, which in turn lowers the plasma level of LDL. The most common side effects of these resins are constipation and bloating, although mild steatorrhea may occur when they are used in high doses.

597. The answer is A. *(Wilson, ed 12. chap 72.)* Weight loss requires caloric deficit: the total number of calories consumed must be exceeded by the total number of calories expended as energy. Notwithstanding the claims for various "fad" diets, there is little evidence to support the efficacy of one type of hypocaloric diet over any other in achieving long-term weight loss. Basically a calorie is a calorie—whether from protein, fat, or carbohydrate. Liquid protein diets have been associated with a variety of adverse developments, including hyperuricemia, hypercholesterolemia, and sudden cardiovascular death. Total starvation diets are simpler to follow and lead to greater weight loss than hypocaloric diets, but adverse effects include increased loss of lean body mass, hypotension, and arrhythmias. Amphetamines act as weak anorexiants but are usually ineffective after several weeks; also, the risks of dependence and abuse are significant. Exercise is a useful adjunct to caloric restriction; it may increase lean body mass and improve the sense of well-being, but moderate exercise does not increase caloric expenditure sufficiently to alter the initial rate of weight loss if caloric restriction is not also undertaken.

598. The answer is A. *(Wilson, ed 12. chap 72.)* Although only a minority of obese persons have diabetes mellitus, more than 80 percent of type 2 diabetics are obese. Obesity appears to be a major contributory factor to the development of diabetes, largely through its effects on insulin sensitivity. A clear relationship also exists between hypertension and obesity in adults, though the mechanism is unclear. Hypertriglyceridemia is associated commonly with obesity and correlates with the degree of obesity; increased hepatic production of very low density lipoproteins (VLDL) from free fatty acids is felt to be the major cause of increased triglyceride levels in obese persons, although peripheral defects in VLDL clearance may be present in some. Weight loss can reduce or reverse all these complications. The prevalence of cholelithiasis is increased with increasing adiposity, but the same cannot be said of hypothyroidism—only a small percentage of hypothyroid persons are obese, and an even smaller fraction of obese persons are hypothyroid.

599. The answer is D. *(Wilson, ed 12. chap 317.)* Primary aldosteronism may be due to an aldosterone-producing adrenal adenoma, bilateral adrenal cortical nodular hyperplasia, or rarely adrenal carcinoma. The diagnosis should be suspected when mild diastolic hypertension, hypokalemia, and metabolic acidosis are present in a patient not taking diuretics. Peripheral edema is uncommon. Plasma renin activity should be suppressed by the chronically elevated aldosterone level, but suppressed renin activity (low after volume depletion maneuvers) also occurs in 25 percent of patients with essential hypertension. To make the diagnosis of primary aldosteronism in a patient with the above clinical features and a low plasma renin, the best test is measurement of plasma aldosterone following an attempt to suppress mineralocorticoid secretion by the infusion of saline. Once failure to suppress aldosterone secretion is demonstrated, then anatomic localization of the adenoma (or documentation of hyperplasia) should be attempted.

600. The answer is C. *(Wilson, ed 12. chap 318. Bravo, N Engl J Med 311:1298, 1984.)* Pheochromocytomas produce and secrete catecholamines, which may lead to paroxysmally high blood pressure. Approximately 80 percent of these tumors are solitary adrenal lesions, but 10 percent are bilateral and 10 percent are extraadrenal. Pheochromocytoma is also associated with familial multiple endocrine neoplasia types IIa and IIb (hyperparathyroidism and medullary carcinoma are the other endocrinologic manifestations). Once the diagnosis is confirmed, usually by documenting excess urinary catecholamine metabolites over a 24-h period plus localization by CT scanning, it is important to prepare the patient for surgery by preventing the effects of catecholamine release by treatment with phenoxybenzamine, a long-acting alpha-adrenergic blocker. Liberal salt intake should also be instituted to help restore the contracted plasma volume to normal prior to surgery. Beta-blockers should not be given before alpha blockade has been established because of the potential for hypertension due to the antagonism of beta-mediated vasodilation in skeletal muscle beds. However, propranolol is useful in treating the reflex tachycardia induced by phenoxybenzamine. While prazosin is an effective agent for the treatment of hypertensive crises associated with pheochromocytoma, its use as a primary agent in the management of this disorder has not been established.

601. The answer is A. *(Wilson, ed 12. chap 313.)* The adrenal glands normally produce hydrocortisone at a rate of approximately 20 to 30 mg/d. As in the treatment of primary adrenal insufficiency, a replacement dose of hydrocortisone, 30 mg/d, should be given to all patients following transsphenoidal removal of an ACTH-secreting microadenoma; treatment should continue until the uninvolved corticotropic cells recover and secrete ACTH at a level sufficient to maintain basal glucocorticoid production. If symptoms of withdrawal from high levels of glucocorticoid develop, a transient increase in glucocorticoid dosage may be necessary. Administration of desmopressin or levothyroxine is required only if diabetes insipidus or hypothyroidism, respectively, develops postoperatively.

602. The answer is C. *(Wilson, ed 12. chap 317.)* The absolute degree of elevation of plasma cortisol concentration is not a reliable criterion in the diagnosis of Cushing's disease. Rather, impaired suppressibility of adrenal cortisol production must be demonstrated by formal dexamethasone testing. Following administration of dexamethasone, 2 mg/d for 2 days, urinary free cortisol excretion may fall in persons with Cushing's disease but not to the degree seen in normal persons (<55 nmol/d [<20 μg/d]). A dexamethasone regimen of 8 mg/d would cause urinary 17-hydroxycorticosteroid excretion to fall to less than 50 percent of baseline in persons with Cushing's disease. Cortisol production never increases in response to metyrapone because this drug inhibits the final enzyme (11β-hydroxylase) in the pathway of cortisol synthesis; however, an exaggerated release of ACTH may follow metyrapone administration and result in a threefold to fivefold increase in urinary excretion of 17-hydroxycorticosteroids (predominantly 11-deoxycortisol). Patients with Cushing's disease characteristically have elevation of urinary 17-ketosteroids in addition to elevation of urinary 17-hydroxycorticosteroids.

603. The answer is E. *(Wilson, ed 12. chap 330.)* Wilson's disease is due to a defect in copper metabolism and is inherited in an autosomal recessive fashion. Excess copper accumulation in the liver and central nervous system accounts for the clinical manifestations and results in an inhibition of ceruloplasmin production. Virtually any variant of hepatitis, in addition to cirrhosis, can be observed among the 50 percent of affected patients who develop liver disease. Kayser-Fleischer rings, green or golden deposits of copper in Descemet's membrane of the cornea, do not interfere with vision but occur in all patients with neuropsychiatric manifestations of Wilson's disease. Penicillamine therapy, which removes and detoxifies copper, should be instituted as soon as the diagnosis is established. Lifelong and continued treatment is required; though sensitivity reactions sometimes require discontinuation of penicillamine therapy, such stoppages should be avoided if possible because interruptions are associated with a risk of irreversible relapse.

604. The answer is D. *(Wilson, ed 12. chap 343.)* Magnesium deficiency may occur as a result of generalized nutritional insufficiency or lack of supplementation in programs of total parenteral nutrition. Other causes include gastrointestinal malabsorption of any cause, chronic diarrhea, chronic alcoholism, increased renal excretion (due to cisplatin, amphotericin B, aminoglycosides, loop diuretics), and various endocrine disorders (e.g., hyperparathyroidism, hypoparathyroidism, diabetic ketoacidosis, Conn's syndrome, syndrome of inappropriate secretion of vasopressin). Clinical sequelae of severe magnesium deficiency (< 0.5 mmol/L [1.0 meq/L]) include anorexia, vomiting, lethargy, paresthesias, muscle cramps, irritability, decreased attention span, and confusion. Hypocalcemia, as a result of diminished responsiveness and release of parathyroid hormone, may be severe enough to produce tetany. About half of patients with hypomagnesemia may become hypokalemic (the mechanism is unclear but secondary hyperaldosteronism may play a role). Low levels of serum calcium, potassium, and magnesium all serve to promote dangerous cardiac arrhythmias, especially in the patient receiving digitalis. Hyponatremia is not a known consequence of hypomagnesemia, although the syndrome of inappropriate secretion of vasopressin may promote a low serum magnesium.

605. The answer is B. *(Wilson, ed 12. chap 313.)* Several features in this woman suggest the presence of hypercortisolism. Although the overnight dexamethasone suppression test (1 mg at midnight) is a useful screening test to rule out Cushing's syndrome, it may be falsely positive (failure to suppress morning cortisol rise) in obese patients. If the patient has Cushing's syndrome on a pituitary basis, the cortisol excretion will be suppressed after 8 mg of dexamethasone daily for 2 days. However, normal patients will also evidence suppression of cortisol in this situation. Measurement of 24-h urinary free cortisol excretion is especially useful in these instances; if results are elevated (> 275 nmol/d [100 μg/d]), a standard 2-day, low-dose dexamethazone suppression test is the next step in the evaluation. Measurement of plasma ACTH levels is usually not useful in the diagnosis of Cushing's syndrome although very high levels suggest ectopic ACTH production. Radiographic examination of the pituitary gland should not be done until a diagnosis of pituitary-dependent Cushing's syndrome has been established by laboratory testing.

606. The answer is B. *(Wilson, ed 12. chap 313.)* A serum prolactin level above 300 μg/L is diagnostic of a pituitary adenoma, even in a nursing woman. In fact, the serum prolactin level only rarely reaches 300 μg/L during pregnancy and declines post partum (with intermittent peaking with each suckling episode). Six months post partum, basal prolactin levels are normal, and the suckling-induced rise is minimal despite continued nursing. Thus, computed tomography or magnetic resonance imaging of the pituitary gland is indicated at this time. Suppressive treatment with bromocriptine would be indicated if the diagnosis of a pituitary adenoma is confirmed. Since bromocriptine suppresses all types of hyperprolactinemia, it cannot be used as a diagnostic test of physiologic versus pathologic hyperprolactinemia. Any delay in evaluation could allow further tumor enlargement and the risk of visual impairment resulting from optic nerve compression. Visual field testing should be done if an adenoma is found.

607. The answer is C. *(Wilson, ed 12. chap 314.)* Because the secretion of growth hormone is episodic and therefore variable, random measurements of plasma growth hormone are not adequate assessments of growth hormone deficiency, and consequently provocative tests to stimulate growth hormone secretion should be utilized. In contrast, measurement of IGF-I/SM-C is a useful indicator of growth hormone status since it turns over more slowly than growth hormone itself, and hence its level reflects the mean level of growth hormone in the blood throughout the day rather than the moment-to-moment level. Measurement of the serum thyroxine concentration is useful in identification of growth retardation associated with hypothyroidism, and assessment of chromosomal karyotype is useful in identifying girls whose growth retardation is associated with gonadal dysgenesis. Assessment of bone age makes it possible to identify discrepancies between bone age and chronologic age.

608. The answer is B. *(Wilson, ed 12. chap 315.)* Patients with lung cancer, particularly small cell carcinoma, frequently present with the syndrome of inappropriate vasopressin (AVP, antidiuretic hormone) secretion. Indeed, more than half of patients with such tumors show evidence of inappropriate secretion of AVP, even when serum sodium concentration remains normal. AVP is produced by the tumor tissue itself and is chemically identical to arginine vasopressin secreted by the neurohypophysis. Central nervous system lesions of infectious, inflammatory, and vascular etiologies can also result in inappropriate AVP secretion, but intracerebral metastases from lung carcinomas are not usually responsible for inappropriate AVP secretion.

609. The answer is E. *(Wilson, ed 12. chap 315.)* Demeclocycline produces reversible renal insensitivity to endogenous vasopressin. The exact mechanism of action is unknown. The drug's effects are more consistent than those of ethanol or phenytoin, and side effects are less than with lithium. Desmopressin, a synthetic analogue of vasopressin, would worsen water intoxication in a person with chronic inappropriate vasopressin secretion.

610. The answer is C. *(Wilson, ed 12. chap 316.)* Impaired peripheral conversion of thyroxine to triiodothyronine (T_4 to T_3) occurs commonly in acute and chronic illnesses, in fasting and starvation, and following the administration of certain drugs. Although propylthiouracil and methimazole act similarly to cause impaired organification of iodine by thyroid glands affected by thyrotoxicosis, propylthiouracil has the additional effect of inhibiting peripheral conversion of T_4 to T_3, a property not shared by methimazole. The recognition of a similar action of dexamethasone in impairing T_4 conversion to T_3 has provided an explanation for the favorable effect of glucocorticoids in the treatment of thyroid storm. Propranolol also has a minor effect in inhibiting the conversion of T_4 to T_3. The degree of impairment of T_4 conversion to T_3 by oral cholecystography dyes is such that a compensatory increase in T_4 to greater than normal levels is frequently noted 1 to 2 weeks after ingestion of the compounds.

611. The answer is E. *(Wilson, ed 12. chap 316.)* Surgical treatment of nontoxic goiter is most commonly undertaken for diagnostic purposes (i.e., to rule out malignancy). Enlarged thyroid glands often have a limited functional reserve capacity, and lobectomy can further compromise hormone production. The thyroid scan presented in the question demonstrates adequate concentration and diffuse distribution of the radionuclide throughout the enlarged remnant, and there is little risk of malignancy. Exogenous hormone administration can prevent or improve postsurgical "compensatory" thyroid hyperplasia, which is the likely explanation for the mass in the woman described. Ultrasonography would be useful if the scan showed irregularities of uptake.

612. The answer is D. *(Wilson, ed 12. chap 316.)* Normal pregnancy can stimulate thyrotoxicosis in regard to increased heart rate, heat intolerance, and anxiety. The level found in the sensitive TSH test is low, but detectable, and therefore does not confirm hyperthyroidism. The test best able to exclude thyrotoxicosis in this patient would be the thyrotropin-releasing hormone (TRH) stimulation test. Testing radioactive iodine uptake (RAIU) is not always useful in diagnosing hyperthyroidism because of the wide range of normal values in the population and is not advisable in pregnancy. Similarly, the T_3 suppression test, although useful in the diagnosis of thyroid autonomy, requires RAIU tests and therefore would be contraindicated. Technetium thyroid scans are not useful in the diagnosis of hyperthyroidism. A serum T_3 level, in the absence of some measure of thyroid hormone binding capacity, is also not useful in excluding hyperthyroidism.

613. The answer is B. *(Wilson, ed 12. chap 316.)* The most appropriate treatment for Graves' disease in the third trimester of pregnancy is propylthiouracil in the minimal dosages sufficient to control the hyperthyroidism. Because levothyroxine crosses the placenta poorly, hypothyroidism may occur in the fetus if levothyroxine is combined with sufficient doses of propylthiouracil to block thyroid function in the fetus. Subtotal thyroidectomy is usually reserved for treating affected women in the second trimester. Use of radioactive iodine is contraindicated during pregnancy because it crosses the placenta and may have deleterious effects on fetal development. Propranolol can cause fetal hypoglycemia and apnea and should not be used in treating thyrotoxicosis of pregnancy, except in emergencies.

614. The answer is C. *(Wilson, ed 12. chap 316.)* Measurement of serum TSH concentration by radioimmunoassay is useful in the diagnosis of both early and advanced primary hypothyroidism. Because of the exquisitely sensitive feedback relationship between TSH secretion and thyroid hormone levels in plasma, TSH levels in serum are increased in patients with untreated hypothyroidism of thyroidal etiology. In contrast, serum T_3 measurement and radioactive iodine uptake tests are generally poor discriminators of hypothyroidism. The TRH stimulation test is of less value in the diagnosis of hypothyroidism than in the diagnosis of hyperthyroidism. Reverse T_3 measurement, when available, is helpful in separating primary hypothyroidism from the "sick euthyroid" syndrome, since results are subnormal in patients with hypothyroidism but normal or high in association with the "sick euthyroid" syndrome.

615. The answer is E. *(Wilson, ed 12. chap 317.)* In the case presented in the question, the development of muscle weakness, arthralgias, fatigue, and fever is likely to be the result of steroid withdrawal. Steroid withdrawal symptoms commonly appear after therapy is switched from a daily to an alternate-day regimen and ordinarily abate after a few days. If the symptoms persist, then it may be necessary to switch back to daily therapy and make the transition to alternate-day steroid treatment in stages.

616. The answer is D. *(Wilson, ed 12. chap 317.)* In the various forms of congenital adrenal hyperplasia, including steroid C-21 hydroxylase deficiency, both pituitary and adrenal regulatory mechanisms function appropriately. The enzymatic defect in cortisol production results in an absence of the product (cortisol) necessary for feedback inhibition of ACTH secretion by the pituitary gland. ACTH in turn causes the production of increased amounts of cortisol precursors such as 17-hydroxyprogesterone, which is converted to androgens by the adrenal gland. Therapy with appropriate doses of glucocorticoid causes suppression of pituitary ACTH and adrenal androgen secretion, indicating that inhibiting and stimulating control mechanisms of the hypothalamic-pituitary-adrenal axis can function normally.

617. The answer is D. *(Wilson, ed 12. chap 317.)* In a single-dose overnight dexamethasone suppression test, which is a screening procedure in the workup of possible cortisol excess, suppression of plasma cortisol concentration to less than 140 nmol/L (5 μg/dL) implies normal hypothalamic-pituitary-adrenal feedback and excludes a diagnosis of Cushing's syndrome. However, failure to suppress plasma cortisol following this procedure is not necessarily diagnostic and must be investigated further. Several factors can affect the validity of screening dexamethasone testing. For example, in 10 to 15 percent of cases obesity interferes with normal suppression of cortisol after the overnight dexamethasone test. However, obese persons uniformly show normal excretion of free cortisol in urine (< 275 nmol/d [< 100 μg/d]). The 2-day low-dose dexamethasone test is necessary to exclude or establish the diagnosis of Cushing's syndrome in all persons with abnormal or equivocal screening tests. The high-dose test, which is reserved for patients with established Cushing's syndrome, serves to delineate the specific cause. Imaging procedures should only be performed once a diagnosis of cortisol excess is established.

618. The answer is B. *(Wilson, ed 12. chap 317.)* Hyporeninemic hypoaldosteronism occurs most commonly in adults with diabetes mellitus in association with mild renal failure, metabolic acidosis, and hyperkalemia. The defect in aldosterone synthesis is almost certainly caused by hyporeninism, since in these patients aldosterone secretion increases promptly after the administration of ACTH but not after salt restriction or postural changes. Most patients respond to the administration of potent mineralocorticoids (fludrocortisone) or diuretics such as furosemide, or both, but in general mineralocorticoids should not be the sole therapeutic agents in patients with hypertension. Furosemide will treat both the hyperkalemia and the acidosis; this diuretic will be more effective if sodium intake is reduced. Hemodialysis may be useful in emergency situations to correct hyperkalemia. Potassium restriction and enhancement of potassium excretion with anion-exchange resins are both likely to predispose to total-body potassium deficits.

619. The answer is A. *(Wilson, ed 12. chap 319. Brownlee, Ann Intern Med 101:527, 1984.)* Hemoglobin A$_{1c}$ (HbA$_{1c}$), the most abundant minor component of human hemoglobin, is a ketoamine formed by the nonenzymatic glycosylation of the N-terminal valine on the β globin chain. Because the rate of HbA$_{1c}$ formation is dependent on the average plasma glucose level during the life span of the red blood cell (nearly 120 days), HbA$_{1c}$ levels reflect the average blood sugar for the previous weeks or months. HbA$_{1c}$ makes up about 5 to 8 percent of the hemoglobin of persons without diabetes, whereas in persons with poorly controlled diabetes it accounts for an average of 10 to 14 percent of hemoglobin. Glycosylated albumin can serve as a monitor of diabetic control over a period up to 2 weeks. Plasma C-peptide may indicate residual beta-cell function but does not relate to diabetic control. Plasma glucose and urinary glucose levels fluctuate widely from day to day, so that measurements, no matter how valuable, reflect control only over a short period of time.

620. The answer is A. *(Wilson, ed 12. chap 319. Coustan, N Engl J Med 319:1663, 1988.)* The prognosis for pregnancies complicated by diabetes mellitus has improved markedly, and perinatal mortality has decreased to the point that infant survival is similar to that in the population at large. This improved outcome is a result of aggressive treatment of maternal hyperglycemia and of advances in the techniques of fetal surveillance and neonatal care. When mean maternal blood glucose levels exceed 8.3 mmol/L (150 mg/dL) in the third trimester, perinatal mortality is almost six times that associated with mean maternal glucose levels below 5.6 mmol/L (100 mg/dL). Congenital malformations, the leading cause of perinatal mortality in infants of diabetic pregnancies, remain an unresolved problem; such abnormalities are thought to be related to poor glucose control early in the first trimester (during early embryogenesis), a time when many women do not yet know they are pregnant. Optimal care of a diabetic woman wishing to become pregnant requires that a major attempt be made to achieve as normal a mean blood glucose concentration as possible before conception and throughout the duration of pregnancy. Hospitalization may be required for education or treatment of complications but should not be necessary for extended periods of time. Multiple subcutaneous injections of insulin or continuous subcutaneous injection of insulin should be considered to provide "tight" control in all diabetic women wishing to become pregnant.

621. The answer is B. *(Wilson, ed 12. chap 319.)* Dot hemorrhages and several larger lesions near the disk (caused by superficial retinal bleeding) are characteristic changes of background diabetic retinopathy. However, the presence of innumerable, fine, frondlike vessels extending around and partly covering the disk is indicative of the neovascularization of proliferative retinopathy, which requires urgent treatment. The therapy of choice is photocoagulation by xenon arc or ruby or argon laser. The Diabetic Retinopathy Study Research Group (DRSRG) has established that photocoagulation significantly improves visual prognosis in proliferative retinopathy. Tighter control of blood sugar levels has not been shown to reverse the lesions of diabetic retinopathy. Hypophysectomy is no longer used to treat proliferative retinopathy because of the morbidity and lack of effectiveness of the procedure. Vitrectomy should be reserved for more advanced cases, such as nonresolving vitreal hemorrhage or retinal detachment.

622. The answer is E. *(Wilson, ed 12. chaps 319, 320. Ferner, BMJ 296:949, 1988.)* Hypoglycemia from oral hypoglycemic agents is less common than with insulin therapy, but when it occurs it can be severe and prolonged and cause confusion or coma. Immediate therapy of serious hypoglycemia requires bolus intravenous administration of a 50% glucose solution followed by constant glucose infusions until the patient can eat a meal. Oral intake of glucose is important, because intravenous glucose alone does not replenish liver glycogen. Sulfonylurea overdosage causes overutilization of glucose, so that affected persons may require considerable amounts of glucose to remain conscious. Mild glycosuria is one indication of adequate infusion rates; frequent capillary glucose measurements also may be helpful. Hypoglycemia from the use of sulfonylurea agents may last for several days, especially with chlorpropamide, and patients may lapse back into coma if glucose infusions are stopped prematurely. Hospitalization is mandatory in cases of serious hypoglycemia.

623. The answer is A. *(Wilson, ed 12. chap 320.)* The catabolic changes that occur during fasting vary with the length of the fast. Early on, a slight drop in plasma glucose concentration causes insulin levels to fall and increases the release of counterregulatory hormones, such as glucagon, cortisol, epinephrine, and growth hormone; in this way, plasma glucose levels are sustained within a safe range. Glucagon increases hepatic cyclic AMP, which activates glycogen phosphorylase (and hence stimulates glycogenolysis) and inhibits glycogen synthetase. It also suppresses glycolysis and enhances gluconeogenesis by blocking phosphofructokinase and stimulating fructose diphosphatase, respectively. The effect is to make the liver an organ of net glucose production; however, because hepatic glycogen stores are limited, glycogen breakdown can sustain plasma glucose levels for only 12 to 24 h. After this period, new glucose must be produced from peripheral precursors, such as glycerol, lactate, and especially amino acids (notably alanine). In adipose tissue, lipolysis of stored triglycerides liberates free fatty acids, which are either used in liver for ketone body production or oxidized in peripheral tissues. Fatty acid oxidation also provides the energy for hepatic gluconeogenesis. The brain continues to metabolize glucose for several days of fasting, after which time ketone bodies become a major substrate.

624. The answer is A. *(Wilson, ed 12. chap 321.)* Testosterone esters are hydrolyzed by esterases in the blood as they are absorbed from the oily depots in which they are administered, and, as a consequence, the esters themselves can rarely be detected in blood. Therefore, effectiveness of therapy with agents such as testosterone cypionate can be monitored by measuring the plasma levels of testosterone itself. In men with recent onset of hypogonadism, plasma LH levels should be suppressed into the normal range by testosterone, but when LH levels have been high for many years, LH secretion becomes semiautonomous and may not return to the normal range for many months or years after the restoration of blood testosterone levels to normal. The frequency of nocturnal erections may or may not reflect plasma testosterone levels on a day-to-day or week-to-week basis, and muscle mass depends on factors in addition to plasma testosterone levels, including exercise level.

625. The answer is C. *(Wilson, ed 12. chap 322. Wilson, ed 7. chap 9.)* The fact that withdrawal bleeding occurred after the administration of progestogen indicates that estrogen was being produced. Women with chronic anovulation who react in this way are said to be in the state of "estrus" because of acyclic production of estrogen. This diagnostic response clearly excludes those causes of amenorrhea associated with suppression of ovarian function, including pituitary disease, either functional or organic, and conditions associated with streak gonads. The most likely cause of amenorrhea in such a situation is polycystic ovarian disease (PCOD) in which the ovaries produce androgens that can be converted to estrogens (largely estrone) in extraglandular tissues. In most women with PCOD, menarche occurs at the expected time, and amenorrhea supervenes after a variable time. However, in some women this disorder has an early onset and may cause primary amenorrhea. Other causes of anovulation in the presence of estrogen include estrogen-secreting tumors of the ovary and adrenal tumors.

626. The answer is B. *(Wilson, ed 12. chap 322.)* Asherman's syndrome, destruction of the endometrium, occurs after vigorous curettage, usually in association with postpartum hemorrhage or therapeutic abortion. The diagnosis is confirmed by hysterosalpingography or by direct visualization of the scarred endometrium using a hysteroscope. Treatment consists of dilation and curettage, followed by the insertion of an intrauterine device for 8 weeks.

627. The answer is D. *(Wilson, ed 12. chap 322.)* Low circulating levels of estrogens coupled with elevated gonadotropin levels exclude the presence of pituitary disease and indicate primary ovarian failure, which is premature at this patient's age. Bilateral tubal obstruction would cause infertility but not amenorrhea. Polycystic ovarian disease is associated with typical physical findings of weight gain and hirsutism, an earlier age of onset, and elevated circulating levels of estrogens. Exogenous administration of estrogens would lead to suppression of gonadotropin secretion.

628. The answer is B. *(Wilson, ed 12. chap 324.)* The clinical situation described in the question is characteristic of congenital adrenal hyperplasia due to deficiency of either C-21 hydroxylase or 3β-ol-dehydrogenase. Urinary 17-ketosteroids are elevated in both disorders, whereas urinary pregnanediol and pregnanetriol and plasma 17-hydroxyprogesterone and androstenedione levels are elevated in association with C-21 hydroxylase deficiency. Plasma 11-deoxycortisol is elevated in C-11 hydroxylase deficiency, a disorder producing hypertension owing to overproduction of mineralocorticoids and consequently not associated with vomiting and volume depletion.

629. The answer is D. *(Wilson, ed 12. chap 324.)* Tumors of the streak gonads are unusual in the common forms of gonadal dysgenesis, including those associated with normal karyotypes (46,XX), X-chromosome deletion (45,X), structurally abnormal X chromosomes (46,XX$_i$), and X chromosome mosaicism (45,X/46,XX). However, malignant tumors of the streaks (so-called gonadoblastomas) are common when gonadal dysgenesis is associated with cell lines containing Y chromosomes or fragments of Y chromosomes. Consequently, the gonadal streaks should be resected whenever a Y chromosome is present in a woman with gonadal dysgenesis.

630. The answer is E. *(Wilson, ed 12. chap 340.)* Persons who have hyperparathyroidism can present with manifestations of hypercalcemia—e.g., peptic ulcer, muscle weakness, kidney stones—or symptoms of osteitis fibrosa cystica, a form of bone involvement characteristic of the disease. However, with the widespread application of biochemical screening as a routine tool in patient evaluation, more and more patients are diagnosed early in the course of the disease, when it is manifested only by asymptomatic hypercalcemia. At present, this is the most common source of diagnoses of hyperparathyroidism.

631. The answer is B. *(Wilson, ed 12. chap 340.)* Unless contraindicated by a history of thromboembolic phenomena, severe hypertension, or breast cancer, estrogen therapy provides a useful means of controlling hypercalcemia and protecting the skeleton in postmenopausal women who have hyperparathyroidism but are not good operative candidates. Plicamycin, though also of benefit, is administered as weekly intravenous injections and has cumulative toxic effects on the kidneys, liver, and bone marrow; however, it would be a good choice for treatment of hypercalcemic emergencies if saline and furosemide were ineffective or contraindicated. Phosphate promotes the deposition of calcium into the skeleton, but long-term use in persons with renal insufficiency would cause a buildup in serum phosphorus levels and thereby promote soft-tissue calcification. Oral diphosphonate has not been demonstrated to have a sustained effect in controlling the hypercalcemia of primary hyperparathyroidism, perhaps because it retards bone formation as well as bone resorption. Thiazides would exacerbate hypercalcemia by increasing renal calcium reabsorption.

632. The answer is E. *(Wilson, ed 12. chap 340.)* Remodeling of bone is physiologically responsive to mechanical forces. The early response to immobilization is an increase in bone resorption; bone formation remains normal or decreases. Prolonged immobilization may lead to hypercalcemia, especially in persons with high rates of bone turnover (e.g., persons who have Paget's disease or young persons undergoing rapid growth). Excess calcium entering the circulation results in both hypercalciuria, which can cause nephrolithiasis, and soft-tissue calcification. Although the reason for enhanced bone resorption following immobilization is not completely understood, secretion of parathyroid hormone is suppressed. Hypercalcemia and hypercalciuria resolve when immobilized subjects become ambulatory; parathyroidectomy is unnecessary.

633. The answer is D. *(Wilson, ed 12. chap 342. Carmichael, Am J Med 76:1137, 1984. Ryan, Am J Med 77:501, 1984.)* A direct effect of ingestion of aluminum in patients with renal failure is severe, unresponsive osteomalacia caused by its deposition at the site of osteoid mineralization. However, aluminum accumulation does not occur in patients with normal renal function, and the effects of long-term ingestion of aluminum hydroxide–containing antacids in such patients are a result of phosphorus depletion—that is, the binding of phosphorus by aluminum within the intestine prevents its absorption. In the absence of more specific symptoms, malnutrition is unlikely. Osteomalacia has been reported in association with benign tumors of mesenchymal origin (oncogenous osteomalacia) but not with gastric carcinomas.

634. The answer is E. *(Wilson, ed 12. chap 340.)* Patients with primary hyperparathyroidism are usually asymptomatic, and mild degrees of hypercalcemia in such patients can usually be managed with adequate hydration. Whether observation alone is appropriate in these patients is controversial, especially when the diagnosis is made at a young age, since surveillance of renal function and bone status is lifelong and cumbersome. On the other hand, definitive treatment is clearly indicated when complications arise. In this patient, hypercalcemia and nephrolithiasis constitute a clear-cut indication for surgical treatment of the hyperparathyroidism. An additional reason would be to prevent bone loss in this young woman that would place her at an increased risk for development of skeletal complications at a later time. Glucocorticoids are usually ineffective in the management of primary hyperparathyroidism and would affect bone metabolism negatively, besides producing other serious side effects when administered on a long-term basis. Thiazide diuretics or calcium supplementation are contraindicated in this patient because of the risk of inducing hypercalcemia.

635. The answer is A. *(Wilson, ed 12. chap 341.)* Osteomalacia and rickets both are characterized by defective mineralization of bone; osteomalacia affects the adult skeleton, and rickets impairs the developing skeleton. Muscle weakness, hypocalcemia, hypophosphatemia, skeletal pain, and pseudofractures are cardinal features of both forms of osteomalacia. Bowing of the tibia, although common in children who have rickets, is not prominent in affected adults.

636. The answer is D. *(Wilson, ed 12. chap 344.)* Paget's disease of bone is relatively common, and the incidence increases with age. An estimated prevalence of 3 percent in persons over the age of 40 years is a generally accepted figure. Most frequently, the disease is asymptomatic and diagnosed only when the typical sclerotic bones are incidentally detected on x-ray examinations done for other reasons or when an increased alkaline phosphatase activity is recognized on routine laboratory measurements. The etiology is unknown, but increased bone resorption followed by intensive bone repair is thought to be the mechanism causing increased bone density and increased serum alkaline phosphatase activity as a marker of osteoblast activity. Since increased mineralization of bone takes place (although in an abnormal pattern), hypercalcemia is not present unless a severely affected patient becomes immobilized. Hypercalcemia, in fact, would be an expected finding in a patient with primary hyperparathyroidism, bone metastases, or plasmacytoma, the last typically producing no increase in the alkaline phosphatase activity. Osteomalacia resulting from vitamin D deficiency is associated with bone pain and hypophosphatemia; normal or decreased serum calcium concentration produces secondary hyperparathyroidism, further aggravating the defective bone mineralization.

637. The answer is D. *(Wilson, ed 12. chap 339.)* The most potent vitamin D metabolite in regulating absorption of calcium by the gastrointestinal tract is $1,25(OH)_2D$. Indeed, it is likely that vitamin D (cholecalciferol) and its 25OH derivative become active only after conversion in the kidney to $1,25(OH)_2D$. The 3-hydroxyl group on dihydrotachysterol enhances its capacity to stimulate calcium absorption, but not as much as 1-hydroxylation. When high serum calcium concentration causes decreased parathyroid hormone secretion or when serum phosphorus concentration is high, $24,25(OH)_2D$ is preferentially synthesized by the kidney. Although present in the serum in concentrations considerably higher than that of $1,25(OH)_2D$, $24,25(OH)_2D$ only weakly stimulates intestinal calcium absorption. However, it may have preferential effects on bone mineralization.

638. The answer is E. *(Wilson, ed 12. chap 341.)* The combination of hypocalcemia, hypophosphatemia, elevated serum parathyroid hormone levels, and bone fractures is consistent with a diagnosis of osteomalacia in this ptaient. In the absence of other gastrointestinal or renal abnormalities leading to malabsorption or increased renal loss of calcium or phosphorus, vitamin D deficiency is likely to be present. Inadequate intake of vitamin D and calcium together with limited exposure to the sun are frequent in this age group. Postmenopausal osteoporosis is associated with vertebral and hip fractures as well, but laboratory abnormalities are not present. Primary hyperparathyroidism is associated with increased serum calcium concentration, as is ectopic parathyroid hormone secretion (although existence of the latter has been questioned). Paget's disease of bone does not produce hypocalcemia, and it causes typical sclerotic changes on x-ray examination.

639. The answer is A. *(Wilson, ed 12. chaps 340, 343.)* In most conditions in which hypocalcemia is present — e.g., osteomalacia, renal failure, and parathyroid hormone-resistance states (pseudohypoparathyroidism) — the concentration of circulating parathyroid hormone (PTH) is increased as assessed by radioimmunoassay. However, the syndrome of hypocalcemia with severe hypomagnesemia (<0.4 mmol/L [<0.8 meq/L] is associated with a state of functional hypoparathyroidism. This severe degree of hypomagnesemia, most commonly associated with alcoholism and steatorrhea, may blunt or totally block PTH secretion. Magnesium deficiency also may be associated with reduced peripheral responsiveness to PTH. Correction of hypomagnesemia over several days restores normal parathyroid secretion and responsiveness.

640. The answer is D. *(Wilson, ed 12. chap 339.)* A major function of parathyroid hormone is to act as a trophic hormone to regulate the rate of formation of $1,25(OH)_2$ vitamin D. The mechanism by which parathyroid hormone exerts this effect may be secondary to its effects on phosphorus metabolism. Other hormones, including prolactin and estrogen, also may play a role in stimulating the production of $1,25(OH)_2$ vitamin D.

641. The answer is A-N, B-N, C-Y, D-Y, E-Y. *(Wilson, ed 12. chaps 53, 322.)* The luteal phase of the menstrual cycle follows ovulation and is characterized by an increase in progesterone secretion by the corpus luteum. With anovulatory cycles the corpus luteum does not form, and progesterone levels remain low. Furthermore, with anovulatory cycles the characteristic surge of LH and FSH at midcycle is absent, and menses are usually painless. Irregular estrogen breakthrough bleeding that occurs with anovulatory cycles is the consequence of persistent ovarian estradiol secretion and an absence of luteal-phase progesterone secretion.

642. The answer is A-Y, B-Y, C-Y, D-Y, E-N. *(Wilson, ed 12. chap 5.)* Since the gene responsible for an autosomally transmitted dominant disorder is located on one of the 22 autosomes, no predilection for either sex exists; on average, both sexes are affected equally, and half the offspring of an affected patient (and hence half the siblings) are affected. For the same reason, male-to-male transmission can occur. Since dominantly inherited disorders are manifested in the heterozygous state, unaffected persons are not carriers of the defective gene and cannot transmit it. Consanguinity among parents of affected offspring is not common, and new mutation seems to be the usual mechanism in affected patients without a family history of the disorder.

643. The answer is A-N, B-Y, C-Y, D-Y, E-N. *(Wilson, ed 12. chaps 68, 340.)* Familial hypocalcemia, short stature, and abnormalities of the metacarpal and metatarsal bones are characteristic features of pseudohypoparathyroidism. The underlying defect is renal resistance to the action of parathyroid hormone; although plasma levels of parathyroid hormone are elevated, urinary cyclic AMP is low, and there is a diminished response of urinary cyclic AMP to the exogenous administration of the hormone. The basal ganglia are frequently calcified. No antibodies to parathyroid tissue can be demonstrated, and, unlike the situation in idiopathic hypoparathyroidism, the frequency of monilial infection is not increased. Hypothyroidism is common in persons with pseudohypoparathyroidism; it is usually the result of resistance to thyroid-stimulating hormone due to the same defect in membrane adenylate cyclase that causes resistance to parathyroid hormone.

644. The answer is A-Y, B-N, C-N, D-N, E-Y. *(Wilson, ed 12. chap 5.)* Many common diseases are known to "run in families," yet are not inherited in a simple mendelian fashion. It is likely that the expression of these disorders depends on a family of genes that can impart a certain degree of risk and then be modified by subsequent environmental factors. The risk of development of disease for a relative of an affected person varies with the degree of relationship; first-degree relatives (parents, siblings, and offspring) have the highest risk, which in itself varies with the specific disease. Many of these multifactorial genetic diseases are inherited in a greater frequency in persons with certain HLA (major histocompatibility system) types. For example, there is a tenfold increased risk of celiac sprue (gluten-sensitive enteropathy) in persons harboring HLA-B8. This genotype also imparts increased risk for chronic active hepatitis, myasthenia gravis, and Addison's disease. The incidence of diabetes mellitus is much higher in those expressing HLA-D3 and HLA-D4. Spondyloarthropathies, psoriatic arthritis (HLA-B27), hyperthyroidism (HLA-DR3), and multiple sclerosis (HLA-DR2) are other examples of diseases with histocompatibility predispositions. On the other hand, Wilson's disease is inherited in autosomal recessive fashion and adult polycystic kidney disease and neurofibromatosis are among those disorders inherited in an autosomal dominant manner.

645. The answer is A-Y, B-N, C-Y, D-Y, E-Y. *(Wilson, ed 12. chap 52.)* The endocrine causes of organic impotence include decreased plasma testosterone and hyperprolactinemia. High serum prolactin, usually due to a pituitary microadenoma, suppresses production of luteinizing hormone–releasing hormone (LHRH). Dopaminergic agonists such as bromocriptine may be useful in reducing prolactin levels and restoring potency. Many antihypertensive agents interfere with the sympathetic nervous system's role in penile erection. Beta-blockers are the major offenders in this regard. The angiotensin-converting enzyme inhibitors, calcium channel blockers such as nifedipine, and peripheral vasodilators are not associated with an increased risk of impotence. Histamine (H-2)-receptor antagonists, including cimetidine, cause impotence by both increasing serum prolactin and directly antagonizing the effect of testosterone. Drugs with significant anticholinergic properties, such as tricyclic antidepressants (including amitriptyline), can prevent erection, which is parasympathetically mediated. Other important causes of impotence include neurogenic disorders and vascular insufficiency (e.g., aortic occlusion, or Leriche syndrome, or distal atherosclerosis). Anatomic abnormalities, such as Peyronie's disease in which penile curvature is associated with fibrosis in the venous sinusoids of the penis, can also cause impotence.

646. The answer is A-N, B-Y, C-Y, D-N, E-Y. *(Wilson, ed 12. chaps 70, 71.)* Whenever caloric intake is deficient, amino acids are utilized as energy substrates and for gluconeogenesis to maintain an adequate blood level of glucose, especially important for metabolism of the brain. Thus, protein synthesis is compromised when energy requirements are not met by nonprotein calories. Stated in another way, energy undernutrition predisposes to protein starvation even when the protein supply is otherwise adequate. Nevertheless, it should be kept in mind that diets deficient in energy are frequently deficient in protein as well. Carbohydrates have a protein-sparing effect if given in sufficient quantities, but this effect does not hold true for fat. Low carbohydrate and fat diets do not produce a selective protein malabsorption, although generalized malabsorption occurs in patients with severe chronic malnutrition.

647. The answer is A-N, B-Y, C-N, D-Y, E-Y. *(Wilson, ed 12. chap 71.)* Several methods are useful in assessing protein undernutrition. Clinically, the ratio of 24-h urinary creatinine excretion to height is the most sensitive and practical measure of muscle mass; it is decreased in the presence of protein malnutrition. Reduced blood levels of proteins synthesized by the liver, such as albumin and transferrin, are also characteristic findings with protein starvation. Anthropometric assessment of midarm circumference and triceps skin-fold thickness are measures of the mass of muscle and adipose tissue, respectively. While in many instances calculation of body weight as a percentage of ideal body weight is a good measure of lean body mass plus adipose tissue, the presence of ascites and edema makes this assessment unreliable. Blood ammonia levels may indicate protein overload from intestinal causes (e.g., gastrointestinal bleeding) but are not helpful in assessing protein nutrition. The combination of a careful clinical history and a thorough examination is also a reproducible and valid technique to evaluate nutritional status; however, many cachectic patients are unable to provide a detailed history.

648. The answer is A-Y, B-N, C-Y, D-N, E-Y. *(Wilson, ed 12. chap 71. Saudek, Am J Med 60:117, 1976.)* Protein-calorie undernutrition affects the function of nearly every organ. Physiologic adaptations to caloric deficiency include a fall in plasma insulin concentration coupled with a rise in glucagon and cortisol levels. This mechanism, which protects against hypoglycemia, permits liberation of amino acids from muscle and of free fatty acids from adipose tissue, thereby providing carbon chains for hepatic gluconeogenesis and ketogenesis, respectively. In addition, ketones and free fatty acids are oxidized directly in many tissues and provide the energy for hepatic gluconeogenesis. Thyroid hormone metabolism is also changed such that T_3 and T_4 are decreased. The 5'-deiodination of reverse T_3 (rT_3) is reduced, causing serum levels of rT_3, which is metabolically inert, to rise significantly. Cell-mediated immunity is impaired (as evidenced by cutaneous anergy), although serum immunoglobulin levels and humoral response to antigens are relatively preserved.

649. The answer is A-N, B-Y, C-Y, D-Y, E-Y. *(Wilson, ed 12. chap 75.)* In most malnourished persons, positive nitrogen balance can be achieved by providing 1 g of amino acids per kilogram of ideal body weight. However, in the presence of abnormal protein losses (e.g., from burn exudates, pancreatic secretions, or gastrointestinal fistula) or hypermetabolic states (sepsis, trauma, hyperthyroidism), additional protein intake must be provided. Likewise, daily protein requirements are increased in the presence of caloric deficiency, because amino acids are used for oxidative metabolism and gluconeogenesis. Renal insufficiency and hepatic insufficiency are examples of "nitrogen accumulation diseases." When the kidneys are unable to excrete urea, ammonia may be used for the net synthesis of nonessential amino acids; thus, the need for nonessential nitrogen is reduced. In hepatic failure, amino acid catabolism is decreased, so that even normal protein intake may be deleterious.

650. The answer is A-Y, B-Y, C-Y, D-N, E-N. *(Wilson, ed 12. chap 75.)* As a general rule, when patients cannot eat a normal diet, cannot absorb an oral diet efficiently, or deteriorate in health with oral feeding, total parenteral nutrition (TPN) is needed to provide partial or complete nourishment. Bowel rest, a frequent indication for TPN, is important in treating exacerbations of inflammatory bowel disease, intestinal fistulas, and pancreatitis. While medium chain triglycerides can be helpful, TPN is the best management for short bowel syndrome (>70 percent resected). Persons who are markedly hypermetabolic from severe trauma, burns, or sepsis, for example, also may be helped by supplemental parenteral nutrition, even when some oral intake is possible. Well-nourished patients who are not expected to be able to eat for 10 to 14 days should receive TPN to avoid excess wasting and malnutrition. It is unclear whether the decrease in negative nitrogen balance that results from administration for a week or less of TPN to otherwise healthy people is of clinical significance. Patients who are unable to swallow for long periods of time (e.g., because of stroke, neuromuscular disorders, or coma) are best treated with enteral feedings.

651. The answer is A-Y, B-Y, C-N, D-N, E-Y. *(Wilson, ed 12. chap 8.)* Several inborn errors of metabolism can be treated successfully by the appropriate dietary restriction of a substrate or its precursors. Mental retardation and other problems associated with galactosemia and phenylketonuria can be prevented by reduced intake of galactose or phenylalanine, respectively, during childhood. Restriction of neutral fats can prevent pancreatitis in persons with lipoprotein lipase deficiency. Neither hyperprolinemia nor Tay-Sachs disease is treatable by dietary management.

652. The answer is A-Y, B-Y, C-Y, D-Y, E-Y. *(Wilson, ed 12. chap 326. Havel, J Clin Invest 81:1653, 1988.)* Appropriate therapy for patients who have familial hypercholesterolemia should begin with a diet that is low in cholesterol and saturated fats and high in polyunsaturated fats. The administration of nicotinic acid and bile acid–binding resins, such as cholestyramine or colestipol, may be required if diet alone is insufficient therapy. Probucol also can be effective in lowering serum cholesterol levels when other measures are inadequate. Drugs such as lovastatin that inhibit 3-hydroxy-3-methyl glutaryl coenzyme A, the rate-limiting step in cholesterol biosynthesis, show great promise in treating patients with hypercholesterolemia.

653. The answer is A-Y, B-N, C-Y, D-Y, E-N. *(Wilson, ed 12. chap 326.)* Genetic analysis of survivors of myocardial infarction indicates that 20 percent of those persons less than 60 years of age have some form of inherited hyperlipidemia. Familial hypercholesterolemia, familial hypertriglyceridemia, and familial combined hyperlipidemia are the three most common primary hyperlipidemias. Inherited in an autosomal dominant manner, these disorders are associated with a fivefold to tenfold increase in the risk of developing premature coronary atherosclerosis. Familial hyperalphalipoproteinemia is characterized by elevated levels of high density lipoprotein (HDL); it is associated with a slightly increased longevity and confers an apparent protection against myocardial infarction. Familial lipoprotein lipase deficiency is a rare autosomal recessive disorder that leads to marked elevations of serum triglyceride.

654. The answer is A-Y, B-Y, C-Y, D-Y, E-Y. *(Wilson, ed 12. chap 326.)* Diabetic patients with insulin deficiency may show massive elevation of the serum level of triglycerides, with the concomitant risk of development of acute pancreatitis, as well as eruptive xanthomas, lipemia retinalis, and hepatomegaly. Adequate insulin replacement restores lipoprotein lipase activity and decreases hepatic production of very low density lipoproteins by impairing fatty acid mobilization from the adipose tissue. However, hypertriglyceridemia also occurs in well-controlled diabetic patients (generally obese) in whom it may be present as an independently inherited trait as shown by family studies. Specific drug therapy may be required in this group of patients when diet and adequate control of the diabetic state fail to return triglyceride levels to normal.

655. The answer is A-N, B-Y, C-Y, D-Y, E-Y. *(Wilson, ed 12. chap 326. Scriver, ed 6. chap 47.)* This patient has familial type 3 hyperlipoproteinemia with typical tuberoeruptive and palmar xanthomas. The basic defect in type 3 hyperlipoproteinemia is an abnormal form of apoprotein E (E_2) with a lower affinity for its liver receptor, thus impairing the rate of clearance of chylomicron remnants and intermediate density lipoprotein (IDL) from the circulation. Heterozygotes for the E_2 allele (e.g., E_4/E_2, E_3/E_2) do not have hyperlipidemia. Since the incidence of the E_2/E_2 genotype in the general population is 1 in 100, but the incidence of type 3 hyperlipoproteinemia is only 1 in 10,000, other factors contribute to the expression of the genetic defect. Thus, obesity, hypothyroidism, and diabetes mellitus must be sought and treated accordingly. Clofibrate or gemfibrozil is usually effective when drug therapy is required in these patients.

656. The answer is A-N, B-N, C-Y, D-N, E-N. *(Wilson, ed 12. chap 72. Bray, Diabetes 26:1072, 1977.)* The failure of traditional medical therapies for morbid obesity has provided the impetus for the development of bypass surgery. The initial common bypass operation was jejunoileal bypass. Although weight loss is usually rapid and long-lasting, there are serious postoperative complications, including wound infection (2 to 5 percent), thromboembolism (1 to 5 percent), and death (4 percent). Medical sequelae include diarrhea in all patients, polyarthritis due to circulating immune complexes (6 percent), progressive liver disease (2 to 4 percent), and nephrolithiasis due to calcium malabsorption with secondary hyperoxaluria (3 to 10 percent). Gastric surgery—either bypass or plication—leads to limitation of food intake by delaying gastric emptying and providing a smaller reservoir, which result in early satiety. Both types of gastric procedures, by maintaining intestinal continuity, can promote significant weight loss without causing malabsorption, diarrhea, or hepatic dysfunction.

657. The answer is A-Y, B-N, C-N, D-N, E-Y. *(Wilson, ed 12. chap 72. Olefsky, Am J Physiol 243:E15, 1982.)* Increased insulin secretion is a characteristic feature of obesity, and the combination of normal or elevated blood sugar concentration with hyperinsulinemia indicates that an insulin-resistant state is present. Tissue insensitivity to insulin is common in obesity and appears to have two components: a decreased number of tissue insulin receptors and, with more severe insulin resistance, a postreceptor intracellular defect in glucose metabolism. Circulating insulin antagonists have not been implicated in the insulin resistance of obesity. Both the formation of insulin and the rate of insulin degradation are normal in obese persons.

658. The answer is A-N, B-Y, C-Y, D-Y, E-N. *(Wilson, ed 12. chap 54.)* Hirsutism is a common complaint of women. The evaluation of this problem should include questions regarding the rate of onset of hair growth, menstrual history, and drug intake. Examination should be directed toward sites of androgen-dependent hair (pubic, chest, extremity) and assessment of virilizing features such as clitoromegaly, coarsened voice, acne, and frontal balding. Rapid onset of frank virilization or elevations in serum dehydroepiandrosterone sulfate greater than 22 nmol/L (6 μg/L) or serum testosterone concentrations > 7 nmol/L (2 ng/dL) suggest the presence of either an adrenal or ovarian tumor. Thus, it is unlikely that the patient had either an adrenal carcinoma or the androgen-producing ovarian tumor called arrhenoblastoma. On the other hand, the patient could have polycystic ovaries (measurement of gonadotropins and pelvic ultrasound might be helpful in this regard), late-onset congenital adrenal hyperplasia (demonstrable by 17-hydroxyprogesterone production after cosyntropin [Cortrosyn] stimulation and treated with synthetic glucocorticosteroids to suppress pituitary ACTH), or idiopathic hirsutism.

659. The answer is A-N, B-N, C-N, D-Y, E-Y. *(Wilson, ed 12. chap 73.)* Anorexia nervosa is an eating disorder usually manifest in teenage girls who markedly restrict nutritional intake and partake in ritualized exercise. Amenorrhea always accompanies this disorder. Presumably because of hypothalamic dysfunction, the episodic pituitary release of LH characteristic of the pubertal state is blunted or absent; basal levels of LH and FSH are low, and the LH response to LHRH is impaired. The skin is dry, scaly, and yellow (due to increased carotene levels). Bradycardia, hypothermia, hypotension, and life-threatening hypokalemia may be present in advanced cases. Growth hormone (GH) levels may be normal or elevated with an acromegalic-type rise in response to injection of thyrotropin-releasing hormone (TRH). Levels of insulin-like growth factor I (IGF-I, somatomedin C) are low, perhaps contributing to the high GH levels because of impaired feedback inhibition. Hypothalamic secretion of corticotropin-releasing hormone is enhanced, resulting in elevated plasma cortisol levels. The thyroid hormone profile is similar to that observed in the "sick euthyroid" state. Decreased activity of the 5'-deiodinase that converts thyroxine (T_4) to triiodothyronine (T_3) and reverse T_3 (rT_3) to diiodothyronine results in reduced serum T_3 and elevated rT_3 concentrations.

660. The answer is A-N, B-N, C-N, D-Y, E-N. *(Wilson, ed 12. chap 72. Stunkard, N Engl J Med 314:193, 1986.)* Basal metabolic rates in obese persons are normal when the results are expressed as a function of fat-free body weight. Similarly, depending on the type of exercise performed, energy expenditure is normal or even increased in obese persons because of extra body mass. Although weight gain does occur in patients with hypothyroidism, the gain is usually modest and is a result of fluid retention in connective tissues rich in mucopolysaccharides. The obesity associated with Cushing's syndrome is centripetal in type and is usually accompanied by other manifestations of the disease such as cutaneous striae, muscle weakness, and hypertension. The genetic background is probably more important than environmental factors in the development of human obesity. Overactivity of lipoprotein lipase rather than its deficiency has been suggested as a pathogenetic mechanism in rodent and human obesity, but the importance of this is still unclear.

661. The answer is A-Y, B-Y, C-N, D-N, E-Y. *(Wilson, ed 12. chap 313.)* The development of a pituitary adenoma in a patient who has undergone bilateral adrenalectomy for the treatment of Cushing's disease is termed *Nelson's syndrome.* This disorder is characterized by hyperpigmentation, erosion of the sella turcica, and high plasma ACTH levels. Because of adrenalectomy, urinary 17-ketosteroid excretion usually is low; plasma cortisol levels are determined by the regimen of replacement therapy.

662. The answer is A-Y, B-N, C-Y, D-Y, E-N. *(Wilson, ed 12. chap 313.)* Hypoglycemia, exercise, administration of levodopa, and intravenous arginine infusion all stimulate growth hormone secretion in normal subjects. These factors commonly serve as the basis for stimulation tests to measure reserve capacities for growth hormone secretion and consequently to assess the functional capacity of the pituitary gland. Hyperglycemia suppresses growth hormone secretion, and thyrotropin-releasing hormone does not release growth hormone in normal subjects; these stimuli, however, may cause a paradoxical increase in plasma growth hormone concentration in persons with acromegaly.

663. The answer is A-Y, B-N, C-N, D-N, E-Y. *(Wilson, ed 12. chap 313. Snyder, Endocr Rev 6:552, 1985.)* Serum prolactin levels correlate with tumor size in patients with macroprolactinomas. Thus, the prolactin level in this patient is lower than that expected in association with a large pituitary prolactinoma, and the modest hyperprolactinemia probably reflects impaired delivery of dopamine from the hypothalamus resulting from mechanical effects of the tumor. Since the patient has no clinical evidence of acromegaly, hyperthyroidism, or Cushing's syndrome, measurement of serum gonadotropin and testosterone levels would be useful to assess the mechanism of the sexual dysfunction or to rule out the presence of a gonadotropin-producing pituitary adenoma, or both. Paradoxically, gonadotropin-secreting tumors usually cause hypogonadotropic hypogonadism because they produce isolated α or β subunits of luteinizing hormone (LH) instead of intact, bioactive LH. Evaluation for other pituitary hormone deficiencies is also indicated. Treatment with desmopressin is not indicated unless diabetes insipidus ensues. The use of bromocriptine would be confusing in this patient because it would suppress the elevated prolactin levels without affecting tumor behavior. Formal visual testing is mandatory in every patient with a pituitary macroadenoma.

664. The answer is A-Y, B-Y, C-N, D-Y, E-Y. *(Wilson, ed 12. chap 316.)* Radioactive iodine uptake (RAIU) is often a useful test in distinguishing among the various causes of hyperthyroidism. Elevation of RAIU above the normal range usually indicates thyroid hyperfunction (some persons with hyperthyroidism have a normal or low RAIU). Painless thyroiditis is a variant of chronic lymphocytic thyroiditis associated with transient thyrotoxicosis from release of preformed hormone. Radiographic contrast studies, such as intravenous pyelography and oral cholecystography, use organic media that release iodide and thus serve as sources for dilution of administered radioactive iodine; as a result, RAIU may be falsely low for as long as 6 months. *Thyrotoxicosis factitia* is the term used to designate thyrotoxicosis resulting from ingestion of thyroid hormones. Ingestion of liothyronine (T_3) results in a low serum thyroxine (T_4) concentration, while ingestion of levothyroxine leads to elevations of both T_4 and T_3. In either case, feedback of exogenous thyroid hormone decreases TSH secretion and lowers RAIU. Struma ovarii, which is an ovarian tumor with thyroid-like tissue that releases thyroid hormone, is a rare cause of thyrotoxicosis. Measurement of RAIU over the thyroid gland would not, of course, detect the abdominal source of increased RAIU in women affected with struma ovarii. Choriocarcinoma releases factors with TSH-like activity that enhance uptake of radioactive iodine.

665. The answer is A-Y, B-Y, C-Y, D-Y, E-Y. *(Wilson, ed 12. chap 316.)* The changes in thyroid hormone economy termed the ''sick euthyroid'' syndrome may be induced by a variety of illnesses, traumas, and stresses. Depending upon the severity and duration of the stress, these changes lead to alterations in the concentrations of the free and, eventually, the total circulating thyroid hormones. Decreased production of T_3 resulting from inhibition of the peripheral 5'-monodeiodination of T_4 is a consistent feature. A decrease in the protein binding of T_4 and T_3 also occurs, and as a consequence the percentage of free T_4 usually increases. In more seriously ill patients, abnormalities of hormone binding to protein increase still further so that serum T_4 concentrations decrease into the hypothyroid range, most commonly the consequence of an inhibition of thyroid hormone binding to protein. Such inhibition is likely to result from an increase in quantity of a circulating fatty acid.

666. The answer is A-N, B-N, C-Y, D-Y, E-Y. *(Wilson, ed 12. chap 316.)* The woman described has subacute thyroiditis, which seems to have a viral etiology. The tenderness may respond to aspirin therapy, and, in more severe cases, the use of glucocorticoids is generally efficacious in treatment, although such therapy is associated with a high recurrence rate. Hyperthyroidism, when it occurs in association with subacute thyroiditis, is usually transient and is best controlled symptomatically with propranolol or phenobarbital, or both. Subtotal thyroidectomy and radioactive iodine therapy are never appropriate therapy for subacute thyroiditis.

667. The answer is A-Y, B-Y, C-N, D-Y, E-N. *(Wilson, ed 12. chap 317.)* Adrenal carcinomas are likely to present as abdominal masses and secrete large amounts of adrenal androgens, which results in markedly elevated urinary 17-ketosteroid excretion. Neoplastic secretion of adrenal steroids characteristically is not suppressed with high doses (2 mg every 6 h) of dexamethasone, because it is not regulated by ACTH. Indeed, ACTH levels are usually immeasurably low in persons with adrenal carcinoma. Testing with metyrapone (750 mg every 4 h for a day) usually does not result in an increase in urinary 17-hydroxycorticosteroids or plasma 11-deoxycortisol because of the prolonged suppression of ACTH secretion by the autonomous adrenal tumor. In contrast, patients with pituitary-dependent Cushing's syndrome show a normal response to metyrapone.

668. The answer is A-Y, B-N, C-Y, D-Y, E-N. *(Wilson, ed 12. chap 317.)* Complications of long-term treatment with high doses of glucocorticoids include the development or acceleration of osteoporosis and depression of immune function. Whether high-dose steroids can induce frank peptic ulceration is not established, but persons with preexisting ulcer disease may have exacerbations while on steroid therapy. Detection of preexisting abnormalities before the start of steroid therapy allows clinicians to institute appropriate treatment concurrently with the institution of steroid therapy. Testing the integrity of the hypothalamic-pituitary-adrenal axis is unwarranted prior to the initiation of chronic high-dose glucocorticoid therapy.

669. The answer is A-Y, B-Y, C-Y, D-Y, E-Y. *(Wilson, ed 12. chaps 317, 324.)* The syndromes of congenital adrenal hyperplasia may result in all the following: virilization in females (due to C-21 hydroxylase or C-11 hydroxylase deficiency); isosexual precocious puberty in males (C-21 hydroxylase or C-11 hydroxylase deficiency); male pseudohermaphroditism (3β-ol-dehydrogenase, C-17 hydroxylase, or 20,22-desmolase deficiency); hypertension due to salt retention (C-11 hydroxylase or C-17 hydroxylase deficiency); and hypotension secondary to renal salt wasting (C-21 hydroxylase, 3β-ol-dehydrogenase, or 20,22-desmolase deficiency).

670. The answer is A-N, B-Y, C-Y, D-Y, E-Y. *(Wilson, ed 12. chaps 317, 324.)* Urinary 17-ketosteroid determination, a venerable procedure in endocrinology, measures the metabolites of weak adrenal and gonadal androgens. It is not a specific test for assessment of gonadal function and is a poor means of assessing the potent testicular androgen testosterone (only about 40 percent of urinary levels of 17-ketosteroids in men comes from production of testosterone). Although it is not the most sensitive indicator of congenital adrenal hyperplasia, urinary excretion of 17-ketosteroids usually is elevated in affected untreated persons.

671. The answer is A-Y, B-Y, C-Y, D-Y, E-Y. *(Wilson, ed 12. chap 319. Foster, N Engl J Med 309:159, 1983.)* The insulin-to-glucagon ratio determines the rate of ketogenesis by the liver. A fall in insulin increases adipose-cell lipolysis, with the resultant liberation of free fatty acids, the substrate for ketone body synthesis. In the liver, carnitine palmitoyltransferase I is the critical mitochondrial enzyme necessary to transport free fatty acids from the cytosol into the mitochondrial matrix, where they are oxidized to ketone bodies. Glucagon stimulates ketogenesis by increasing hepatic carnitine levels and decreasing liver malonyl CoA concentrations. Carnitine is required for this movement of free fatty acids into the mitochondria, and malonyl CoA, the first committed intermediate in the synthesis of fatty acids from glucose, is a powerful competitive inhibitor of carnitine palmitoyltransferase I.

672. The answer is A-N, B-N, C-Y, D-Y, E-Y. *(Wilson, ed 12. chap 319. Harrison, Diabetes 38:815, 1989.)* There is considerable disagreement regarding the genetics of diabetes mellitus, but certain aspects appear to be clear-cut. Genetic factors are probably permissive for the development of type 1 (immune-mediated) and related more directly to the development of type 2 (non–immune-mediated) diabetes. The genetic locus for diabetes appears to be located near the HLA genes on the sixth chromosome. The presence of HLA antigens B8 or B15 increases the risk for developing type 1 diabetes nearly threefold, antigens DR3 and DR4 fourfold to fivefold, and antigen combinations (e.g., B8/B15) up to tenfold. However, homozygosity for a high-risk allele (e.g., DR3/DR3) does not increase the risk further. Evidence implicates positions 45 and 57 of the DQ_β chain as having importance in determining genetic susceptibility to type 1 diabetes. The concordance rate for monozygotic twins under 40 years of age is less than 50 percent. Pedigree analysis has shown a very low prevalence of vertical transmission for type 1 diabetes. The onset of juvenile diabetes has a seasonal variation and may follow mumps, hepatitis, or Coxsackie virus infections, among others. These infections in genetically predisposed persons are theorized to produce an immune response with the development of cytotoxic islet-cell antibodies, which complete the destruction of the beta cells. This theory would explain why circulating islet cell antibodies are usually detectable soon after the onset of type 1 diabetes. In some cases anti-islet-cell antibodies have been demonstrated in twins of diabetics destined to develop the disease even before glucose tolerance became abnormal.

673. The answer is A-Y, B-N, C-Y, D-Y, E-N. *(Wilson, ed 12. chap 319. Arieff, Medicine 51:73, 1972. Carroll, Diabetes Care 6:579, 1983.)* Diabetic hyperosmolar nonketotic coma is a medical emergency usually occurring as a complication of maturity-onset diabetes. Typically, affected persons are elderly (often living alone or in a nursing home), have a history of recent stroke or infection, and are unable to drink sufficient water to balance urinary fluid losses. These factors combine to cause sustained hyperglycemic diuresis with profound volume depletion and decreased urine output. Presenting features often include signs of circulatory compromise as well as central nervous system manifestations ranging from confusion or seizures to coma. Ketoacidosis is absent, perhaps because portal-vein insulin concentration is high enough to prevent full activation of hepatic ketogenesis. Serum levels of free fatty acids are generally lower than in diabetic ketoacidosis, and although hypertonicity is marked, measured serum sodium concentration is kept from being significantly elevated by the profound hyperglycemia. Infections are common, and disseminated intravascular coagulation can occur as a result of elevated plasma viscosity (both bleeding and in situ thrombosis have been reported). Although administration of free water eventually becomes necessary, the treatment of salt deficits has highest initial therapeutic priority. Several liters of isotonic saline should be given over the first 2 h, followed by half-normal saline, and then a 5% glucose solution when blood glucose levels approach normal. Hypotonic fluids should not be used initially, because most of the water enters the intracellular compartment—possibly leading to cerebral edema—rather than remaining in the plasma and interstitial spaces, where it is needed to support the circulation. Insulin also is required but usually in lower doses than in diabetic ketoacidosis.

674. The answer is A-N, B-Y, C-Y, D-N, E-Y. *(Wilson, ed 12. chap 319.)* The occurrence of hyperglycemic ketoacidosis or hyperglycemic hyperosmolar coma is diagnostic of diabetes mellitus. Similarly, persistent fasting hyperglycemia (glucose concentration greater than 7.8 mmol/L [140 mg/dL]), even if asymptomatic, has been recommended by the National Diabetes Data Group as a criterion for the diagnosis of diabetes. On the other hand, abnormal glucose tolerance—whether after eating or occurring after a standard "glucose tolerance test"—can be caused by many factors (e.g., anxiety, infection or other illness, lack of exercise, or inadequate diet). Likewise, glycosuria may have renal as well as endocrinologic causes. Therefore, these two conditions cannot be considered diagnostic of diabetes.

675. The answer is A-Y, B-N, C-N, D-N, E-Y. *(Wilson, ed 12. chap 319. Kahn, J Clin Invest 82:1151, 1988. Kurtz, Diabetologia 19:329, 1980.)* Chronic insulin resistance is defined as a need for more than 200 units of insulin per day for several days in the absence of infection or ketoacidosis. This definition was based on the assumption that the normal human pancreas produces this much insulin daily; in fact, normal daily insulin production is probably 30 to 40 units, so that relative resistance is present when more than this amount is required to control blood sugar levels. The most common causes of insulin resistance are obesity and anti-insulin antibodies of the IgG type. Antibodies develop within 60 days of initiation of insulin therapy in nearly all diabetic persons. It is assumed that the binding of insulin by these antibodies is the major cause of severe insulin resistance, but the correlation between antibody titer and resistance is not always close. Uncontrolled hyperglycemia is the major consequence of insulin resistance, though ketoacidosis also may result. A history of discontinuous insulin use is frequent, and concomitant insulin allergy occurs in a minority of affected persons. Most patients require high doses of steroids, which frequently begin to take effect in a few days.

Acanthosis nigricans is a cutaneous disorder associated with two types of insulin resistance: type A, in which young women show accelerated growth, evidence of virilization, and decreased numbers of insulin receptors; and type B, in which older women have anti-insulin-receptor antibodies and other symptoms and signs of autoimmune disease (arthralgias, positive assay for antinuclear antibody, and others). The absence of acanthosis nigricans in the woman described in the question makes it unlikely that decreased numbers of insulin receptors or the presence of anti-insulin-receptor antibodies is playing a role in her insulin resistance.

676. The answer is A-Y, B-Y, C-Y, D-N, E-N. *(Wilson, ed 12. chap 319.)* Approximately 40 percent of patients with type 1 diabetes mellitus sustain diabetic nephropathy. Progression of renal disease is markedly accelerated by hypertension, and even mild degrees of hypertension in diabetic patients should be treated aggressively. A hallmark of diabetic nephropathy is the presence of so-called macroproteinuria (excretion of more than 0.55 g/d), and once this phase is reached there is a steady decline in renal function. So-called microalbuminuria, the excretion of 0.03 to 0.3 g/d of albumin, is also statistically predictive of progression of renal disease. In contrast, nocturia is usually a manifestation of undertreatment of diabetes and is an indication not of renal failure but of an osmotic diuresis. There is no clear-cut relation between insulin requirement and the development of any of the long-term complications of diabetes, including nephropathy; the development of these complications correlates better with the duration rather than the severity of diabetes mellitus.

677. The answer is A-N, B-Y, C-Y, D-N, E-N. *(Wilson, ed 12. chap 320.)* Because factitious hypoglycemia due to insulin injection or sulfonylurea ingestion is common, the finding of hyperinsulinemia associated with a low blood sugar concentration can no longer be considered diagnostic of an islet cell tumor (insulinoma). Suspicion of factitious disease should be especially high in medical personnel and in families of diabetics. The alpha and beta subunits of insulin are cleaved from proinsulin in the beta cell and released in equimolar amounts with the connecting (C) peptide; elevation of plasma C-peptide levels signifies endogenous hyperinsulinemia, because exogenous insulin administration suppresses beta-cell function. Therefore, the triad of fasting hypoglycemia, hyperinsulinemia and elevated plasma C-peptide levels is consistent with either endogenous hyper-insulinemia or ingestion of a sulfonylurea; documentation of the latter in urine or plasma would be diagnostic. Proinsulin usually is released into the circulation in small quantities. However, in patients with insulinoma, proinsulin concentration frequently exceeds 20 percent of total insulin; ingestion of a sulfonylurea, on the other hand, does not cause a disproportionate elevation of plasma proinsulin levels. Insulin antibody measurements in this case would not be expected to be helpful—antibodies may not develop for several months after the start of insulin injections, and the high C-peptide levels essentially rule out an exogenous source of insulin. However, under some circumstances antibodies to specific species of insulin can be identified and hence establish that exogenous insulin has been taken. Attempts to localize an islet cell tumor by radiologic means should only be done once factitious types of hypoglycemia are excluded.

678. The answer is A-Y, B-Y, C-Y, D-N, E-N. *(Wilson, ed 12. chap 320.)* Hypoglycemia due to overutilization of glucose can be associated either with high or low insulin levels. Hypoglycemia associated with hyperinsulinism can occur in persons who have pancreatic insulinoma or who take exogenous insulin or ingest sulfonylurea drugs. Low plasma insulin levels can be associated with overutilization of glucose; examples include large, solid extrapancreatic tumors (e.g., hepatoma and sarcoma), in which high levels of insulin-like growth factors may play a role, and systemic carnitine deficiency, in which peripheral tissues are unable to use free fatty acids for energy production and the liver cannot synthesize ketone bodies. Underproduction of glucose may occur with acquired liver disease, such as hepatic congestion due to right-sided heart failure or viral hepatitis, or with hormone deficiencies, such as adrenal insufficiency and hypopituitarism.

679. The answer is A-N, B-N, C-Y, D-N, E-Y. *(Wilson, ed 12. chap 321.)* Klinefelter syndrome is frequently not diagnosed in patients until the time of expected puberty or during adult life when incomplete virilization or some other manifestation of androgen deficiency first becomes apparent. Testosterone replacement is likely to promote virilization and to restore potency in these patients. However, if gynecomastia is already present, testosterone replacement therapy does not produce regression of the breast tissue, and it may even aggravate the gynecomastia. Surgical resection of the breast is usually necessary in this situation. Since the basic testicular lesion consists of progressive hyalinization of the seminiferous tubules, spermatogenic function is irreversibly impaired, and no form of hormonal therapy is effective in maintaining spermatogenesis. Even in normal persons, testosterone treatment produces hypospermia because of the inhibition of gonadotropin production. Although antisocial behavior may be a part of Klinefelter syndrome, it is unlikely to be a manifestation of androgen deficiency and is not correctable by testosterone replacement.

680. The answer is A-Y, B-Y, C-N, D-Y, E-Y. *(Wilson, ed 12. chap 77.)* Deficiencies of trace elements (metals present at concentrations less than one microgram per gram of tissue) can be due to dietary deficiency, malabsorption (as in chronic diarrhea), or administration of total parenteral nutrition. Iron, copper, selenium, and zinc form stable complexes with enzymes. Selenium, for example, is a component of glutathione peroxidase and therefore functions as an antioxidant. Selenium deficiency results in myocardial necrosis. Zinc is required in tissues with a high cellular turnover, such as the gonads, and pregnant women and the developing fetus are at particular risk for zinc deficiency. Zinc deficiency dermatitis includes hyperkeratotic lesions and alopecia. Since cobalt is a component of vitamin B_{12}, deficiencies of this metal result in megaloblastic anemia. Copper deficiency may result in anemia, pigmentation abnormalities, hypothermia, and scurvy-like skeletal changes.

681. The answer is A-Y, B-N, C-N, D-Y, E-Y. *(Wilson, ed 12. chap 311.)* The first step in hormone-mediated responses is binding of the hormone to a specific receptor. Hormone receptors exist on the cell membrane or, as in the case of steroid hormones, vitamin D, and triiodothyronine, the receptors (which bear homology to the *erbA* oncogene) are present in the cytoplasm, the nucleus, or both. In the case of intracellular receptors, the hormone-receptor complex binds to specific regions of the genome and participates in the control of messenger RNA transcription. The cell membrane hormone receptors may be divided into several classes. The insulin receptor, for example, is related to the *src* tyrosine kinase family of proto-oncogenes. Binding of insulin to its receptor leads to phosphorylation of a number of substrate proteins on tyrosine residues, resulting in further biologic effects. LH and TSH bind to so-called G proteins, which upon activation bind GTP, beginning a cascade of events involved in the control of intracellular mediators such as cyclic AMP. The growth hormone receptor, which is a protein of 600 amino acids, is found in the membrane and has homology with the prolactin receptor; these hormone receptors are dissimilar to G proteins or tyrosine kinases.

682. The answer is A-Y, B-N, C-Y, D-N, E-N. *(Wilson, ed 12. chaps 322, 324.)* In persons with testicular feminization, estradiol secretion by the testes is markedly increased (but not to the level produced by normal ovaries); the mechanism is lack of suppression of luteinizing hormone by testosterone and consequent increased stimulation of gonadal testosterone and estradiol secretion. Ovaries containing follicle cysts may be a source of increased estrogen production, particularly during the postmenopausal years, when gonadotropin levels are very high. The increase in estrogen production characteristic of polycystic ovarian disease is the consequence of peripheral conversion of androstenedione to estrogen and not of direct gonadal production. During the third trimester of pregnancy estrogen production is increased because of formation of estrogen by the placenta rather than by the ovary. Arrhenoblastoma is a virilizing ovarian tumor and does not secrete estrogen.

683. The answer is A-Y, B-Y, C-N, D-Y, E-Y. *(Wilson, ed 12. chaps 322, 324.)* The pathogenesis of hot flashes is uncertain, but in some manner it is related to estrogen deprivation. There is a close temporal relationship between the timing of the hot flash and the onset of pulses of luteinizing hormone (LH) secretion, and suggestions have been made that the flash itself is caused by alterations in metabolism of catecholamines, endorphins, or neurotensin. However, the most striking feature is that the symptoms are preceded by a decrease in estrogen secretion, so that the hot flashes commonly result after the removal of estrogen-secreting tissues, including estrogen-secreting testes in patients with testicular feminization, normal ovaries from premenopausal women, and estrogen-secreting tumors of the ovaries (dysgerminomas). Likewise, menopause at all ages commonly causes symptoms that include hot flashes, whereas removal of gonads or gonadal streaks in women who have never had estrogen secretion from the ovaries, as in women with gonadal dysgenesis, does not cause hot flashes.

684. The answer is A-Y, B-Y, C-Y, D-N, E-Y. *(Wilson, ed 12. chap 322. Judd, Ann Intern Med 98:195, 1983.)* In this young woman with surgical castration, estrogen replacement therapy is indicated to relieve the vasomotor instability and to prevent the atrophy of estrogen target tissues such as the breast and urogenital epithelium. The beneficial effects of estrogens on bone metabolism and calcium balance constitute another indication for replacement therapy, especially in patients at high risk for postmenopausal development of osteoporosis (menopause at a young age in thin, white women). Hirsutism is a manifestation of androgen excess rather than of estrogen deficiency. Treatment with estrogen at physiologic or pharmacologic doses should be cyclic and include administration of progestogen during the last 10 days of the cycle to diminish the risk of development of endometrial hyperplasia and carcinoma of the uterus.

685. The answer is A-Y, B-Y, C-Y, D-N, E-N. *(Wilson, ed 12. chap 323.)* Pathologic gynecomastia develops when the effective testosterone-to-estrogen ratio is decreased, owing to either diminished testosterone production (as in primary testicular failure) or increased estrogen production. The latter may arise from direct estradiol secretion by a testis stimulated by luteinizing hormone or human chorionic gonadotropin or from an increase in peripheral aromatization of precursor steroids, most notably androstenedione. Elevated androstenedione levels may result from increased secretion by an adrenal tumor (leading to an elevated level of urinary 17-ketosteroids) or decreased hepatic clearance in patients with chronic liver disease. A variety of drugs, including diethylstilbestrol, heroin, digitalis, spironolactone, cimetidine, isoniazid, and tricyclic antidepressants, also can cause gynecomastia. In the case presented in the question, the history of paternity and the otherwise-normal physical examination speak against the necessity of obtaining a karyotype, and the bilateral breast enlargement essentially excludes the presence of carcinoma and, thus, the need for biopsy.

686. The answer is A-N, B-Y, C-Y, D-N, E-Y. *(Wilson, ed 12. chap 324.)* Ambiguous genitalia results when androgen production (or action) is defective in a male fetus or when androgen production is enhanced in a female fetus. Such aberrations can arise from a variety of causes. The most common cause is congenital adrenal hyperplasia, followed by mixed gonadal dysgenesis, which is a nonfamilial aberration of the sex chromosomes that interferes with normal sexual development, including 45,X/46,XY mosaicism. Examples of single gene mutations leading to abnormal sexual differentiation are the Reifenstein syndrome, in which genetic males have incompletely developed male genitalia because of androgen resistance, and 5α-reductase deficiency, in which testosterone cannot be converted to dihydrotestosterone. The use in the past of progestational agents to treat pregnant women presenting with threatened abortion was associated with variable degrees of hypospadias in male offspring. Hypogonadotropic hypogonadism is associated with microphallus in male infants but not with hypospadias or abnormal sexual differentiation. Men whose chromosome pattern is 47,XYY are anatomically normal.

687. The answer is A-Y, B-Y, C-N, D-N, E-Y. *(Wilson, ed 12. chap 324.)* Phenotypic men who have two or more X chromosomes have Klinefelter syndrome. Although the diagnosis of Klinefelter syndrome may be suspected prepubertally owing to the increased length of the lower body segment, most affected persons first present postpubertally with signs of decreased testosterone production and small testes. The risk of breast cancer is 20 times that of normal men (and one-fifth that of women), presumably the consequence of long-term estrogen stimulation of the breast. Mosaic chromosome patterns (46,XY/47,XXY) are found in 10 percent of affected persons, 70 percent of whom display the mosaicism only in the testes, which may be normal in size. Hypospadias is not increased in incidence in affected persons. Although mental deficiency and social maladjustment occur with increased frequency in persons with Klinefelter syndrome, most patients with the disorder have normal mental and social competence.

688. The answer is A-Y, B-Y, C-Y, D-Y, E-Y. *(Wilson, ed 12. chap 342.)* Persistent hypophosphatemia is characterized by varying degrees of anorexia, dizziness, bone pain, proximal muscle weakness, cardiomyopathy, and waddling gait. Severe hypophosphatemia may result in rhabdomyolysis, which is heralded by a sharp elevation in serum creatine phosphokinase concentration. A consequence of reduced levels of 2,3-diphosphoglycerate and ATP in erythrocytes is reduced tissue oxygenation. Leukocyte dysfunction resulting in defective phagocytosis makes the hypophosphatemic patient more susceptible to bacterial and fungal infection. Nervous system dysfunction, manifested by irritability and apprehension progressing to obtundation, may occur upon refeeding. Persons with alcoholism may develop severe hypophosphatemia shortly after hospitalization, probably related to the combined effects of glucose administration and phosphorus deficiency due to diminished intake. Correction of phosphorus deficits leads to prompt reversal of the abnormalities.

689. The answer is A-Y, B-Y, C-Y, D-Y, E-N. *(Wilson, ed 12. chap 342.)* Because dietary phosphorus is so ubiquitous and its absorption is so efficient, phosphorus deficiency from poor intake alone is unusual. However, hypophosphatemia can arise if absorption is prevented by some means, such as the administration of nonabsorbable antacids, which bind phorphorus and block its absorption from the gastrointestinal tract. Significant but rapidly reversible hypophosphatemia may accompany the respiratory alkalosis of hyperventilation. Insulin, by driving phosphate into cells, may induce hypophosphatemia. In the kidney, phosphorus is reabsorbed efficiently in the proximal tubule; therefore, diuretics that act proximally are phosphaturic (their use may result in hypophosphatemia), whereas distally acting diuretics are not. Though chronic renal failure is associated with hyperphosphatemia, severe hypophosphatemia may be seen in acute renal failure.

690. The answer is A-Y, B-Y, C-N, D-Y, E-Y. *(Wilson, ed 12. chap 339.)* Measuring the serum concentration of 25OH vitamin D, the major circulating form of vitamin D, can be used to assess the adequacy of dietary intake and absorption of the vitamin. (Vitamin D also is made in the skin in the presence of sunlight.) Once ingested or synthesized, vitamin D is metabolized to 25OH vitamin D in the liver. This reaction is not tightly regulated, and an increase in dietary intake or endogenous production of vitamin D is reflected by linear elevations of serum 25OH vitamin D levels. Levels are reduced in severe chronic parenchymal and cholestatic liver disease but usually are normal in renal failure. Anticonvulsant drugs and glucocorticoids induce hepatic microsomal enzymes, which metabolize vitamin D and 25OH vitamin D into inactive products; this phenomenon, along with other complex effects on calcium metabolism, helps to explain why these drugs cause osteopenia.

691. The answer is A-N, B-N, C-Y, D-Y, E-N. *(Wilson, ed 12. chaps 339, 340.)* Vitamin D toxicity generally occurs after chronic ingestion of large doses of vitamin D_2 or D_3 (usually in excess of 50,000 to 100,000 IU daily for months). Ingestion of a single large dose of vitamin D_2 or D_3 does not cause acute toxicity, because excessive quantities are stored in body fat and released slowly into the bloodstream. Some vitamin D metabolites, such as $1,25(OH)_2$ vitamin D, could conceivably cause toxicity after a single overdose. Hypervitaminosis D has not been reported following prolonged sun exposure, partly because the vitamin is released slowly from the skin after conversion from previtamin D. Hypervitaminosis D causes hypercalcemia, hypercalciuria, and soft-tissue calcification, particularly in the kidneys. It is believed that high circulating levels of 25OH vitamin D directly stimulate intestinal calcium absorption and bone resorption, since toxicity can occur in anephric persons.

692. The answer is A-N, B-N, C-Y, D-Y, E-N. *(Wilson, ed 12. chap 341.)* The presenting findings in both primary hyperparathyroidism and multiple myeloma can include hypercalcemia and vertebral compression fractures. The absence of several key features—anemia, elevated erythrocyte sedimentation rate, abnormal serum protein electrophoresis, and Bence Jones proteinuria—is helpful in eliminating the possibility of multiple myeloma. If doubt remains as to the diagnosis of myeloma, a marrow aspiration should be performed. The presence of hypercalcemia makes unlikely the diagnoses of osteomalacia, which is associated with hypocalcemia, and of osteoporosis and Paget's disease, which are associated with normal blood calcium values.

693. **The answer is A-Y, B-Y, C-N, D-Y, E-Y.** *(Wilson, ed 12. chap 313.)* The enlarged pituitary gland of pregnancy is particularly vulnerable to ischemic necrosis (Sheehan's syndrome) should hypotension occur in the postpartum period. Symptoms and signs of panhypopituitarism even several years after a difficult childbirth are consistent with this condition. Continued amenorrhea, decreased libido, cold intolerance typical of hypothyroidism, and loss of hair should therefore prompt an evaluation for anterior pituitary hypofunction. Lowering the blood sugar by giving a small amount of IV insulin normally triggers release of counterregulatory hormones, including growth hormone and cortisol. The urinary free cortisol itself is not helpful, since a normal or low value is compatible with a stressless period and not just panhypopituitarism. Since the patient probably has central hypothyroidism, the TSH will be inappropriately low in the face of low peripheral hormone. The response to ACTH stimulation should be blunted because the adrenal glands are not "primed" to respond to the pituitary release. Treatment of panhypopituitarism consists of hydrocortisone and thyroid hormone. Growth hormone injections are rarely required.

694. **The answer is A-Y, B-N, C-N, D-Y, E-Y.** *(Wilson, ed 12. chap 316.)* Hypothyroidism should be suspected in the setting of certain laboratory findings not clearly associated with an obvious explanation. In addition to an increased ratio of preejection period to left ventricular ejection time on cardiac systolic time intervals, decreased QRS amplitude on electrocardiographic examination is common. Elevated creatine phosphokinase and lactic dehydrogenase serum values may mimic a myocardial infarction. Hypothyroidism is also typically associated with macrocytic red blood cell indices, due either to coexistent pernicious anemia or to unknown causes. Serum cholesterol is elevated in many patients with primary hypothyroidism.

695. **The answer is A-N, B-Y, C-N, D-Y, E-Y.** *(Wilson, ed 12. chap 317.)* Weakness, hypotension, weight loss, nausea, and vomiting are each present in over 80 percent of patients with adrenal insufficiency, as documented by a failure of exogenously administered ACTH to effect a rise in the serum cortisol level. Hyperpigmentation, resulting from the melanocyte stimulating hormone released in excess along with ACTH in cases of primary adrenal failure, is not seen in cases of secondary failure that occur because of suppressed ACTH. The best example of the latter condition is long-term steroid administration, which depresses ACTH release. Any cause of panhypopituitarism, such as brain tumor invading the sellar region, could also lead to adrenal failure on a secondary basis. Measurement of serum ACTH will distinguish between primary and secondary adrenal insufficiency. Destruction of the adrenal glands may occur as a consequence of infection with mycobacteria, cytomegalovirus, histoplasmosis, coccidioidomycosis, or cryptococcosis. Noninfectious causes of adrenal gland failure include bilateral tumor metastasis, bilateral hemorrhage, amyloidosis, sarcoidosis, autoimmune disease, and administration of certain medications (e.g., rifampin, ketoconazole, and phenytoin).

696. **The answer is A-Y, B-N, C-N, D-Y, E-N.** *(Wilson, ed 12. chap 319. Foster, N Engl J Med 309:159, 1983. Kitabchi, Diabetes Metab Rev 5:337, 1989.)* Insulin must be supplied to the patient with diabetic ketoacidosis to inhibit production of ketone bodies that can cause life-threatening levels of acidosis. While low-dose insulin infusions are now commonly employed, it is generally believed appropriate to use 25 to 50 units/h until the acidosis is reversed. Since there are no known toxic effects of excess insulin in the carefully monitored patient, such an approach will saturate insulin receptors and circumvent the problem of insulin resistance. Insulin therapy should be directed to the pH and the calculated anion gap, not to the plasma ketone value. Tests for ketones measure acetone and acetoacetate but fail to measure β-hydroxybutyrate, which is converted to acetoacetate as tissue oxygenation is restored. Thus, plasma ketones may increase as the patient improves clinically and not mandate an increase in the insulin dosage. When the plasma glucose approaches normal levels, some glucose should be added to the intravenous solutions to prevent cerebral edema. However, since plasma glucose falls more rapidly than plasma ketones, insulin therapy should not be discontinued as glucose levels return to normal; the pH and anion gap remain the most important determinants. Potassium should be given if the admission serum potassium is normal or low, since total body potassium is invariably low and serum potassium will fall as a consequence of insulin therapy. However, it is recommended that potassium initially be given in the form of potassium phosphate because of the severe phosphate depletion associated with ketoacidosis.

697. **The answer is A-Y, B-Y, C-Y, D-N, E-N.** *(Wilson, ed 12. chap 322.)* Death rates associated with oral contraceptive use in women under age 40 are lower than those in women using no contraception. The increased death rate in those not taking oral contraceptives is probably due to the higher pregnancy rate and the consequent risks associated with pregnancy. However, even with the low estrogen dose in current contraceptive pills, there are risks. The most serious are due to the tendency toward hypercoagulability induced by these agents and the increased relative risk for deep venous thrombosis, pulmonary embolism, and thromboembolic stroke. Smoking and advanced age both increase the incidence of these complications. Five percent of women taking oral contraceptives develop significant hypertension, which is possibly due to an estrogen-induced rise in angiotensinogen synthesis. Rare complications involving the liver include peliosis hepatitis (blood-filled venous lakes) and cholestatic jaundice. There is no convincing evidence to implicate the oral contraceptive as a cause of increased risk of breast cancer; its use may be associated with a decreased risk of endometrial and ovarian cancer.

698. The answer is A-N, B-Y, C-Y, D-N, E-Y. *(Wilson, ed 12. chap 324.)* Congenital deficiencies of the enzymes catalyzing the final two steps in testosterone biosynthesis, namely 17,20-desmolase and 17β-hydroxysteroid dehydrogenase, result in ambiguous genitalia from lack of embryologic exposure to testosterone. LH levels are high owing to the deficiency of testosterone, but adrenal hyperplasia does not occur because glucocorticoid production is normal. Defects in testosterone synthesis proximal to these two enzymes also lead to ambiguous genitalia in males, but ACTH levels are high, and associated salt loss or hypertension will occur. In 5α-reductase deficiency, testosterone formation is normal, but an inability to convert this compound to dihydrotestosterone impairs development of external genitalia (although partial virilization may occur at puberty). Severe androgen receptor defects cause testicular feminization and phenotypical females who have a male genotype. Less severe defects of the androgen receptor can lead to a male with cryptorchidism, severe hypospadias, and gynecomastia (Reifenstein syndrome). In cases of defective or insufficient androgen receptor, levels of testosterone tend to be elevated, since the hypothalamic-pituitary axis cannot recognize the presence of the testosterone and continues to secrete LH in large quantities.

699. The answer is A-Y, B-N, C-N, D-N, E-Y. *(Wilson, ed 12. chap 328.)* The porphyrias represent disorders of heme biosynthesis. The biochemical abnormalities and clinical manifestations depend on the step that is blocked and accumulation of precursor metabolites. Congenital erythropoietic porphyria is a rare autosomal recessive disorder due to a defect in the enzyme uroporphyrinogen II cosynthase, which is expressed solely in maturing erythroid cells. Porphobilinogen is preferentially converted to uroporphyrinogen I and then to coproporphyrinogen I. These latter metabolites account for the red urine observed in children with this disorder, but excretion of porphobilinogen is normal. Intermittent acute porphyria, characterized by attacks of recurrent neurologic and psychiatric dysfunction, is an autosomal dominant deficiency of porphobilinogen deaminase, the enzyme that converts porphobilinogen to uroporphyrinogen I. Thus, urinary levels of porphobilinogen are high during attacks. Hereditary coproporphyria is a similar disease caused by partial deficiency of coproporphyrinogen oxidase. A deficiency of protoporphyrinogen oxidase, the next-to-last enzyme involved in heme synthesis, leads to variegate porphyria manifested by attacks of neuropsychiatric dysfunction and photosensitivity and overexcretion of the proximal metabolite, porphobilinogen. Porphyria cutanea tarda, which is inherited or acquired deficiency of hepatic uroporphyrinogen decarboxylase, is not associated with excess porphobilinogen production, probably because aminolevulinic acid synthase activity is not enhanced. Mild skin photosensitivity is the major manifestation of protoporphyria, which is due to a deficiency of ferrochelatase, the final enzyme in heme biosynthesis. Protoporphyrins may accumulate in erythrocytes, but urinary porphobilinogen is normal.

700. The answer is A-N, B-Y, C-N, D-N, E-Y. *(Wilson, ed 12. chaps 331, 332, 334–336.)* In Niemann-Pick disease accumulation of sphingomyelins occurs usually because of sphingomyelinase deficiency. Organomegaly and neurologic involvement are clinical features, but there is highly variable expression depending on the subtype. The most common lysosomal storage disease, adult Gaucher's, is characterized by splenomegaly, pancytopenia, hepatic dysfunction, and bone pain. Accumulation of glucosylceramides presumably accounts for the clinical manifestations and for the distinctive Gaucher cell observed on bone marrow examinations. Tay-Sachs disease, caused by a deficiency of hexosaminidase A with concomitant accumulation of sphingolipids, presents as rapidly progressive neurologic deterioration during infancy and with a characteristic macular cherry-red spot. Heterozygote detection programs (enzyme assays in Ashkenazi Jews) have reduced the incidence of this disease in North America.

   Diseases of glycogen metabolism can result in disorders whose pathophysiology is based either on hepatic hypoglycemia, as in von Gierke disease (glucose 6-phosphatase deficiency), or on muscle-energy deficiency, as in McArdles disease (muscle phosphorylase deficiency). Muscle-energy diseases generally result in painful cramping or myoglobinemia after exercise, so strenuous exercise should be avoided. These diseases are otherwise compatible with a normal life.

A defect in the phenylalanine hydroxylase enzyme complex leads to accumulation of phenylalanine in blood and urine with associated brain damage. The plasma phenylalanine concentration does not usually rise until the institution of protein feedings but is abnormal by the fourth day of life. A diet low in phenylalanine, if instituted during the first month of life, can avert mental retardation. Screening all newborns for blood phenylalanine concentration has been beneficial in this regard.

Excessive urinary excretion of the dibasic amino acids cysteine, lysine, arginine, and ornithine due to impaired tubular reabsorption is the pathophysiologic hallmark of cystinuria, the most common inborn error of amino acid transport. Due to the insolubility of cysteine, the primary clinical manifestation of this disorder is cysteine nephrolithiasis.

Dermatologic Disorders

DIRECTIONS: Each question below contains five suggested responses. Select the **one best** response to each question.

Questions 701–702

After several weeks of tetracycline treatment for acne, an obese 20-year-old man develops a scaling groin rash with satellite pustules. He has been applying non-prescription ointments for "jock itch" without relief. A potassium hydroxide preparation of the pustules and scales reveals budding yeasts and nonseptate and non-branching pseudohyphae.

701. The most likely diagnosis in the case described above is

(A) tinea cruris
(B) tinea versicolor
(C) nonspecific intertrigo
(D) intertriginous psoriasis
(E) moniliasis

702. All of the following therapeutic measures might be appropriate for the man presented EXCEPT

(A) hydrocortisone cream (1%)
(B) nystatin cream
(C) miconazole cream
(D) clotrimazole cream
(E) discontinuation of tetracycline therapy

703. A 7-year-old girl is brought to the local emergency room after having a generalized seizure during which she lost consciousness. No history of head trauma can be elicited from her family and friends. A paternal uncle is mentally retarded and has had seizures. On examination, numerous brown spots—each greater than 3 cm and similar to those in Color Plate J—are present on the torso and extremities; one spot is 5 cm in size. Many smaller lesions (1 mm or less) are noted, especially in the axillary areas. The most likely diagnosis is

(A) Peutz-Jeghers syndrome
(B) Gardner's syndrome
(C) neurofibromatosis
(D) xeroderma pigmentosum
(E) hemochromatosis

704. A 25-year-old man presents with crusting, pruritic lesions of both hands (see Color Plate K). He has a history of asthma, hay fever, and skin problems as a child. All the following represent appropriate therapies EXCEPT

(A) triamcinolone ointment
(B) limited use of soap
(C) oral dicloxacillin
(D) patch testing to determine ingested or environmental allergens
(E) oral diphenhydramine

705. A 55-year-old Japanese businessman visiting the United States has been in excellent health until 6 months ago, when he first noted mild upper abdominal fullness after meals. On examination the man is noted to have hyperpigmented, heaped-up velvety lesions (as shown in Color Plate L) confined to the neck, axillae, and groin. All the following conditions have been associated with the skin findings presented EXCEPT

(A) Cushing's syndrome
(B) massive obesity
(C) acromegaly
(D) adenocarcinoma of the stomach
(E) Addison's disease

706. A 35-year-old man began intensive induction chemotherapy with daunorubicin and cytosine arabinoside for acute myeloid leukemia 3 weeks ago. He is febrile and profoundly neutropenic. The skin lesion seen on Color Plate M is noted. The cause of this lesion could be any of the following EXCEPT

(A) *Pseudomonas aeruginosa*
(B) *Escherichia coli*
(C) *Staphylococcus aureus*
(D) *Candida*
(E) *Aspergillus*

707. A 17-year-old girl complains of pain during chewing and tender lesions on the sides of her fingers. Shallow yellow-to-gray ulcerations with erythematous halos are present on her tongue, hard palate, and buccal mucosa. On the dorsal and lateral surfaces of her fingers are oval vesicles with a surrounding ring of erythema (as shown in Color Plate N). Her 5-year-old sister had a similar eruption last week and is now well. The most likely diagnosis is

(A) bullous erythema multiforme
(B) herpes simplex
(C) hand-foot-and-mouth disease
(D) Behçet's syndrome
(E) gonococcemia

708. For the last 2 days, a 24-year-old woman has had fever and pain in the left wrist, right ankle, and left knee. Nine painful skin lesions are present on the distal extremities, predominantly about the joints (as shown in Color Plate O). The most likely diagnosis is

(A) herpes simplex
(B) meningococcemia
(C) gonococcemia
(D) erythema multiforme
(E) anthrax

Questions 709–710

A 42-year-old, obese man is admitted to the hospital for severe right-upper-quadrant pain suggestive of cholecystitis. During the first 2 days of hospitalization he is afebrile and has normal white blood cell counts, liver function tests, and oral cholecystogram. On the third day clusters of small vesicles are noted on the right upper abdomen extending laterally around to the right side of his back (as shown in Color Plate P). His right-upper-quadrant pain became more intense.

709. A helpful diagnostic test to determine the cause of his pain would be

(A) percutaneous liver biopsy
(B) right-upper-quadrant ultrasound
(C) Giemsa stain of cellular material from the base of a vesicle
(D) endoscopic retrograde cholangiopancreatography (ERCP)
(E) exploratory laparotomy

710. Appropriate therapy for his condition would include

(A) cholecystectomy
(B) intravenous antibiotic therapy
(C) topical acyclovir
(D) topical fluorinated steroids
(E) none of the above

711. A 21-year-old woman is hospitalized for the treatment of a painful ulcer that has been present on her right lower leg for the last 4 weeks. The lesion began as a painful, reddish-purple nodule, then rapidly broke down and enlarged (see Color Plate Q). Bacterial cultures did not yield a significant pathogen, and a 2-week course of oral dicloxacillin, 250 mg four times daily, was not helpful. The lesion border now is undermined with a violaceous rim; biopsy is consistent with pyoderma gangrenosum. The lesion described is associated with all the following disorders EXCEPT

(A) ulcerative colitis
(B) regional enteritis
(C) multiple myeloma
(D) rheumatoid arthritis
(E) pernicious anemia

Questions 712–713

A 26-year-old man from Cape Cod sees his physician because of a 3-week history of an expanding, slightly burning ring of redness (as shown in Color Plate R) that first surrounded a red papule on the posterior neck. He complains of headaches, generalized muscle aches, anorexia, and malaise. On examination, he is noted to be febrile (38.3°C—101°F); his rash is slightly raised and slightly tender and displays central clearing but no scaling, even after vigorous scraping.

712. Which of the following vectors has been strongly associated with the type of rash described above?

(A) Kissing bug
(B) Spider
(C) Flea
(D) Tick
(E) Housefly

713. After 6 weeks of observation without treatment, the rash and systemic signs and symptoms disappear. Two months later, however, the man develops acute arthritis of his shoulders and knees. Joint and bone x-rays are normal, and serologic studies for systemic lupus erythematosus and rheumatoid arthritis are negative. The man's joint complaints resolve without therapy in a week, but during the next 3 months he has three similar episodes of asymmetrical arthritis of the knees, elbows, and shoulders, each episode lasting 5 to 7 days and responding to therapy with aspirin. Between episodes, he has been entirely asymptomatic, and neither joint deformities nor persistent synovitis has occurred.

Appropriate therapies could include all the following EXCEPT

(A) intravenous penicillin G
(B) oral doxycycline
(C) oral amoxicillin and probenecid
(D) intravenous ceftriaxone
(E) oral chloroquine

714. A homosexual male develops a violaceous nodule on his right forearm (as shown in Color Plate S). Biopsy reveals spindle cell infiltration in the dermis with erythrocyte-containing vascular channels. Which of the following statements about this man's condition is true?

(A) It is caused by retroviral infection of dermal mesenchymal cells
(B) Extracutaneous involvement is uncommon
(C) The entity is seen most frequently in association with intravenous drug abuse
(D) α-Interferon is a useful treatment modality
(E) Standard cytotoxic chemotherapy is absolutely contraindicated because of the low response rate and enhancement of immunosuppression

DIRECTIONS: Each question below contains five suggested responses. For **each** of the five responses listed with every question, you are to respond either YES (Y) or NO (N). In a given item **all, some, or none of the alternatives may be correct**.

715. A 50-year-old man has had 3 months of stiffness and pain in both wrists, his right knee, left elbow, back, and the distal interphalangeal joints of several fingers of both hands. On examination, he has the skin findings shown in Color Plate T. This case is accurately described by which of the following statements?

(A) An oral psoralen compound plus long-wave ultraviolet light would likely be effective therapy for the skin lesions
(B) Weekly oral methotrexate administration would likely be effective therapy for both the skin lesions and arthritis
(C) Treatment with prednisone, 40 mg daily for 4 weeks, would likely be effective
(D) Pitting of the nails is often associated with this syndrome
(E) The prevalence of arthritis in persons with this disease is higher than that in the unaffected population

716. A 35-year-old woman visits her doctor for her yearly checkup. Physical examination is unremarkable except for white patches (as shown in Color Plate U) involving her face, hands, torso, anus, and genitalia. The white spots have been present for 2 years. This dermatologic condition has been associated with which of the following diseases?

(A) Alopecia areata
(B) Pernicious anemia
(C) Addison's disease
(D) Hyperthyroidism
(E) Hypothyroidism

717. A 9-month-old baby has a generalized seizure at home. Emergency examination and laboratory studies are unremarkable, with the exception of three hypopigmented macules on the back. Family history of genetic or neurologic disorders is negative. Follow-up examination of the parents and two older siblings is unremarkable. The baby's physician should inform the parents that

(A) the child most likely will have normal mental development
(B) the child may develop an acne-like condition
(C) the child will develop neurofibromas
(D) subsequent children, if they have them, probably would be normal
(E) they should seek genetic counseling

718. A 35-year-old man has had recurrent diarrhea for at least 5 years. About 7 years ago many reddish-brown macules appeared on his torso and extremities (see Color Plate V). Rubbing these lesions gently results in the formation of a wheal. He also has been bothered by severe generalized itching, which is made worse when he takes aspirin for his frequent headaches. He has loss 11.4 kg (25 lb) in the last few months. Reasonable measures in his management would include

(A) reassurance that his disease is likely to disappear spontaneously
(B) bone survey and liver scan for evaluation of systemic involvement
(C) prescription of oral cromolyn for diarrhea
(D) prescription of codeine for his headaches
(E) genetic counseling

719. An 18-year-old man (pictured in Color Plate W) presents because of unsightly facial inflammation. Correct statements concerning this patient include which of the following?

(A) Closed comedones (whiteheads) are less commonly associated with the inflammatory lesions than are open comedones (blackheads)
(B) Glucocorticoids, although not indicated except in the most severe cases, would likely result in improvement
(C) Vigorous scrubbing of the face, which will eliminate surface oils, is indicated
(D) Systemic antibiotic therapy is unlikely to be helpful
(E) Patients on systemic retinoic acid may experience very dry skin and hypertriglyceridemia

Questions 720–721

A 55-year-old female noted the onset of skin fragility on the back of her hands 6 months ago. Occasional tense blisters are noted at these sites (see Color Plate X). The blisters heal with the formation of tiny inclusion cysts (milia). Increased facial hair on the upper cheeks and a violaceous color periocularly is noted. The skin appears entirely normal in non–sun-exposed areas. She has smoked two packs of cigarettes per day for 20 years and has consumed a six-pack of beer daily for years.

720. Laboratory findings might include

(A) elevated AST (SGOT)
(B) elevated serum iron
(C) elevated urinary uroporphyrin and coproporphyrin
(D) elevated immunoglobulin E
(E) anemia

721. Effective treatments might include

(A)   oral ferrous sulfate
(B)   serial phlebotomy
(C)   oral estrogens
(D)   oral hexachlorobenzene
(E)   oral chloroquine

722. Known cutaneous reactions to specific drugs include

(A)   aspirin-induced photosensitivity
(B)   phenytoin-induced skin necrosis
(C)   propylthiouracil-induced vasculitis
(D)   thiazide-induced photosensitivity
(E)   gold-induced hyperpigmentation

723. A 70-year-old man of Eastern European origin presents with easily rupturing, painful blisters on much of his body, including the face, trunk, and oral cavity. Manual pressure on the skin causes a separation of the dermal and epidermal layers. He has no other significant medical conditions nor was he taking any drugs prior to the onset of the eruption. True statements about this man's condition include

(A)   biopsy of the lesions would demonstrate a linear band of C3 at the basement membrane zone
(B)   the disease has a greater than 50 percent mortality if untreated
(C)   after confirmation of the diagnosis, the patient should be started on glucocorticoid therapy
(D)   blister cavities contain detached epidermal cells
(E)   involvement of the rectum and esophagus can be seen

Dermatologic Disorders

Answers

701. The answer is E. *(Wilson, ed 12. chap 56.)* Moniliasis commonly occurs in warm, moist areas, such as the axillae, groin, and beneath the breasts. Predisposing factors include obesity, diabetes mellitus, pregnancy, and use of broad-spectrum antibiotics, oral contraceptives, or local and systemic steroids. The presence of satellite pustules distinguishes moniliasis from tinea cruris. Potassium hydroxide preparations assist in the differential diagnosis—budding yeast and pseudohyphae are diagnostic for moniliasis.

702. The answer is A. *(Wilson, ed 12. chap 56.)* Nystatin, a polyene antibiotic, is quite effective in eradicating monilial infection. Clotrimazole, one of the new imidazoles, has broad-spectrum activity against both yeast and fungi and is useful if mixed infection is present or if the diagnosis is in doubt. A related drug, miconazole, also is an effective treatment of moniliasis. Use of hydrocortisone would allow yeast to flourish. In the case described, stopping the tetracycline would eliminate one of the predisposing factors.

703. The answer is C. *(Wilson, ed 12. chap 59. Fitzpatrick, ed 3. chap 79.)* Flat, brown spots, called *café au lait spots,* are areas of increased pigmentation produced by clones of genetically programmed melanocytes. Café au lait spots, which can vary in size from several millimeters up to 1 cm in diameter, occur in both neurofibromatosis (von Recklinghausen's disease) and Albright's disease (polyostotic fibrous dysplasia with precocious puberty in females), as well as in some normal persons. One or two spots at least 0.5 cm in diameter appear in 25 percent of normal children, but three or more spots of the same size occur in only 0.6 percent. About 9 percent of college-age persons have at least one spot 1.5 cm in size or greater. Of those persons with neurofibromatosis, 95 percent have at least one spot 1.5 cm or larger, and 78 percent have six or more spots. Because persons with Albright's disease rarely have more than four macules, the presence of six or more spots 1.5 cm or greater in size, especially in the presence of axillary freckling, is strongly suggestive of neurofibromatosis. Furthermore, the café au lait spots in Albright's disease tend to be larger and more irregular than those in neurofibromatosis.

704. The answer is D. *(Wilson, ed 12. chap 56.)* A diagnosis of atopic eczematous dermatitis can be made in the presence of a family history of atopic disorders (present in 70 percent), a personal history of asthma, allergic rhinitis, or childhood eczema, and characteristic cutaneous involvement. In the adult such involvement is manifested by intensely pruritic, crusting, or weeping lesions on the hands, neck, face, or genitalia. Secondary infection with *Staphylococcus aureus* or *Streptococcus pyogenes* is common. All cutaneous irritants should be avoided, as should excessive hand washing, which further dries the skin. The patient should bathe in lukewarm water, use soap sparingly, and apply a mid-to-low-potency topical steroid, such as triamcinolone or fluocinolone. An oral antistaphylococcal antibiotic is appropriate because the weepy lesions are probably secondarily infected. Antihistamines may help to control the associated severe pruritus. Allergy testing is of limited usefulness. Food allergy is implicated in infantile eczema, but not in the adult forms. Given the strong atopic history, searching for a contact allergen would probably provide a very low yield.

705. The answer is E. *(Wilson, ed 12. chap 59.)* Acanthosis nigricans is a skin disease associated with a number of disorders. The skin, which is thrown up into folds, appears velvety and hyperpigmented (brown to black) grossly and papillomatous microscopically. The lesions appear on the flexural areas of the neck, axillae, groin, antecubital fossae, and occasionally around the areolae, periumbilical and perianal areas, lips, buccal mucosa, and over the surfaces of the palms, elbows, knees, and interphalangeal joints. The disorder may be hereditary or appear in association with obesity or an endocrinopathy (acromegaly, Stein-Leventhal syndrome, diabetes mellitus, Cushing's syndrome, but *not* adrenal insufficiency). Drugs such as nicotinic acid also can produce the condition. When acanthosis nigricans develops in a nonobese adult, neoplasia, particularly gastric adenocarcinoma, must be suspected.

706. The answer is C. *(Wilson, ed 12. chaps 59, 111.)* Patients who are profoundly neutropenic are at risk of developing disseminated infections due to skin flora such as *Staphylococcus aureus* and *Staphylococcus* *epidermidis,* as well as enteric gram-negative rods, *Candida,* and *Aspergillus.* Although *Pseudomonas aeruginosa* is the classic etiologic agent, blood stream infection with any of these organisms, except those typically inhabiting the skin, can produce the centrally necrotic lesion termed *ecthyma gangrenosum.* This lesion, representing a localized necrotizing vasculitis due to invasion with microorganisms, may begin as an erythematous papule.

707. The answer is C. *(Wilson, ed 12. chaps 59, 144. Fitzpatrick, ed 3. chap 188.)* Although hand-foot-and-mouth disease usually affects children under the age of 10 years, especially preschoolers, the disease has been noted in adults with or without contact with affected children. The responsible agent is a coxsackievirus. The differential diagnosis includes aphthous ulcers, herpangina, herpes simplex, and erythema multiforme. Characteristically, the prodromal phase of hand-foot-and-mouth disease features malaise and upper-respiratory-tract symptoms; then, acute ulcerative stomatitis, mild pyrexia, and vesiculation of hands, feet, and buttocks occur. Vesicles in the oral cavity rapidly become ulcerated; tongue, gums, buccal mucous membrane, palate, and pharynx can all be involved. The cutaneous vesicles frequently are oval in shape and have an erythematous halo. Recovery occurs without specific treatment in 7 to 10 days.

708. The answer is C. *(Wilson, ed 12. chap 110. Hook, Ann Intern Med 102:229, 1985.)* The skin lesions of disseminated gonococcal infection occur on the distal extremities, usually around joints, and appear within a week of the onset of joint symptoms. The lesions, which may number as many as 20 (average: 4 or 5), often are painful, and each crop of new lesions is associated with a temperature rise. Lesions begin as a red macule or purpuric spot and then develop into a papule, a vesicle, and, finally, a pustule. Organisms rarely are cultured from the skin lesions; they can be demonstrated occasionally on Gram stain and more regularly with immunofluorescent techniques. Herpes simplex typically occurs as grouped vesicles. Skin lesions of meningococcemia consist of red macules that quickly become petechial or purpuric; migratory polyarthralgias and tenosynovitis are atypical. Erythema multiforme requires "iris" lesions for diagnosis. Anthrax consists of a single pimple or papule on exposed parts of the body; the lesion rapidly enlarges, developing into a vesicle that is surrounded by edema and later undergoes hemorrhagic necrosis, ulceration, and eschar formation.

709. The answer is C. *(Wilson, ed 12. chaps 59, 136.)* The differential diagnosis of grouped vesicular eruptions includes contact dermatitis and herpetic infections. Microscopic examination of the cellular material from the base of a fresh vesicle (less than 2 days old is best) stained with Giemsa reveals pathognomonic multinucleated giant cells diagnostic of a herpesvirus infection (varicella, zoster, or simplex). Unilateral dermatomal involvement establishes the diagnosis of shingles (herpes zoster). Neuralgia associated with zoster may precede the appearance of the cutaneous eruption and mimic myocardial infarction or acute cholecystitis.

710. The answer is E. *(Wilson, ed 12. chap 136.)* Herpes zoster will not respond to topical acyclovir. Oral or intravenous acyclovir may be helpful if dissemination occurs. Antibiotic therapy is indicated only for significant secondary bacterial infection. There is no evidence that fluorinated topical steroids are of help although systemic steroids are sometimes employed in the hope that the frequency of postherpetic neuralgia might be reduced. Most patients will respond to conservative therapy, which should include adequate oral pain medication and topical wet-to-dry saline or aluminum acetate (Domeboro) soaks to help dry up the vesicles and reduce the likelihood of secondary bacterial infection.

711. The answer is E. *(Wilson, ed 12. chap 59.)* Pyoderma gangrenosum is most closely associated with ulcerative colitis and regional enteritis. Its association with rheumatoid arthritis also is well recognized, and it can accompany a variety of hematologic disorders, such as acute and chronic myelogenous leukemia, myeloma, myeloid metaplasia, and polycythemia vera. Bacterial cultures and skin biopsies should be done in an evaluation for sepsis, vasculitis, or leukemia cutis. However, diagnosis of pyoderma gangrenosum is not made by biopsy.

712. The answer is D. *(Wilson, ed 12. chaps 59, 132. Steere, N Engl J Med 321:586, 1989.)* An expanding erythematous rash not associated with scaling is characteristic of erythema chronicum migrans. The disease first appears weeks to months after a tick bite. The lesion begins as a red macule at the site of the bite; the borders of the lesion then expand to form a red ring, with central clearing, as wide as 20 to 30 cm or more in diameter. Occasionally, secondary rings may occur within the original one. The lesion may itch or burn and may be accompanied by fever, headache, vomiting, fatigue, and regional adenopathy.

713. The answer is E. *(Wilson, ed 12. chaps 59, 132. Steere, N Engl J Med 321:586, 1989.)* Acute recurrent arthritis not associated with joint damage should suggest the possibility of Lyme arthritis. The spirochete *Borrelia burgdorferi* is the causative agent. The arthritis is sometimes monoarticular, often asymmetric and migratory; the knee joints most commonly are involved. Attacks are separated by gradually lengthening intervals: 1 to 3 weeks at first, later as much as 1 to 3 years. Acute attacks, which may be associated with fever, sometimes are preceded by a few days to several weeks by erythema chronicum migrans. For the arthritis characteristic of stage 3 Lyme disease, 100 mg of doxycycline twice daily or amoxicillin and probenecid, each 500 mg four times a day, are effective. Alternatively, or in the case of therapeutic failures, intravenous penicillin or ceftriaxone may be given. Chloroquine is a disease-modifying agent used for rheumatoid arthritis, which is not the diagnosis in this case because of the short-lived, intermittent nature of the man's symptoms.

714. The answer is D. *(Wilson, ed 12. chaps 59, 264.)* AIDS-associated Kaposi's sarcoma, which is present in this man, is a much more fulminant disease than the variant of the disease seen in elderly, non–HIV-infected patients. There is no evidence to implicate direct HIV-induced transformation as the etiology. For unknown reasons, the disease is much more common in homosexuals with AIDS than in heterosexuals with AIDS. While the lesions begin as papules or plaques on the face and upper extremities, they typically evolve into nodules and may be present in any location, most commonly the lungs, lymph nodes, and gastrointestinal tract. Treatment strategies include watchful waiting in low-volume, cosmetically acceptable disease, electron-beam (superficial) radiation therapy for local disease requiring palliation, and carefully administered chemotherapy (VP-16, doxorubicin, vinblastine, and bleomycin have activity) for disseminated disease. A promising approach involves the use of α-interferon, which is associated with a 30 percent rate of complete remission in those with Kaposi's sarcoma and relatively well-preserved circulating helper T cells (CD4+ cells).

715. The answer is A-Y, B-Y, C-N, D-Y, E-Y. *(Wilson, ed 12. chaps 56, 283.)* Psoriasis is manifested by silvery and scaly thick red plaques. Serum uric acid levels are elevated in 10 to 20 percent of affected persons, probably as a result of the high epidermal turnover rate, which causes accelerated synthesis and degradation of nucleoproteins. There are several forms of psoriatic arthritis, including asymmetric interphalangeal joint involvement similar to that seen in rheumatoid arthritis and a severe destructive polyarthritis often associated with spondylitis. Oral methoxsalen, a psoralen compound, in conjunction with long-wave ultraviolet light (PUVA) offers the possibility of excellent control of the skin lesions. Methotrexate, which also is effective in treating psoriasis, is reserved for adults with severe disease. Treatment with systemic corticosteroids is contraindicated. About one-half of the patients have fingernail involvement, which frequently manifests as pitting of the nailbeds or thickening of the nails.

716. The answer is A-Y, B-Y, C-Y, D-Y, E-Y. *(Wilson, ed 12. chap 59.)* The photographed skin lesions are depigmented macules of vitiligo. Vitiliginous macules are completely lacking in pigment and are histologically devoid of melanocytes. This disorder is believed to be transmitted as an autosomal dominant trait with incomplete penetrance. Although the majority of cases of vitiligo are not associated with other disease processes, an association has been described between vitiligo and several disorders, including diabetes mellitus, pernicious anemia, hyperthyroidism, hypothyroidism, Addison's disease, alopecia areata, and hypoparathyroidism. The polyglandular autoimmune syndromes, which may involve several of the aforementioned endocrine abnormalities, are also associated with vitiligo.

717. The answer is A-N, B-Y, C-N, D-Y, E-Y. *(Wilson, ed 12. chaps 59, 358.)* Tuberous sclerosis is a relatively uncommon disorder (5 to 7/100,000) in which a diverse combination of features is noted (seizures, mental retardation, adenoma sebaceum, periungual fibromas, connective tissue nevi, and hypopigmented macules). The hypopigmented macules, present in 98 percent of cases, may be the earliest and only physical finding at initial presentation. Wood's lamp examination (with long-wave ultraviolet light) of affected children and their families may make previously unrecognized hypopigmented areas discernible. Although inherited as an autosomal dominant gene, tuberous sclerosis usually is the result of spontaneous mutations.

718. The answer is A-N, B-Y, C-Y, D-N, E-Y. *(Wilson, ed 12. chap 59.)* Urticaria pigmentosa is a disorder of mast cells. The development of a wheal on gentle stroking of a pigmented macule (Darier's sign) is a useful diagnostic maneuver. Prognosis is said to worsen with age of onset: half the patients who develop multiple lesions by 4 years of age are disease-free by adolescence. Onset in adulthood is more ominous, with active lesions persisting indefinitely; systemic mastocytosis, which may have a fatal outcome, occurs frequently in affected adults. Symptomatic improvement has been reported with oral cromolyn. Affected persons should be warned to avoid substances and environmental factors known to cause mast-cell degranulation (e.g., cold, heat, trauma, or the ingestion of alcohol, aspirin, or morphine-opium alkaloid drugs). Although the disorder is usually an isolated event, familial disease occurs, indicating autosomal dominant inheritance in some cases.

719. The answer is A-N, B-N, C-N, D-N, E-Y. *(Wilson, ed 12. chap 56.)* Acne vulgaris is a self-limited disease mainly of young adults that causes inflamed cysts (comedones), which sometimes result in scarring. Closed comedones, or whiteheads, seen as white lesions of 1 to 2 mm, are often accompanied by inflammatory papules, pustules, or nodules as a consequence of the extrusion of oily and keratinous cyst debris. On the other hand, blackheads, or open comedones, which are filled with easily expressible dark material, do not usually cause serious problems. Vigorous facial scrubbing is contraindicated since this trauma could lead to rupture of comedones. Other predisposing factors include the use of systemic glucocorticoids, phenytoin, isoniazid, or phenobarbital. Treatment strategies include oral tetracycline or erythromycin therapy to decrease cyst colonization. Severe acne may be treated with a 20-week course of oral retinoic acid therapy, which may prevent formation of comedones by altering the pattern of epidermal desquamation. Pregnant patients should avoid retinoic acid given the teratogenic nature of this compound; this drug also causes extremely dry skin and hypertriglyceridemia.

720. The answer is A-Y, B-Y, C-Y, D-N, E-N. *(Wilson, ed 12. chaps 60, 328.)* Porphyria cutanea tarda results from a derangement in the synthesis of heme usually induced by an ingestion (e.g., of alcohol or estrogens). There is decreased activity of the enzyme uroporphyrinogen decarboxylase. Laboratory findings usually include elevation of hematocrit, serum iron, hepatic transaminases, and urinary uro- and coproporphyrins. The elevation of porphyrins in the circulation leads to the development of phototoxic tense blisters in sun-exposed areas, which heal with milia formation. Increased facial hair, increased skin fragility in sun-exposed areas, and periocular violaceous skin coloration are also frequently found.

721. The answer is A-N, B-Y, C-N, D-N, E-Y. *(Wilson, ed 12. chaps 60, 328.)* Porphyria cutanea tarda should be treated by removal of inciting agents. The use of phlebotomies or chelation therapy will reduce the potentially dangerous buildup of iron stores. Intermittent low doses of antimalarials, such as chloroquine and hydroxychloroquine, may also be useful.

722. The answer is A-N, B-N, C-Y, D-Y, E-Y. *(Wilson, ed 12. chap 57.)* It is well recognized that drugs can produce virtually any cutaneous reaction. Drug-induced urticaria, for example, may be induced via IgE release, immune complexes, or nonimmunologic means. Aspirin, penicillin, and blood products are commonly associated with urticaria, but virtually any drug can cause this particular reaction. Photosensitivity reactions may be due to phototoxicity, which is predictable, dose-related, and tends to produce sunburn-like changes, or to photoallergy, in which an immune response plus light is required to produce a wide variety of skin manifestations. The list of drugs producing photosensitivity is long and includes chlorpromazine, tetracycline, and thiazides. Hyperpigmentation is either secondary to drug-induced melanocyte stimulation (estrogens) or to direct skin deposition as in the case of the phenothiazines or heavy metals, including arsenic, gold, silver, bismuth, and mercury. Immune-complex formation is probably the mechanism of drug-induced palpable purpura as a manifestation of vasculitis. In addition to propylthiouracil, which can cause splenomegaly and lymphadenopathy plus cutaneous lesions, other drugs able to produce vasculitis include allopurinol, thiazides, penicillin, and phenytoin. Phenytoin is associated with a particular hypersensitivity reaction that occurs 1 to 3 weeks after starting the drug. It is characterized by purpuric eruption accompanied by fever, edema, lymphadenopathy, and hepatitis. Some patients, usually women, develop a sharply demarcated erythematous eruption 3 to 10 days after warfarin or heparin therapy has been started. The eruption progresses to hemorrhagic bullae and skin necrosis. Such a phenomenon is seen in patients with protein C deficiency. In such patients, the warfarin-induced drop in low baseline levels of this vitamin K–dependent antithrombotic protein leads to hypercoagulability and thrombosis in dermal vessels.

723. The answer is A-N, B-Y, C-Y, D-Y, E-Y. *(Wilson, ed 12. chap 58. Korman, J Am Acad Dermatol 18:1219, 1988.)* Pemphigus vulgaris is a bullous skin disease of autoimmune origin typically seen in elderly Jewish patients. Acantholysis, or the loss of cohesion between neighboring keratinocytes, is the mechanism by which the blisters occur. The blisters can occur anywhere on the body, but involvement of the oral mucosa and face is most common. The disease has a greater than 60 percent mortality if untreated and can include involvement of virtually any mucosal surface, such as the esophagus, rectum, larynx, and vulva. Nikolsky's sign, whereby manual pressure on the skin causes epidermal sliding, is another manifestation of the failure of cohesion of the epidermal cells. Rounded-up epidermal acantholytic cells are present inside the blisters. IgG or the third component of complement or both may be found on the keratinocyte surface, in contrast to the deposition of these proteins on the epidermal basement membrane in a related disorder, bullous pemphigoid. Circulating antibodies to monkey esophagus can be demonstrated in most cases of pemphigus vulgaris. Glucocorticoids will lead to good control in most patients, although it is frequently necessary to add azathioprine or cyclophosphamide.

Disorders of the Nervous System and Muscles

DIRECTIONS: Each question below contains five suggested responses. Select the **one best** response to each question.

724. Brain abscess can be best identified by which of the following diagnostic tests?

(A) CT scanning
(B) Radionuclide scanning with technetium 99m
(C) Gallium-labeled neutrophil scanning
(D) Ultrasonography
(E) Arteriography

725. A 70-year-old man complains of loss of energy, trouble concentrating, decreased appetite, and insomnia. He has lost considerable weight since his last visit and appears disheveled. It would be most appropriate initially to

(A) suspect that he has depression, and inquire whether he has frequent crying spells and has thought about suicide
(B) examine his stool for occult blood and schedule tests to search for a malignancy
(C) order tests to determine reversible causes of dementia
(D) refer the patient to a psychiatric clinic
(E) engage a social worker to help with basic home skills

726. Biologic factors associated with depression include

(A) derangement in pituitary-adrenal function
(B) a higher-than-normal incidence of epileptiform activity on electroencephalography
(C) abnormalities of dopamine metabolism reflected in elevated dopamine β-hydroxylase levels
(D) increased levels of γ-aminobutyric acid (GABA) in the cerebrospinal fluid after probenecid loading
(E) long-lasting suppression of serum cortisol levels with small doses of dexamethasone

727. The function of the muscle spindle is to furnish the central nervous system with information concerning

(A) muscle tension
(B) muscle length
(C) muscle tone
(D) joint flexion
(E) joint extension

728. For the last 5 weeks, a 35-year-old woman has had episodes of intense vertigo lasting several hours. Each episode is associated with tinnitus and a sense of fullness in her right ear; during the attacks, she prefers to lie on her left side. Examination during an attack shows that she has fine rotatory nystagmus, which is maximal on gaze to the left. There are no ocular palsies, cranial-nerve signs, or long-tract signs. An audiogram shows a high-tone hearing loss in the right ear, with recruitment but no tone decay.

The most likely diagnosis in the case described is

(A) labyrinthitis
(B) Ménière's disease
(C) vertebral-basilar insufficiency
(D) acoustic neurinoma
(E) multiple sclerosis

729. A 29-year-old woman who uses oral contraceptives comes to the emergency room because when she looked in the mirror this morning, her face was twisted. It felt numb and swollen. Eating breakfast, she found that her food tasted different and drooled out of the right side of her mouth when she swallowed. Neurologic examination discloses only a dense right facial paresis equally involving the frontalis, orbicularis oculi, and orbicularis oris. Finger rubbing is appreciated as louder in the right ear than in the left. The physician should

(A) instruct the patient in using a patch over the right eye during sleep
(B) recommend that she discontinue use of oral contraceptives
(C) order brainstem auditory evoked potentials to assess her hearing asymmetry
(D) inform her that her chances of substantial improvement within several weeks are only about 40 percent
(E) order an echocardiogram to rule out mitral valve prolapse as a source of emboli

730. The distinctive tetrad of symptoms of the narco-lepsy-cataplexy syndrome includes all the following EXCEPT

(A) uncontrollable daytime sleepiness
(B) sudden brief episodes of loss of muscle tone
(C) paralysis upon falling asleep
(D) confusional episodes
(E) hallucinations at the onset of sleep or wakening

731. A man brought into an emergency room is unresponsive and is displaying posturing. Pupils are 4 mm in size and react to light. No eye movements occur with head turning (oculocephalic maneuver) or with ice-water irrigation of the ear canals. The most likely diagnosis is

(A) brain death
(B) hysteria-conversion coma
(C) brainstem hemorrhage
(D) drug ingestion
(E) bilateral internal carotid artery occlusion

732. A patient with previous spells of diplopia, ataxia, dysarthria, and dizziness becomes acutely comatose. The most likely cause is

(A) basilar artery thrombosis
(B) subarachnoid hemorrhage
(C) carotid occlusion
(D) cerebellar hemorrhage
(E) pontine hemorrhage

733. Evoked-potential testing is most useful in diagnosing

(A) brainstem involvement in stroke
(B) a clinically occult lesion in multiple sclerosis
(C) large hemispheral strokes
(D) spinal cord compression
(E) shearing of white matter tracts after head injury

734. A normal pattern-shift visual evoked response is most useful and specific in diagnosing

(A) malingering
(B) Creutzfeldt-Jakob disease
(C) pituitary tumor
(D) brainstem glioma
(E) temporal arteritis

735. All the following statements are true of typical absence seizures in children EXCEPT

(A) they frequently present as learning disability
(B) they are associated with a characteristic electroencephalographic pattern
(C) they generally are not associated with other neurologic abnormalities
(D) phenytoin is the treatment of choice
(E) one-third of affected children outgrow the condition

736. A 25-year-old weight lifter comes to the emergency room frightened by recent headaches. He recently read a newspaper article about cerebral aneurysms. He reports 5 to 10 sudden, severe headaches, all occurring during coitus, each lasting about 1 h. The physician should

(A) recommend that the patient seek psychiatric help for his sexual dysfunction
(B) perform a CT scan with contrast and schedule four-vessel cerebral angiography to search for an aneurysm or arteriovenous malformation
(C) inform the patient that coital headache is a benign clinical syndrome that may be helped by administration of propranolol, 20 mg three times a day
(D) tell the patient to report back to the emergency room for a cerebrospinal fluid examination and CT scan without contrast to search for subarachnoid blood
(E) determine whether other members of his family have a history of migraine

737. While wrestling with his young son, a 32-year-old man suddenly develops a severe headache, then lapses into unconsciousness. Examination in the emergency room reveals retinal hemorrhages, nuchal rigidity, and normal eye movements on passive head rotation. The best initial diagnostic measure would be

(A) lumbar puncture
(B) skull x-rays
(C) CT scan of the head
(D) radionuclide brain scan
(E) bilateral carotid and vertebral angiography

738. The most common site for hypertensive brain hemorrhage is the

(A) pons
(B) central white matter
(C) cerebellar hemispheres
(D) putamen
(E) thalamus

739. Depression may be mistaken for dementia because of the hypokinetic state, poor attention span, and loss of impulse control common to both conditions. However, a major distinguishing feature of dementia would be

(A) anorexia
(B) headache
(C) multiple somatic complaints
(D) impaired performance on memory tests
(E) prominent release reflexes

740. A 65-year-old man with advanced pancreatic cancer complains of increasing abdominal pain. He is taking codeine 60 mg every 4 h. Examination reveals an alert man with a benign abdomen and normal neurologic function. The best step at this point would be to

(A) add amitriptyline
(B) add indomethacin
(C) increase the dose of codeine
(D) refer the patient for a celiac block
(E) add sustained-release morphine sulfate and use the codeine as circumstances require (prn)

741. A 55-year-old woman presents because of intermittent, brief, extreme stabbing pains in her lips and right cheek. The pain can be brought on by touching her face. The results of examination of the structures of the face and cranial nerves are entirely normal. Appropriate initial treatment for this condition would be

(A) ergotamine
(B) amitriptyline
(C) propranolol
(D) carbamazepine
(E) referral to an otolaryngologist for nerve block

742. A patient is evaluated for anisocoria. The right pupil is small and round compared with the left pupil in room light; this difference is magnified when the room is darkened. The right pupil responds briskly to light, constricts when pilocarpine is placed in the eye, and dilates when atropine is placed in the eye. Minimal dilation is produced by 4% cocaine. This patient has a lesion in the

(A) right optic nerve
(B) right iris
(C) right third nerve
(D) right sympathetic chain
(E) left occipital lobe

743. Which of the following would help to confirm the diagnosis of syncope in a patient with sudden loss of consciousness?

(A) A brief period of tonic-clonic movements at the time of falling
(B) An aura of a strange odor prior to falling
(C) Sudden return to normal mental function upon awakening, though feeling physically weak
(D) Urinary incontinence
(E) Laceration of the tongue

744. A physician confronted with a comatose patient with a severe head injury would be best advised to

(A) perform a skull and neurologic examination, obtain a CT scan of the head, and recommend burr holes if the pupils are enlarged
(B) stabilize the neck, administer mannitol and steroids, and obtain a CT scan
(C) treat hypotension, ensure airway patency, perform a skull and neurologic examination, and obtain a CT scan
(D) treat hypoxia and hypotension, raise the head, and obtain a CT scan
(E) stabilize the neck, obtain neck and skull x-rays, and recommend burr holes if the pupils are enlarged

745. A 65-year-old man presents with severe right-sided eye and facial pain, nausea, vomiting, colored halos around lights, and loss of visual acuity. His right eye is quite red and his pupil is dilated and fixed. Which of the following diagnostic tests would confirm the diagnosis?

(A) CT scan of the head
(B) MRI scan of the head
(C) Cerebral angiography
(D) Tonometry
(E) Slit-lamp examination

746. A patient who complains of imbalance is found to walk with a wide-based gait and to sway forward and backward upon standing. Balance cannot be maintained when standing with the feet together when the eyes are open or closed. No limb ataxia or nystagmus can be elicited. These findings are most consistent with a lesion or lesions in the

(A) vestibular apparatus
(B) midline cerebellar zone
(C) intermediate cerebellar zone
(D) lateral cerebellar zone
(E) left frontal cortex

747. Which of the following brain tumors tends to occur in immunosuppressed persons, arise in periventricular regions, and respond both clinically and radiographically to corticosteroid therapy?

(A) Glioblastoma
(B) Ependymoma
(C) Meningioma
(D) Medulloblastoma
(E) B-cell lymphoma

748. Septic cerebral emboli can be described by which of the following statements?

(A) Anaerobes commonly predominate
(B) Staphylococci commonly predominate
(C) Meningitis commonly is present
(D) Microbiologic diagnosis can be made by Gram stain of cerebrospinal fluid
(E) None of the above

749. A person who has right hemiparesis from stroke would be LEAST likely to display

(A) left facial weakness
(B) left-gaze paresis
(C) inability to calculate
(D) left-right confusion
(E) ignoring of the deficit

750. Lumbar back pain may be caused by all the following EXCEPT

(A) metastatic carcinoma of the prostate
(B) retroperitoneal hemorrhage in a patient on a regimen of warfarin
(C) expanding abdominal aneurysm
(D) pancreatitis
(E) diphtheritic polyneuropathy

751. For the last several days a college student has had back pain in the midlumbar area, difficulty in starting urination, and paresthesias in the feet. On examination, temperature is 38.3°C (101°F); straight leg raising produces pain, slight hip weakness is present, and Babinski signs are absent. The physician should

(A) perform a lumbar puncture
(B) obtain spine films and a bone scan
(C) obtain blood cultures and start antibiotic therapy
(D) obtain urinalysis and retroperitoneal ultrasound
(E) arrange for emergency myelography or CT scan of the spine

752. Elevated levels of gamma globulin in cerebrospinal fluid are associated with

(A) subacute sclerosing panencephalitis
(B) Creutzfeldt-Jakob disease
(C) progressive multifocal leukoencephalopathy
(D) paracarcinomatous encephalopathy
(E) western equine encephalitis

753. For the last 6 weeks, a 64-year-old woman has had a headache and difficulty reading. Her husband has noted a mild but progressive intellectual decline in his wife during this period. On examination, she has grasping reactions and myoclonic jerks when loud noises occur. CT scan and cerebrospinal fluid examination are normal. The most likely diagnosis is

(A) multiple sclerosis
(B) Alzheimer's disease
(C) bilateral subdural hematoma
(D) Creutzfeldt-Jakob disease
(E) subacute sclerosing panencephalitis

754. The most common presenting finding or symptom of multiple sclerosis is

(A) internuclear ophthalmoplegia
(B) transverse myelitis
(C) cerebellar ataxia
(D) optic neuritis
(E) urinary retention

755. A 28-year-old woman complains of horizontal diplopia. Examination shows only a lag in adduction of the left eye with nystagmus in the abducting right eye. The most appropriate workup would include

(A) electroencephalography and CT scan with contrast infusion
(B) cerebral angiography and formal visual-field testing
(C) lumbar puncture and evoked potentials
(D) electronystagmography and electroencephalography
(E) none of the above

756. A comatose patient is being evaluated by caloric stimulation of the vestibular apparatus. Cold-water irrigation of the right external auditory canal leads to deviation of both eyes to the right for 2 min followed by a slow drift back to the midline. This finding is most consistent with a lesion in the

(A) right labyrinth
(B) midbrain
(C) medulla
(D) pons
(E) cerebral hemispheres

757. A 69-year-old man is brought to the doctor by his wife because she complains that he has been "talking strangely." The patient enunciates words slowly and with difficulty. The melody of speech is abnormal. The speech is agrammatic in the sense that many prepositions and articles are omitted. When a word can be discerned, it is usually appropriate for the conversation and the patient appears to comprehend what is said to him. The lesion accounting for this problem is most likely to be in the

(A) left frontal lobe
(B) right frontal lobe
(C) left parietal lobe
(D) right parietal lobe
(E) bilateral temporal lobes

758. Initial therapy for persons with increased intracranial pressure would include

(A) beta-adrenergic blockers
(B) phenytoin
(C) mechanical ventilation to achieve high airway pressures
(D) hyperosmolar dehydration
(E) intravenous fluids

759. A 59-year-old man who has alcoholic cirrhosis but has been abstinent for 10 years has progressive dysarthria, tongue dystonia, shuffling gait, and fast tremor that worsens as his hand moves toward a target. The disease process causing these symptoms most likely is

(A) Wilson's disease
(B) acquired hepatocerebral degeneration
(C) Wernicke's disease
(D) Marchiafava-Bignami disease
(E) paracarcinomatous syndrome

760. The most likely diagnosis for a patient with impotence and urinary incontinence who, over years, sustains a tremor at rest, bradykinesia, rigidity, severe orthostatic hypotension, and anhidrosis is

(A) an autonomic form of the Landry-Guillain-Barré syndrome
(B) the Shy-Drager syndrome
(C) guanethidine intoxication
(D) micturition syncope
(E) Parkinson's disease

761. Lower brachial plexus injuries commonly occur during certain surgical procedures or in association with apical lung tumors. These injuries most typically cause

(A) weakness of thumb abduction and apposition
(B) ulnar hand numbness and a "claw hand" deformity
(C) ulnar hand numbness and inability to flex the elbow
(D) weakness of shoulder abduction and a patch of numbness over the triceps
(E) wrist drop and numbness over the dorsal hand between the thumb and index finger

762. A 42-year-old man, who has had difficulty concentrating on his job lately, comes to medical attention because of irregular, jerky movements of his extremities and fingers. A sister and an uncle died in mental institutions, and his mother became demented in middle age. The most likely diagnosis is

(A) alcoholic cerebral degeneration
(B) Huntington's chorea
(C) Wilson's disease
(D) Hallervorden-Spatz disease
(E) Gilles de la Tourette's disease

763. A 67-year-old woman appears to have parkinsonian rigidity but no tremor. In addition, she is completely unable to look down and has difficulty looking up. No improvement is seen after treatment with carbidopa-levodopa (Sinemet). The most likely diagnosis is

(A) atypical parkinsonism
(B) postencephalitic parkinsonism
(C) drug-induced parkinsonism and oculogyric crisis
(D) striatonigral degeneration
(E) progressive supranuclear palsy

764. Syringomyelia is characterized by all the following EXCEPT

(A) thoracic scoliosis
(B) ataxia
(C) muscle atrophy in the hands
(D) loss of pain sensation in the shoulders
(E) preservation of sense of touch

765. A 30-year-old man comes to the emergency room because for the last 3 days he has had progressive weakness of his legs, sensory loss ascending from his toes to the level of his umbilicus, and urinary retention. Examination reveals a central scotoma, absent knee and ankle jerks, and diminished pinprick sensation in the legs and abdomen up to the umbilicus. Cerebrospinal fluid contains 40 lymphocytes per cubic millimeter and a protein concentration of 0.72 g/L (72 mg/dL).

This clinical picture is LEAST consistent with which of the following diagnoses?

(A) Acute idiopathic polyneuritis
(B) Acute necrotizing myelitis
(C) Postvaccinal myelitis
(D) Postinfectious myelitis
(E) Multiple sclerosis

766. Bitemporal hemianopsia is most commonly due to

(A) saccular aneurysm of the distal internal carotid artery
(B) craniopharyngioma
(C) meningioma
(D) metastatic carcinoma
(E) suprasellar extension of a pituitary tumor

767. Magnetic resonance imaging (MRI) offers advantages over computed tomography (CT) in the diagnosis of all the following conditions EXCEPT

(A) subarachnoid hemorrhage
(B) multiple sclerosis
(C) arteriovenous malformation
(D) vertebral osteomyelitis
(E) syringomyelia

768. A 70-year-old man is brought in by his wife because of increased drowsiness and generally confused thinking over the past 2 months. Prior to a seemingly minor motor vehicle accident about 2 months ago, the patient had been running a small business without difficulty. There are no focal or lateralizing signs on neurologic examination. A noncontrast CT scan of the brain is normal except that there are no cortical sulci and the ventricles are small. The most likely diagnosis is

(A) Alzheimer's disease
(B) metabolic encephalopathy
(C) subdural hematoma
(D) cerebrovascular accident
(E) depression

769. A 60-year-old, mildly obese woman complains of a very bothersome burning pain on the anterolateral aspect of her right thigh from the groin almost as far distally as the knee. Examination shows reduction of sensation to touch and pinprick in the affected area. There is no loss of muscle strength and reflexes are normal. The most likely diagnosis is

(A) ruptured intervertebral disk
(B) femoral hernia
(C) nutritional neuropathy
(D) compression of the lateral femoral cutaneous nerve
(E) disruption of the lumbosacral plexus

770. The major pathologic feature of idiopathic inflammatory polyneuropathy (Guillain-Barré syndrome) is

(A) loss of anterior horn cells
(B) destruction of axons
(C) inflammation of sensory ganglia
(D) wallerian degeneration
(E) segmental demyelination

771. Cataracts, frontal baldness, testicular atrophy, and muscle weakness and wasting occur in association with

(A) myotonic dystrophy
(B) limb-girdle dystrophy
(C) pseudohypertrophic dystrophy
(D) facioscapulohumeral dystrophy
(E) myotonia congenita

772. The form of muscular dystrophy most likely to be encountered in persons older than 50 years of age is

(A) facioscapulohumeral dystrophy
(B) oculopharyngeal dystrophy
(C) myotonic dystrophy
(D) Duchenne's dystrophy
(E) limb-girdle dystrophy

773. Delayed relaxation of a muscle after voluntary contraction is characteristic of certain dystrophic diseases and periodic paralysis. This phenomenon is called

(A) myokymia
(B) myoedema
(C) myotonia
(D) contracture
(E) fibrillation

774. A 65-year-old woman with diabetes mellitus has a 3-month history of sacral pain. In the last month a burning pain progressively developed over the lateral aspect of her left foot and was followed by loss of sensation and weakness of plantar flexion and dorsiflexion. Electromyography showed fibrillations in left gastrocnemius, extensor hallucis, and quadriceps muscles. Nerve conduction was normal in the legs. A myelogram showed normal results. Now she complains that her knee "gives out" while walking; she has an absence of left knee and ankle jerks.

Her physician should

(A) inform the patient that normal results on her myelogram make a diabetic neuropathy the most likely diagnosis
(B) arrange for a pelvic examination and schedule a CT scan of the pelvis to search for a malignancy compressing or infiltrating the lumbar-sacral plexus
(C) arrange for a repeat myelogram because of new quadriceps weakness
(D) arrange for a CT scan of the head to search for an expanding mass over the right sensorimotor strip that would affect the foot and leg
(E) reexamine her at 2-month intervals to determine progression of her condition

775. The weakness associated with myasthenia gravis is due to which of the following disorders in the neuromuscular junction?

(A) Reduced acetylcholine in presynaptic vesicles
(B) Presynaptic block in release of acetylcholine
(C) Presence of antibodies against presynaptic membranes
(D) Degradation and blockage of postsynaptic receptors
(E) Damage of postsynaptic membranes by T lymphocytes

776. A 49-year-old man with long-standing hypertension presents with right-sided weakness involving the face, arm, and leg, which has evolved over the past 6 h. Neurologic examination is remarkable only for a right-sided hemiparesis without associated aphasia, papilledema, or sensory loss. A CT scan done after several days would most likely reveal

(A) small infarction in the left internal capsule
(B) large infarction in the left cerebral cortex
(C) left internal capsule hemorrhage
(D) left cerebral cortical hemorrhage
(E) normal findings

777. A 54-year-old woman with metastatic breast cancer and extensive bony involvement presents with headache and diplopia. Neurologic examination reveals no evidence for increased intracranial pressure and the only new abnormalities are slight disorientation and inability to abduct the right eye. Head CT without contrast is negative. Lumbar puncture reveals a mononuclear pleocytosis and elevated protein, but the results, including those of cytologic examination, are otherwise unremarkable. Of the following studies, which is most likely to establish a diagnosis?

(A) Contrast CT of the head
(B) MRI of the head
(C) CT of the right orbit, performed with bone windows
(D) Retinal angiography
(E) Repeat lumbar puncture

778. A 35-year-old man comes to the emergency room at midnight because he has awakened from sleep three nights in a row with severe pain in and above his left eye. In addition he noted unusual tearing, nasal stuffiness, and a sense of swelling over his left cheek. Neurologic evaluation reveals left ptosis and miosis that disappear after the headache resolves. The most appropriate action is to

(A) obtain an emergency CT scan and, if results are normal, perform a lumbar puncture to search for evidence of subarachnoid hemorrhage
(B) reassure the patient that he has a characteristic clinical syndrome called *cluster headache*. It is benign and frequently responds to administration of ergotamine or lithium
(C) refer the patient to an ophthalmologist for evaluation of eye pain and pupillary change
(D) inform the patient that he has "classic migraine" and administer ergotamine, 1 mg four times a day
(E) evaluate diabetes mellitus in the patient

779. A 27-year-old man seeks advice because he has noticed fasciculations in his calf muscles. He has no other complaints. Examination shows that muscle bulk and strength, tendon and plantar reflexes, and sensory function are all normal. He should undergo

(A) muscle biopsy
(B) sural nerve biopsy
(C) myelography
(D) electromyography
(E) none of the above

780. Which of the following statements concerning porphyric neuropathy is true?

(A) It is rarely associated with confusion or seizures
(B) It predominantly involves the sensory system
(C) It is symmetrical, and weakness is often more proximal than distal
(D) It causes elevated protein concentration in cerebrospinal fluid
(E) It is associated with inflammation of nerves

781. A patient has a total right hemianesthesia at the time of cerebral infarction. One year later he complains of constant severe burning pain with occasional sharp jabs of pain in the left side of his face and left arm. The chronic pain syndrome is most likely

(A) part of a biologic depressive syndrome secondary to a right parietal lobe stroke
(B) caused by a lesion in the spinal cord affecting the right spinothalamic tract
(C) a debilitating sequela of right thalamic infarction known as the Déjerine-Roussy syndrome
(D) secondary to a shoulder-hand syndrome involving the side affected by the stroke
(E) tic douloureux

782. Which of the following is the most frequent manifestation of neurologic abnormality in AIDS patients?

(A) Aseptic meningitis
(B) Myelopathy
(C) Peripheral neuropathy
(D) Subacute encephalitis
(E) Mass lesions

783. A 55-year-old man is evaluated for weakness. Over the past few months he has noted slowly progressive weakness and cramping of his left leg. Lately he has also had some trouble swallowing foods. He is awake and alert. Findings on the neurologic examination are normal except for marked atrophy with fasciculations in the muscles of both legs, hyperactive reflexes in the upper and lower extremities, a diminished gag reflex, and a positive extensor plantar response. Which of the following represents the most likely diagnosis?

(A) Cervical spondylosis
(B) Guillain-Barré syndrome
(C) Lambert-Eaton syndrome
(D) Vitamin-B$_{12}$ deficiency
(E) Amyotrophic lateral sclerosis

784. Duchenne's muscular dystrophy is characterized by

(A) autosomal dominant inheritance
(B) onset in second decade of life
(C) normal cardiac muscle
(D) universal elevation of serum creatine kinase
(E) the requirement in prenatal diagnosis of family studies for analysis of restriction fragment length polymorphisms (RFLPs)

785. A 68-year-old, previously healthy woman develops a lilac-colored rash in a butterfly distribution about the eyes, on the bridge of the nose, and on the cheeks. She has a similar rash on her knuckles. She has had an associated muscle weakness manifested by difficulty arising from a chair or climbing stairs. She takes no medicines. Other than the rash and proximal muscle weakness, the woman's examination is unremarkable. The most appropriate subsequent procedure would be

(A) barium enema, upper-GI series, intravenous pyelography, mammography, and chest x-ray
(B) hemogram, serum chemistries, Pap smear, urinalysis, mammography, and chest x-ray
(C) biopsy of an affected muscle
(D) electromyography (EMG)
(E) glucocorticoid treatment

DIRECTIONS: Each question below contains five suggested responses. For **each** of the five responses listed with every question, you are to respond either YES (Y) or NO (N). In a given item **all, some, or none of the alternatives may be correct.**

786. Weakness is a prominent symptom in which of the following disorders?

(A) Polymyositis
(B) Polymyalgia rheumatica
(C) Polyneuritis
(D) Botulism
(E) Subacute combined degeneration

787. Progressive gait disability in elderly persons may be due to

(A) normal-pressure hydrocephalus
(B) cervical spondylosis
(C) subdural hematoma
(D) carotid stenosis
(E) subacute combined degeneration

788. Which of the following elements would be involved in the appreciation of pain due to an injurious stimulus?

(A) Spinocerebellar tract
(B) Spinothalamic tract
(C) Dorsal horn of the spinal cord
(D) Red nucleus
(E) Nucleus ventralis posterolateralis

789. A patient complains of hearing loss in the right ear. A 256-Hz tuning fork is placed in the middle of the forehead; the patient reports that he hears the tone in his right ear. He also notes better perception of a tone when the tuning fork is placed in contact with the right mastoid process than when it is placed outside of his right ear. Lesions in which of the following structures could account for these findings?

(A) Eighth nerve
(B) Central auditory pathways
(C) Cochlea
(D) External auditory canal
(E) Middle ear

790. In the acute workup of newly comatose persons, CT scanning would be helpful in establishing a diagnosis of

(A) subarachnoid hemorrhage
(B) brain death
(C) brainstem infarction
(D) middle cerebral artery infarction
(E) subdural hematoma

791. Seizure discharges in the temporal lobe may manifest as

(A) facial paresthesias
(B) foot twitching
(C) vertigo
(D) intense fear
(E) déjà vu

792. Useful tests for myasthenia gravis would include which of the following?

(A) Repetitive motor-nerve stimulation
(B) Single-fiber electromyography
(C) Muscle biopsy
(D) Nerve conduction studies
(E) Curare challenge testing

793. Which of the following would be consistent with a diagnosis of muscle spasm in a patient with low back pain?

(A) Limitation of flexion of the spine
(B) Scoliosis or straightening of the normal lordosis as noted on x-ray films
(C) Urinary retention and obstipation
(D) Sudden onset while bending over shoveling snow
(E) Absence of ankle reflex with radiating pain

794. The destruction of all motor nerves supplying a muscle would result in

(A) fasciculations
(B) fibrillations
(C) hypotonia
(D) atrophy
(E) loss of response to electrical stimulations of short duration (faradic stimuli)

795. A lesion in the corticospinal tract rather than in an anterior horn neuron projecting to muscle cells is suggested by

(A) spasticity
(B) marked atrophy
(C) fasciculations
(D) involvement of individual muscles
(E) presence of an extensor plantar reflex

796. The tremor associated with Parkinson's disease is characterized by

(A) worsening with voluntary movement
(B) occurrence with flexed posture
(C) occurrence at a rate of 5 Hz
(D) association with rigidity
(E) abolition by moderate intake of alcohol

797. Treatment can reverse or cease progression of which of the following causes of dementia?

(A) Alzheimer's disease
(B) Binswanger's disease
(C) Creutzfeldt-Jakob disease
(D) Chronic subdural hematoma
(E) Infection by human immunodeficiency virus

798. Conditions associated with highly characteristic (specific) findings on electroencephalography include

(A) hypoglycemia
(B) Creutzfeldt-Jakob disease
(C) delirium tremens
(D) multiple sclerosis
(E) herpes simplex encephalitis

799. Dialysis encephalopathy can be described by which of the following statements?

(A) It is a progressive disorder
(B) Dysarthria is a characteristic sign
(C) Dementia is a key feature
(D) Myoclonus can be treated with clonazepam
(E) Cerebrospinal fluid analysis reveals characteristic abnormalities

800. Peripheral nerve damage caused by diabetes may result in

(A) relapsing weakness
(B) distal sensory neuropathy
(C) incontinence
(D) foot drop
(E) ophthalmoplegia

801. Chronically progressive spinal cord disease with sensory and motor signs evolving over years may be due to

(A) spinocerebellar degeneration
(B) multiple sclerosis
(C) cervical spondylosis
(D) lumbar disk disease
(E) amyotrophic lateral sclerosis

802. A person with long-standing alcoholism develops bilateral lateral-rectus (sixth-nerve) palsies. Diagnostic considerations would include

(A) brainstem hemorrhage
(B) subdural hematoma
(C) orbital fractures
(D) neurosyphilis
(E) Wernicke's encephalopathy

803. Which of the following disorders will usually produce a sensory level on neurologic examination?

(A) Myelopathy due to vitamin-B_{12} deficiency
(B) Neoplastic cord compression
(C) Vertebral dislocation and cord compression
(D) Acute myelitis
(E) Spinal epidural abscess

804. A 60-year-old man comes to the emergency room with sudden onset of a neurologic deficit. After examining the patient the physician orders cerebral angiography. Results show occlusion of the left vertebral artery from its origin to where it joins the basilar. The right vertebral artery, basilar artery, and both carotid arteries are patent. Examination in the emergency room probably disclosed

(A) left hemiparesis sparing the face
(B) deviation of the uvula to the right on phonation
(C) left appendicular ataxia
(D) left internuclear ophthalmoplegia
(E) diminished pain and temperature sensation in the right arm and leg

805. Which of the following may occur ipsilateral to a disease process within the cavernous sinus?

(A) Ptosis
(B) Numbness of the brow
(C) Numbness of the chin
(D) Marked decrease in visual acuity
(E) Inability to elevate the eye

806. Favorable prognostic factors for a patient's remaining seizure-free when anticonvulsants are stopped after 2 years on therapy include

(A) a normal EEG before drug withdrawal
(B) complex partial seizures with secondary generalization
(C) simple partial seizures
(D) requirement of a single drug for seizure control
(E) few seizures prior to becoming seizure-free

807. Correct statements concerning Wernicke's encephalopathy include which of the following?

(A) The most prominently affected area is the frontal cortex, bilaterally
(B) Most patients present with the triad of encephalopathy, ophthalmoplegia, and ataxia
(C) In the absence of response to glucose, thiamine should be administered
(D) After the patient responds to emergent treatment, profound amnesic psychosis may supervene
(E) Intake of alcohol is required to produce the full-blown syndrome

808. The following drugs are used in the treatment of Parkinson's disease. The functions lost by the neurotransmitter deficiency resulting from the primary pathologic change associated with this disorder are directly restored by

(A) benztropine
(B) metoprolol
(C) amantadine
(D) carbidopa
(E) bromocriptine

809. Correct statements concerning the use of lithium in psychiatry include

(A) lithium is effective for treating acute manic/hypomanic episodes but has no role in prophylaxis against future attacks
(B) hyperthyroidism is an important long-term complication
(C) nephrogenic diabetes insipidus is common
(D) gastrointestinal complaints and thirst are common side effects
(E) during acute mania, lithium can be administered with behavior control as the sole end point

810. True statements regarding hypokalemic periodic paralysis include

(A) it is inherited in an autosomal recessive fashion
(B) patients exhibit myotonia between attacks
(C) proximal musculature is involved more than distal musculature
(D) deranged renal handling of potassium accounts for the pathogenesis
(E) prophylactic administration of potassium is effective

DIRECTIONS: Each group of questions below consists of five lettered headings followed by a set of numbered items. For each numbered item select the **one** lettered heading with which it is **most** closely associated. Each lettered heading may be used **once, more than once, or not at all.**

Questions 811–814

For each clinical syndrome described below, select the most likely site of disk protrusion.

   (A) L2-L3 interspace
   (B) L3-L4 interspace
   (C) L4-L5 interspace
   (D) L5-S1 interspace
   (E) S1-S2 interspace

811. Sciatica, inability to walk on toes, and depressed ankle tendon reflex

812. Sciatica, weakness of foot inversion, and hallux extensor weakness

813. Sciatica, foot drop, and normal reflexes

814. Hip flexion weakness, knee extension weakness, and diminished knee tendon reflex

Questions 815–819

For each of the following conditions, select the region of the brain most likely affected by a pathologic process.

   (A) Frontal lobe
   (B) Temporal lobe
   (C) Dominant parietal lobe
   (D) Nondominant parietal lobe
   (E) Occipital lobe

815. Wernicke's aphasia

816. Apathy and lack of initiative and spontaneity

817. Acalculia

818. Inability to recognize faces

819. Dense homonymous hemianopia

Questions 820–824

Match each anatomic landmark with the appropriate sensory dermatomal level.

   (A) C2
   (B) T2
   (C) T4
   (D) T10
   (E) L5

820. Posterior scalp

821. Nipple

822. Axilla

823. Umbilicus

824. Great toe

Questions 825–830

For each systemic side effect listed below, choose the anticonvulsant drug with which it is most likely to be associated.

   (A) Phenobarbital
   (B) Phenytoin
   (C) Carbamazepine
   (D) Valproic acid
   (E) Clonazepam

825. Hirsutism

826. Gum hyperplasia

827. Leukopenia

828. Osteomalacia

829. Lymphadenopathy

830. Acute hepatic failure

Questions 831–835

For each abnormality of eye movement listed below, select the associated lesion.

   (A) Lesion in the low pons surrounding the left abducens (sixth-nerve) nucleus, including the left pontine gaze center
   (B) Lesion in the right frontal lobe
   (C) Lesion in the left upper pons affecting the medial longitudinal fasciculus
   (D) Unilateral left labyrinthine dysfunction
   (E) Midbrain lesion affecting the rostral interstitial nucleus of the medial longitudinal fasciculus

831. Absence of vertical gaze

832. Inability to move the eyes to the left of midline

833. Tendency to keep the eyes to the right of midline

834. Saw-toothed jerk nystagmus with slow phase to the left and quick corrective movements to the right

835. Inability to adduct the left eye past the midline and nystagmus in the right eye when abducted

Disorders of the Nervous System and Muscles

Answers

724. The answer is A. *(Wilson, ed 12. chap 354.)* Computerized tomography scanning is the best test to identify a brain abscess and has largely supplanted arteriography in this setting. Radionuclide scanning is also quite reliable, if CT facilities are not available. Generally, a CT or radionuclide scan is sufficient to rule out the diagnosis of brain abscess; rarely are both a scan and an arteriogram needed to rule out this diagnosis. The somewhat increased sensitivity of MRI scanning is usually clinically insignificant.

725. The answer is A. *(Wilson, ed 12. chap 368.)* None of the actions listed is inappropriate. Malignancy, endocrine disorders, and Alzheimer's disease are frequent causes of depressive symptoms. The majority of depressed patients present to their physicians with the somatic complaints listed. In a major depression the most immediate threat to the patient's health is suicide. The risk needs to be assessed by direct questioning, and appropriate safety precautions then taken.

726. The answer is A. *(Wilson, ed 12. chap 368.)* Endogenous depression can be distinguished from reactive depression in some cases by the dexamethasone suppression test. In this procedure, the integrity of the hypothalamic-pituitary-adrenal axis is tested by response to low doses (1 or 2 mg) of dexamethasone. Normally, suppression of endogenous cortisol production would be expected to last at least 24 h; in endogenous depression, however, suppression is overcome rapidly. Retesting after treatment has produced clinical improvement typically is associated with reversion to a suppression response. Biochemical theories of depression mainly involve deficiencies of norepinephrine and its metabolites. Dopamine metabolism appears to be normal. No EEG abnormalities have been associated with depression.

727. The answer is B. *(Wilson, ed 12. chap 25.)* Muscle spindles are bundles of small striated muscle fibers encased in a connective-tissue capsule around which are coiled specialized sensory nerve endings. Dispersed throughout each muscle, spindles send subliminal afferent impulses that aid the central nervous system in monitoring changes in muscle length. Joint capsule receptors are responsible for conscious proprioception; muscle tension is monitored by Golgi tendon organs.

728. The answer is B. *(Wilson, ed 12. chap 22.)* The symptoms and signs described in the question are most consistent with Ménière's disease. In this disorder, paroxysmal vertigo due to labyrinthine lesions is associated with nausea, vomiting, rotatory nystagmus, tinnitus, high-tone hearing loss with recruitment, and, most characteristically, fullness in the ear. Labyrinthitis would be an unlikely diagnosis in the case presented because of the hearing loss and multiple episodes. Vertebral-basilar insufficiency and multiple sclerosis typically are associated with brainstem signs. Acoustic neuroma only rarely causes vertigo as its initial symptom, and the vertigo it causes is mild and intermittent.

729. The answer is A. *(Wilson, ed 12. chap 360.)* The abrupt appearance of an isolated peripheral facial palsy, which may include ipsilateral hyperacusis resulting from involvement of fibers to the stapedius and loss of taste on the anterior two-thirds of the tongue resulting from involvement of the fibers of the chorda tympani, is most often idiopathic, i.e., Bell's palsy. If the patient is unable to close the eye, artificial tears may be helpful during the day to prevent drying, and the eye should be patched at night to prevent corneal abrasion. Excellent recovery occurs in 80 percent of such cases. Oral contraceptives and mitral valve prolapse are not associated with causes of such a clinical picture. Evoked potentials are not helpful diagnostically.

730. The answer is D. *(Wilson, ed 12. chap 34.)* Narcolepsy is uncontrollable daytime sleepiness, and cataplexy is sudden, brief loss of muscle tone. Sleep paralysis and hypnagogic hallucinations are common in persons with narcolepsy. A properly performed sleep electroencephalogram is useful in supporting a diagnosis of narcolepsy—REM sleep occurs much earlier in sleep than normal in affected persons. (False-positive tests can occur if the subject has recently been sleeping, awakens briefly, and then falls asleep again for the test.) Confusion and epileptic disorders are not part of the narcolepsy-cataplexy syndrome.

731. The answer is D. *(Wilson, ed 12. chap 31.)* In a comatose person, reactive pupils and the absence of eye movements in response to head turning or ice-water irrigation of the ear canals signify metabolic suppression of brainstem neurons. The major distinction that must be made is between true unresponsiveness and a "locked-in" stroke state, in which eye movements also may be obliterated. In brain death, pupils are unreactive. A person unresponsive because of a conversion reaction cannot voluntarily suppress the nystagmus induced by caloric irrigation, although tonic eye movements can be suppressed by gaze fixation. Pontine hemorrhage is associated with small pupils. Bilateral infarcts in a carotid distribution may cause coma, but oculocephalic movements are normal.

732. The answer is A. *(Wilson, ed 12. chap 31.)* Patients with basilar artery stenosis frequently have spells of ischemic brainstem dysfunction prior to a catastrophic stroke caused by arterial thrombosis. Timely anticoagulation and allowing a higher blood pressure can arrest the progression of this potentially fatal stroke. Acute coma can occur in association with each of the cerebrovascular accidents mentioned except carotid occlusion. Subarachnoid hemorrhage causes an acute increase in intracranial pressure that reduces blood flow to the brain. Unilateral cortical infarction does not cause coma, but damage to brainstem structures via infarction or compression will cause coma.

733. The answer is B. *(Wilson, ed 12. chap 349.)* The testing of evoked potentials is of greatest utility in detecting subclinical spinal cord and optic nerve lesions. Up to two-thirds of persons who have multiple sclerosis have neurologic deficits evident on visual or peroneal somatic evoked potentials but *not* on physical examination. Such a "second lesion" frequently establishes the diagnosis of multiple sclerosis. Evoked potentials may be abnormal in the other conditions listed in the question.

734. The answer is A. *(Wilson, ed 12. chap 349.)* Because visual acuity even as poor as 20/200 would not produce an abnormal pattern-shift visual evoked potential, the test may be used to support a diagnosis of hysterical blindness or malingering. By alteration of the check sizes on the displayed pattern and variation in the pattern's distance from the eyes, the technique can be refined to provide an accurate measure of acuity. Papilledema does not affect the test, unless it causes severe optic atrophy. Temporal arteritis and pituitary tumor may be associated with an abnormal evoked response if the optic nerve is affected.

735. The answer is D. *(Wilson, ed 12. chap 350.)* Absence, or petit mal, seizures are distinguished from complex partial seizures in a number of ways, including lack of an aura, a characteristic 3-Hz rhythmic EEG pattern during a spell, and immediate recovery. Because of their brevity and subtlety, absence seizures frequently go unrecognized until an affected child begins school and performs poorly. The prognosis is good: one-third outgrow the disorder, one-third have a milder form in adulthood, and one-third have easily controlled generalized seizures. Ethosuximide and valproic acid, not phenytoin, are the drugs of choice.

736. The answer is C. *(Wilson, ed 12. chap 18.)* Errors made in the investigation of patients with sudden onset of severe headache can result in catastrophic subarachnoid hemorrhage from a ruptured aneurysm. Patients frequently have "warning" bleeding that causes severe headache and brings them for medical attention. Sudden headache during physical exertion is a presentation of ruptured intracranial aneurysm. A careful cerebrospinal fluid examination is the most sensitive test, but a noncontrast CT scan may show the subarachnoid blood and make the lumbar puncture unnecessary. A patient with a reasonable suspicion for aneurysmal bleeding should not be sent home to wait for other symptoms because the next symptom is often a catastrophic subarachnoid hemorrhage. In the patient described, however, the repeated onset of headache with coitus is characteristic of a benign coital headache syndrome. If faced with only a single sudden coital headache, then an investigation for a cerebral aneurysm would be appropriate. The family history of migraine is usually not helpful for the diagnosis of coital headache.

737. The answer is C. *(Wilson, ed 12. chap 351.)* The clinical picture presented in the question suggests acute subarachnoid hemorrhage, either from a ruptured saccular aneurysm or from an arteriovenous malformation. A

CT scan of the head, done initially without infusion of contrast material, would be more likely than the other procedures listed to demonstrate the presence of blood in the subarachnoid space and possibly in the ventricles as well. In addition, a CT scan also can detect the presence of hydrocephalus and intracerebral hematoma, two conditions that, in the presence of coma, may require surgical intervention. Skull films are not likely to be informative in this case, although in the presence of a large arteriovenous malformation they may show intracranial calcification. Lumbar puncture as a means of establishing the presence of intracranial bleeding is rendered less useful and is possibly dangerous in this instance by the finding of retinal hemorrhages, a sign of acute intracranial hemorrhage. A radionuclide scan would have little to offer in this set of circumstances, and angiography would be premature.

738. The answer is D. *(Wilson, ed 12. chap 351.)* Half of all episodes of hypertensive intracerebral hemorrhage occur in the putamen and the adjacent internal capsule. Other sites, in decreasing order of frequency, are the thalamus, cerebellar hemispheres, and pons. Hemorrhages in the subcortical white matter are not generally associated with hypertension and should prompt a search for a bleeding diathesis or an underlying brain lesion. The diagnosis of brain hemorrhage is suggested by clinical signs and confirmed by CT scan; lumbar puncture no longer is recommended.

739. The answer is E. *(Wilson, ed 12. chap 30.)* Grasp or suck responses, though not diagnostic of dementia, do indicate a loss of neurons and thus support the diagnosis of dementia. Somatic complaints, including headache, are common in both dementia and depression, although they tend to be more persistent in depression. Memory may be impaired in persons with depression because of lack of attention to tasks, as well as in persons with dementia; immediate recall is usually poor in severe depression, whereas it is often good in dementia.

740. The answer is E. *(Wilson, ed 12. chap 15.)* The patient is already on maximal doses of a relatively weak narcotic analgesic that also has quite a few side effects. Increasing the dose of codeine or adding a nonsteroidal anti-inflammatory drug such as indomethacin is likely to be of little benefit. Neuropathic pain, unlike the somatic pain afflicting the patient, might be managed with the help of a tricyclic antidepressant such as amitriptyline. Since the patient has not yet failed an adequate trial of narcotics, referral for a nerve-altering intervention is premature. One should now institute a sustained release preparation of morphine, with another narcotic to be taken in between doses of morphine until a sufficient level of analgesia is achieved.

741. The answer is D. *(Wilson, ed 12. chaps 18, 360.)* A disease of middle-aged and elderly patients, particularly women, paroxysmal facial pain (tic douloureux, trigeminal neuralgia) is usually of idiopathic origin. It may occur in association with multiple sclerosis, herpes zoster, or a tumor. Brief, intense, lancinating pains brought on by manipulation of trigger zones in the lips or face, without motor or sensory paralysis, characterize this disorder. The treatment of first choice is the anticonvulsant carbamazepine, which is effective in most patients. In cases of nonresponse or intolerance to carbamazepine, radiofrequency ablation of the gasserian ganglion of the trigeminal nerve may be beneficial.

742. The answer is D. *(Wilson, ed 12. chap 23.)* The features described are consistent with sympathetic denervation of the right eye, the so-called Horner pupil. This lesion, frequently produced by pulmonary neoplasms of the superior sulcus, is usually associated with ipsilateral ptosis and anhidrosis. Pupillary light responses should be normal, as should the response to mydriatics (substances causing pupillary dilation [e.g., anticholinergics]) and miotics (drugs causing pupillary constriction [e.g., cholinergics, beta-adrenergic blockers]). However, since the sympathetic nerve endings are depleted, cocaine is unable to cause local release of sympathomimetic substances and is a poor mydriatic. An oculomotor palsy would also produce ipsilateral ptosis, but a dilated pupil that is poorly reactive to light on that side would be the cause of anisocoria.

743. The answer is C. *(Wilson, ed 12. chap 21.)* Patients with loss of consciousness resulting from a seizure usually have mental confusion, headache, and drowsiness postictally, whereas the patient with a brief syncopal spell recovers fully as soon as the blood pressure returns to normal. Auras, urinary incontinence, and a laceration of the tongue are clues that the cause of the loss of consciousness was a seizure.

744. The answer is C. *(Wilson, ed 12. chap 352.)* Treatment of hypotension, control of the airway, and a search for lesions that raise intracranial pressure are the first priorities in managing persons with severe head trauma. Skull x-rays have been largely replaced by CT scans because contusions and hemorrhages are better seen by CT scanning. Although stabilization of the neck is very important, the other treatment choices mentioned in the question are not.

745. The answer is D. *(Wilson, ed 12. chap 23.)* The patient in question is suffering from acute angle-closure glaucoma, the result of obstruction of outflow of aqueous humor at the iris. The buildup of intraocular pressure can be confirmed by measurement and requires urgent treatment by the use of hyperosmotic agents. Permanent treatment requires laser or surgical iridotomy. Angle-closure glaucoma is less common than primary open-angle glaucoma, which is asymptomatic and usually detectable only through measurements of intraocular pressure at routine eye examination.

746. The answer is B. *(Wilson, ed 12. chap 26.)* Alcoholic cerebellar degeneration is an example of a disease primarily of the midline area of the cerebellum (vermis). A characteristic cerebellar gait disorder will be manifested by a wide-based walk and stance and inability to stand with the feet together even with the eyes open. Patients complain of imbalance and frequently try to hold on to other objects as they walk. However, unlike more diffuse cerebellar disease, there is no associated limb ataxia or nystagmus.

747. The answer is E. *(Wilson, ed 12. chap 353. Hochberg, J Neurosurg 68:835, 1988.)* Lymphoma of the brain (usually diffuse large cell) is increasingly common as a sporadic tumor and occurs frequently in immunosuppressed patients, especially in those with AIDS. Its clinical sensitivity to corticosteroids can mistakenly suggest a diagnosis of multiple sclerosis, and its complete disappearance or dramatic improvement on CT scan after steroid therapy is baffling. Radiosensitivity is a well-known feature of most primary CNS lymphomas, which are almost always of B-cell origin.

748. The answer is A. *(Wilson, ed 12. chap 354.)* Septic cerebral emboli usually originate in infected lung tissue (if right-to-left intracardiac shunt is present), liver abscesses, and other similar lesions. More than one type of organism generally are involved, and anaerobes, such as *Streptococcus, Bacteroides, Fusobacterium, Veillonella, Proprionibacterium,* and *Actinomyces,* are common. Although culture from a resulting abscess may be negative, Gram stain of pus (not cerebrospinal fluid) can be useful.

749. The answer is E. *(Wilson, ed 12. chap 351.)* Before assuming that a stroke is due to hemispheral disease, clinicians should search for contralateral brainstem signs. Right hemiparesis with either left facial weakness or left-gaze paresis indicates a pontine stroke, which generally is due to basilar artery branch disease. Inability to calculate (acalculia) and left-right confusion with dysgraphia are part of the Gerstmann syndrome of left parietal stroke and may occur with right hemiparesis. Minimizing or ignoring the deficit is most typical of a right-brain lesion and is associated with a left hemiparesis.

750. The answer is E. *(Wilson, ed 12. chap 19.)* Lumbar back pain is frequently associated with each of the first four medical conditions described. The patient with lumbar back pain should therefore be given careful abdominal and pelvic examinations; spine films are necessary to detect destructive bone lesions that may cause referred pain to the buttock or leg. Laboratory evaluation should include blood count and determinations of serum calcium, alkaline phosphatase, and acid phosphatase (in elderly men) concentrations. Diphtheria toxin causes a painless, demyelinative neuropathy that can simulate the Landry-Guillain-Barré syndrome. Aching muscular pain occurs commonly in Landry-Guillain-Barré patients.

751. The answer is E. *(Wilson, ed 12. chaps 354, 361.)* Spinal epidural abscess, a neurologic emergency, is currently best diagnosed by myelography, which would demonstrate a blocked flow of dye in the spinal subarachnoid space. Lumbar puncture would show a high protein content and cell count but would not establish the diagnosis and may in fact be harmful. Babinski signs are absent in the case described because lumbar pain indicates an abscess overlying the cauda equina, which is made up of peripheral nerves, rather than the spinal cord.

752. The answer is A. *(Wilson, ed 12. chap 355. Dyken, Neurol Clin 3:179, 1985.)* An increase in the gamma globulin fraction of cerebrospinal fluid (CSF) protein is commonly, but not invariably, associated with multiple sclerosis and occurs in nearly all cases of subacute sclerosing panencephalitis, which is due to persistent measles infection. Slow-virus infections, such as Creutzfeldt-Jakob disease, do not alter CSF chemistries. Viral encephalitis may cause elevated levels of total protein, but CSF gamma globulin levels generally are normal.

753. The answer is D. *(Wilson, ed 12. chap 355.)* Very few diseases cause rapid dementia, noticeable in a period of weeks. Among them are depression, metabolic encephalopathy, encephalitis, poisoning, Binswanger's disease (white-matter infarction), and Creutzfeldt-Jakob disease. (Alzheimer's disease has a more insidious onset.) Creutzfeldt-Jakob disease is a slow-virus infection that causes a spongiform change in the cerebral cortex; it is characterized by rapid dementia, startle myoclonus, and, frequently, signs of occipital and cerebellar disease. CT scan and cerebrospinal fluid examination are nearly always normal in affected persons; after a period of time electroencephalography shows rapid, synchronous sharp waves, a diagnostic finding.

754. The answer is D. *(Wilson, ed 12. chap 356.)* Optic neuritis is the initial symptom in approximately 40 percent of persons who eventually are diagnosed as having multiple sclerosis. This rapidly developing ophthalmologic disorder is associated with partial or total loss of vision, pain on motion of the involved eye, scotoma affecting macular vision, and a variety of other visual-field defects. Ophthalmoscopically visible optic papillitis occurs in about half of cases.

755. The answer is C. *(Wilson, ed 12. chap 356.)* By far the most common cause of unilateral internuclear ophthalmoplegia is multiple sclerosis. Preferred diagnostic tests for multiple sclerosis are lumbar puncture to check particularly for an elevated immunoglobulin G fraction and evoked potentials to search for an occult second lesion in the nervous system (the demonstration of a second lesion makes the diagnosis of multiple sclerosis definite). The workup can be performed on an outpatient basis. Magnetic resonance imaging may also reveal occult white matter lesions.

756. The answer is E. *(Wilson, ed 12. chap 31.)* Bilateral conjugate eye movement to the side of the caloric stimulation indicates integrity of the brainstem pathways from the medulla to the midbrain (where the third nerve originates), as do full conjugate oculocephalic motions (doll's eye maneuvers). The absence of the rapid corrective phase manifested by nystagmus-like leftward eye gazing indicates a bilateral hemispheric lesion. Failure of an eye to adduct properly in the initial phase of the caloric response indicates a lesion in the ipsilateral third nerve (midbrain) or in the medial longitudinal fasciculus producing an internuclear ophthalmoplegia. In the former case, the pupil would be dilated and the eye abducted at rest.

757. The answer is A. *(Wilson, ed 12. chap 33.)* Most lesions that lead to aphasia, a disturbance in the production or comprehension of speech and language, occur in the dominant cerebral hemisphere. Ninety percent of people are right-handed; the left hemisphere is dominant in 95 percent of right-handed people, and in 50 percent of those who are left-handed. Broca's, or major motor, aphasia denotes a syndrome in which the praxis of speech is severely disturbed. This problem usually results from a large lesion in the posterior frontal lobe along the insula and sylvian fissure, not simply Broca's area in the inferior frontal lobe. Patients have great difficulty in articulation, grammar, and writing, though comprehension and fluency are relatively well preserved. Emboli of the superior division of the left middle cerebral artery are the most common cause of this syndrome.

758. The answer is D. *(Wilson, ed 12. chap 31.)* Hyperosmolar dehydration with mannitol or an equivalent agent reduces abnormally elevated intracranial pressure (ICP). Using intravenous fluids to support blood pressure, especially if they are hypoosmolar, would exacerbate cerebral edema and raise ICP still further. Similarly, high airway pressures are transmitted by way of the thoracic venous system and cerebrospinal fluid to the intracranial cavity and thus may worsen ICP elevation. The administration of phenytoin or beta blockers would be ineffective.

759. The answer is B. *(Wilson, ed 12. chap 357.)* Acquired hepatocerebral degeneration is a neurologic syndrome composed mainly of extrapyramidal signs. A well-known consequence of chronic liver disease, this disorder simulates Wilson's disease in many ways, including the presence of neuropathologic lesions in the cortex, basal ganglia, and other deep nuclei. Many cases become evident after a bout of hepatic encephalopathy, but others occur insidiously in persons who never have had encephalopathy.

760. The answer is B. *(Wilson, ed 12. chap 359.)* The combination of autonomic insufficiency and parkinsonian symptoms is known as the Shy-Drager syndrome. The autonomic form of the Landry-Guillain-Barré syndrome causes acute autonomic paralysis but does not cause the parkinsonian symptoms of tremor at rest, bradykinesia, and rigidity. A number of antihypertensive agents cause orthostatic hypotension, but none cause parkinsonism. Micturition syncope is a condition in which syncope occurs because of vagal surge at the time of release of intravesicular pressure.

761. The answer is B. *(Wilson, ed 12. chap 363.)* Lower brachial plexus injuries predominantly produce C8 and T1 deficits. Typically, ulnar border sensory loss affects the hand, and a Horner's syndrome may develop from damage to sympathetic nerve roots exiting at C8. Wasting of the intrinsic hand muscles leads to a "claw hand" deformity.

762. The answer is B. *(Wilson, ed 12. chap 359. Martin, N Engl J Med 315:1267, 1986.)* Huntington's chorea, which is inherited as an autosomal dominant trait, is characterized by dementia and choreiform movements. The motor disorder may include grimacing, respiratory spasms, speech irregularity, and a dancing, jangling quality of the gait. Laboratory workup is normal except that atrophy of the caudate may be seen on a carefully evaluated CT or MRI scan. Through the use of DNA linkage analysis, patients can be tested before disease development, if this is appropriate from a psychosocial standpoint.

763. The answer is E. *(Wilson, ed 12. chap 359.)* Several illnesses produce parkinsonian symptoms—rigidity, bradykinesia, and masked facies—but at the same time are not associated with tremor and do not respond to typical antiparkinsonism drugs. The most common of these diseases is progressive supranuclear palsy, which is characterized by vertical ophthalmoplegia, speech difficulty (hypophonia), and anxiety. No form of therapy has been consistently successful in controlling the symptoms of this disorder.

764. The answer is B. *(Wilson, ed 12. chap 361.)* The most characteristic symptom of syringomyelia is loss of pain sense with preservation of touch. This phenomenon occurs most commonly over the shoulders in a cape-like distribution. Tissue loss in the central gray matter of the spinal cord, where pain fibers cross to join the contralateral spinothalamic tract, is the neuropathologic process involved. Other characteristic features of syringomyelia include thoracic scoliosis and muscle atrophy of the hands. Ataxia does not occur unless the syrinx extends into the brainstem.

765. The answer is A. *(Wilson, ed 12. chap 361.)* Neuromyelitis optica (Devic's disease) usually occurs in association with necrotizing myelitis but also is seen in persons who have multiple sclerosis and postinfectious and postvaccinal myelitis. Neuromyelitis optica is characterized by both transverse myelitis and optic neuritis; affected persons can display such signs and symptoms as progressive sensorimotor deficits, central scotoma, and elevated protein concentration and cell count in cerebrospinal fluid. In the case presented in the question, the presence of optic nerve involvement and the finding of a sensory level on the trunk rule out acute idiopathic polyneuritis, although analysis of cerebrospinal fluid is not inconsistent with polyneuritis in its early stages. A diagnosis of acute spinal epidural abscess is made less likely by the presence of optic neuritis.

766. The answer is E. *(Wilson, ed 12. chap 360.)* Any lesion impinging on the optic chiasm produces a bitemporal hemianopsia by interfering with images projected onto the nasal retina. The most common cause of bilateral hemianopsia is suprasellar extension of pituitary tumors. Suprasellar aneurysms of the carotid artery are common enough that many neurosurgeons perform angiography before removing apparent pituitary tumors. The best initial diagnostic technique is CT scan with contrast infusion. Other causes of bitemporal hemianopsia include craniopharyngioma, meningioma, and metastatic disease.

767. The answer is A. *(Wilson, ed 12. chap 348.)* CT scanning still remains the procedure of choice in the acute setting when rapid information about a suddenly deteriorating patient is required. It has a high specificity for demonstrating acute hemorrhage, and in that respect is superior to MRI. Calcifications within the brain and bony lesions are also better delineated on CT than on MRI. However, MRI has added diagnostic potential in a number of circumstances, including screening for metastatic disease (particularly if gadolinium enhancement is used), imaging demyelinating diseases, and identifying the presence of aneurysms and arteriovenous malformations as well as developmental malformations, posterior fossa lesions, and almost all spinal cord lesions—including vertebral osteomyelitis, epidural abscess, herniated disks, and syringomyelia.

768. The answer is C. *(Wilson, ed 12. chap 352.)* The cause of chronic subdural hematoma may be a trivial or unapparent injury, such as might be sustained by a sudden deceleration experienced in a motor vehicle accident. Symptoms are relatively nonspecific, usually characterized by an intermittent headache accompanied by some degree of personality change, drowsiness, or confusion. This condition is easily confused with drug intoxication, stroke, dementia, and depression. For the patient in the question, however, the lack of focal findings argues against stroke and the rapidity of onset would be unusual for dementia. The CT scan does not define the hematomas because they have become isodense with the passage of time (2 to 6 weeks since injury); however, the absence of sulci and the small size of the ventricles coupled with the clinical scenario are highly suggestive of bilateral subdural hematomas. Surgical evacuation of the hematomas is the treatment of choice.

769. The answer is D. *(Wilson, ed 12. chap 363.)* Entrapment of the lateral femoral cutaneous nerve, which can occur where it enters the thigh beneath the inguinal ligament near the anterior superior iliac spine, causes a sensory neuropathy known as ''meralgia paresthetica.'' Symptoms of this disorder, which typically occurs in obese persons, include pain and decreased tactile sensation over the lateral aspect of the thigh. Treatment is infiltration with a local anesthetic or, if this procedure proves ineffective, surgical sectioning of the nerve.

770. The answer is E. *(Wilson, ed 12. chap 363.)* The inflammatory response in Guillain-Barré syndrome strips myelin between the nodes of Ranvier in peripheral nerves. This phenomenon explains both the slowing of nerve conduction and the potential for recovery. Axons are only destroyed in extensively involved areas as a secondary phenomenon. To date, no convincing evidence has emerged to support the contention that the central nervous system is involved in Guillain-Barré syndrome.

771. The answer is A. *(Wilson, ed 12. chap 365.)* Myotonia, muscle wasting, cataracts, testicular atrophy, and frontal baldness characterize the hereditary disorder myotonic dystrophy. Onset usually is in early adulthood. In affected persons, mental retardation is common, atrial arrhythmia is a frequent complication, and diabetes mellitus is more prevalent than in the general population. Myotonic dystrophy is the type of muscular dystrophy most commonly observed in hospitalized patients.

772. The answer is B. - *(Wilson, ed 12. chap 365.)* Oculopharyngeal dystrophy is a dominantly inherited disease occurring in families of French-Canadian or middle-European ancestry. Because it causes late-onset progressive ptosis and difficulty with swallowing, it may be difficult to distinguish from myasthenia gravis, which is not a dystrophic muscle disease. Proximal weakness and ophthalmoplegia suggest the presence of a progressive external ophthalmoplegia.

773. The answer is C. *(Wilson, ed 12. chap 365.)* Myotonia is the phenomenon in which brief, persistent contractions of a muscle occur after voluntary contraction or, sometimes, percussion. Myokymia is continuous, small-muscle movement that is frequently difficult to distinguish from fasciculations. Fibrillation is the electromyographically detected spontaneous firing of muscle fibers and is not visible except in the tongue. Myoedema is a poorly defined sign similar to myotonia in which a ridge of percussed muscle remains contracted for 5 to 8 s. It was once thought to be related to hypoalbuminemia, but this relationship probably does not exist.

774. The answer is B. *(Wilson, ed 12. chap 19.)* Malignancy in the pelvis not infrequently causes compression or infiltration of nerves exiting the spinal cord en route to the leg. This results in stepwise progression of sensory and motor deficits in areas supplied by the involved nerve roots or trunks. Continuous pain in the distribution of a specific nerve or root is also common. In this patient the neurologic deficits began in an S1 distribution but then progressed to L5 and, finally, L4 roots, suggesting an expanding paravertebral mass. Isolated, spontaneous activity of muscle fibers called *fibrillations* is characteristic of denervation. Nerve conduction will be normal in the leg if the lesion is proximal to the measuring electrodes, i.e., in the pelvis. An expanding cortical mass might also cause progressive numbness in the foot and leg and might be missed on a CT scan that does not take cuts all the way up to the vertex. Back pain and neuropathic pain would not occur with a cortical lesion, and the reflexes under such circumstances should be hyperactive.

775. The answer is D. *(Wilson, ed 12. chap 366.)* More than three-quarters of patients with myasthenia have circulating antibodies against components of the postsynaptic membrane, including acetylcholine receptors. Antibody action leads to an unfolding, or ''simplification,'' of the membrane and, consequently, a reduced number of acetylcholine receptors. As a result, existing acetylcholine in the synapse is less effective in producing muscle contraction.

776. The answer is A. *(Wilson, ed 12. chap 351. Fisher, Neurology 32:871, 1982.)* A pure motor hemiparesis on one side (with ipsilateral face and body involvement) and no other cortical deficits (aphasia or cortical sensory loss) suggests an internal capsular lesion. The major differential diagnosis in this setting is between a hypertensive hemorrhage or an internal capsular lacunar infarct. Both entities may present with a fluctuating course over hours; however, hemorrhages tend to produce some manifestation of increased intracranial pressure. Lacunar infarctions result from atherothrombotic and hyalinization changes in the penetrating branches of the circle of Willis, middle cerebral artery stem, and vertebrobasilar system. Other than the internal capsule, common locations for lacunar infarctions include the thalamus, where they produce pure sensory deficit, and the base of the pons, where they produce hemiparesis and dysarthria with a clumsy hand. CT scanning can document most supratentorial lacunar infarctions, whose size usually ranges from 0.5 to 2 cm.

777. The answer is E. *(Wilson, ed 12. chap 353.)* Typical symptoms of neoplastic meningitis include headache, confusion, radiculopathy, and cranial nerve abnormalities in patients with a variety of tumors, including non-Hodgkin's lymphoma, leukemia, melanoma, breast cancer, lung cancer, and stomach cancer. Given these symptoms, especially in the face of a negative CT, MRI, or both, the diagnosis of leptomeningeal metastases from breast cancer is quite likely. A single lumbar puncture is a relatively insensitive test; repeat examinations of cerebrospinal fluid are often required to establish the diagnosis of cancer that has spread to the meninges. Especially in cases where the cancer cells are "caked" onto the inferior portion of the brain, eradication by chemotherapy alone (usually methotrexate, thio-TEPA, or cytosine arabinoside) is difficult and radiation therapy should be administered as well.

778. The answer is B. *(Wilson, ed 12. chap 18.)* The patient had cluster headache. Cluster headache occurs over the orbit, usually within 2 h of falling asleep. The key to diagnosis is a history of associated lacrimation, nasal stuffiness, and swelling and erythema over the cheek. The headaches may occur every night for weeks and are quite severe. Ergotamine taken at bedtime is often the first preparation to prevent the headache. Lithium is frequently effective, but its use warrants monitoring of the patient's serum electrolytes and renal function. Alcohol frequently precipitates headache in these patients. Note that the dose of ergotamine in Choice D is dangerously excessive. Ergotamine should be limited to a maximum of about 12 mg per week.

779. The answer is E. *(Wilson, ed 12. chaps 25, 362.)* Fasciculations may occur in a variety of metabolic and toxic disorders, including amyotrophic lateral sclerosis, progressive bulbar palsy, ruptured intervertebral disk, and peripheral neuropathy. However, they should not be viewed with alarm in the absence of weakness, muscle atrophy, or loss of tendon reflexes. The best treatment a physician could offer a person who is asymptomatic except for fascicular twitches is reassurance and, if appropriate, advice to reduce coffee intake.

780. The answer is C. *(Wilson, ed 12. chap 363.)* Although porphyric neuropathy may occur without central nervous system involvement, with acute paralysis there is frequently a history of confusion or coma. Predominantly a motor neuropathy, porphyric neuropathy can cause significant sensory loss in some persons. In this respect it may simulate inflammatory polyneuropathy, though inflammation does not occur. Curiously, protein concentration in CSF is usually normal in affected persons.

781. The answer is C. *(Wilson, ed 12. chaps 15, 28.)* One of the most distressing sequela of thalamic damage is a chronic pain syndrome that occurs months to a few years after the initial lesion. The findings of total hemianesthesia and loss of all sensory modalities in the face, arm, and leg are characteristic of thalamic infarction. Lesions of the spinothalamic tract may also cause neuropathic pain syndromes, but hemianesthesia of the face does not occur with spinal cord lesions. Parietal lobe lesions usually affect the cortical senses (i.e., two-point discrimination, graphesthesia, or stereognosia) rather than cause a total hemianesthesia. Depression is not commonly associated with burning pain. Tic douloureux is not associated with sensory loss.

782. The answer is D. *(Wilson, ed 12. chap 355. Gabuzda, Ann Intern Med 107:383, 1987.)* Infected macrophages are probably the Trojan horse by which the human immunodeficiency virus (HIV) enters the central nervous system. AIDS dementia, which is the chief manifestation of subacute encephalitis, the most common neurologic abnormality in this group of patients, is insidious and slowly progressive. The initial CT or MRI scan is normal; the CSF is nonspecifically abnormal (mild pleocytosis and protein rise). Zidovudine (AZT) may be effective if given early in this tragic complication of HIV infection. CNS toxoplasmosis or lymphoma, occurring as a result of the immunocompromised state, can produce mass lesions in AIDS patients. Direct HIV infection is also responsible for the myelopathy, neuropathy, and aseptic meningitis that occur in AIDS patients.

783. The answer is E. *(Wilson, ed 12. chap 359. Tandan, Ann Neurol 18:271, 1985.)* Amyotrophic lateral sclerosis (ALS) is an untreatable disease that results in progressive loss of upper and lower motor neuron function.

Other components of the nervous system remain intact, including the neurons required for ocular motility. Limb weakness and cramping is the first symptom, followed by muscular atrophy, fasciculations, and loss of function of cranial nerve musculature. Early in the disease, upper-tract signs may predominate, resulting in spasticity. Pneumonia due to failure of clearance of secretions is usually the terminal event. Treatable causes of motor neuron disease, such as cervical spondylosis (no bulbar involvement) and lead poisoning, should be excluded whenever the diagnosis of ALS is considered. Guillain-Barré syndrome produces an ascending, rapidly developing paralysis. B_{12} deficiency should lead to abnormalities in posterior column function. Lambert-Eaton syndrome is a paraneoplastic neuromuscular disorder that would not feature upper-tract signs.

784. The answer is D. *(Wilson, ed 12. chap 365. Koenig, Cell 50:509, 1987.)* Duchenne's muscular dystrophy is an X-linked recessive disorder in which affected boys develop progressive weakness of limb girdle muscles beginning at age 5 or earlier. By age 12 walking is impossible and patients usually succumb to respiratory failure by age 25. Most muscular tissues, including cardiac, are involved. An abnormally high creatine kinase level is found in all patients before disease onset and in many female carriers. The responsible gene has been identified. This 2000-kilobase gene codes for a product termed *dystrophin,* a 400-kilodalton protein localized to the muscle plasma membrane. Since about 60 percent of patients have an exon deletion or duplication in the dystrophin gene, it is possible to test directly for these genetic abnormalities in utero, thus obviating the need for more cumbersome family studies to determine RFLPs for linkage.

785. The answer is B. *(Wilson, ed 12. chap 364.)* This patient displays the characteristic heliotropic rash, with knuckle involvement and proximal muscle weakness typical of dermatomyositis. Although a biopsy could be done, the disease is patchy and the absence of a lymphocytic infiltration would not rule out the diagnosis. EMG will be diagnostic in about 40 percent of affected persons. Since the diagnosis is straightforward and dermatomyositis is frequently associated with malignancy in those over age 60, it is quite reasonable to screen for cancer. In addition to the common epithelial malignancies, myeloproliferative disorders can be heralded by dermatomyositis. However, an unfocused radiological diagnostic attack should definitely be suspended in favor of the simple and cost-effective tests outlined in choice B. Although steroids will probably be symptomatically beneficial even in those with malignancies, their use should probably be delayed until the screening is completed. If an early neoplasm can be found and treated, the dermatomyositis could respond without the need of resorting to the dangers of high-dose glucocorticoid therapy.

786. The answer is A-Y, B-N, C-Y, D-Y, E-N. *(Wilson, ed 12. chap 25.)* Polymyalgia rheumatica is characterized by aching pain, but, unlike polymyositis, weakness is minimal or absent. Subacute combined degeneration due to vitamin-B_{12} deficiency is predominantly a sensory syndrome associated with spasticity; weakness is absent until the disease is far advanced. Botulism is fundamentally a paralytic disorder resulting from presynaptic neuromuscular blockade. Like botulism, polyneuritis causes paralysis, although a pure sensory neuropathy is not associated with weakness.

787. The answer is A-Y, B-Y, C-N, D-N, E-Y. *(Wilson, ed 12. chap 26.)* Normal-pressure hydrocephalus and cervical spondylosis typically present with gait difficulty: short steps (sometimes mistaken for parkinsonism), and leg stiffness and slowness of step, respectively. Subacute combined degeneration may produce spasticity of gait as part of its lateral column (corticospinal) damage. Subdural hematoma generally does not cause isolated gait difficulty, and carotid stenosis causes either transient ischemic attacks or strokes but not a progressive syndrome of any sort.

788. The answer is A-N, B-Y, C-Y, D-N, E-Y. *(Wilson, ed 12. chap 15.)* Owing to release of substances from damaged tissue (e.g., histamines, prostaglandins) or from the circulation (e.g., bradykinin), sensory stimuli activate free nerve endings in the skin. Such nerves terminate in the segmental dorsal horn of the spinal cord. Substance P and other neurotransmitters released from terminals stimulate transmission via long axons composing the spinothalamic tract that terminate in the nucleus ventralis posterolateralis (VPL). VPL fibers project to the cerebral somatosensory cortex. Descending pathways that mediate analgesia project from the periaqueductal gray region in the midbrain to the medullary midline raphe nuclei. Raphe nuclei neurons in turn project to dorsal horn nuclei, where painful afferent impulses may be modified. This system contains many opiate receptors. Another descending pain inhibitory pathway, which projects from the pontine locus ceruleus to the dorsal horn of the spinal cord, mediates its effects by alpha-adrenergic signals.

789. The answer is A-N, B-N, C-N, D-Y, E-Y. *(Wilson, ed 12. chap 24.)* Localization of the tone in the affected ear when the tuning fork is placed in the midline position (Weber's test) suggests unilateral conductive loss (external or middle ear), while perception in the unaffected ear would suggest sensorineural hearing loss. A tone heard louder by bone conduction compared with air conduction (Rinne's test) also suggests conductive rather than sensorineural hearing loss. Assuming that the patient's bone conduction is normal (since he did perceive the tone when the fork was at the mastoid process) and that only his air conduction was diminished, we can presume that the lesion is either in the external auditory canal or the middle ear. A common cause of conductive hearing loss in the elderly is otosclerosis (stapes footplate fusion), which is potentially treatable by surgical reconstructive procedures involving the middle ear.

790. The answer is A-Y, B-N, C-N, D-N, E-Y. *(Wilson, ed 12. chap 31.)* For most comatose persons seen in a general hospital setting, CT scanning is not helpful because nonstructural causes—i.e., metabolic or exogenous toxins—are at fault. A lesion appears on CT scan only when there is a difference in density compared with adjacent areas of the brain. An area of infarction generally takes at least a day to become lower in density than normal brain; thus, a CT scan performed acutely would be expected to be normal. Acute unilateral middle cerebral artery infarction does not cause coma. Brain death is a clinical, not a radiologic, diagnosis.

791. The answer is A-N, B-N, C-Y, D-Y, E-Y. *(Wilson, ed 12. chap 350.)* So-called simple partial seizures are due to epileptic discharges in a focal brain region. Most often these are in the temporal lobe, where they cause psychologic phenomena, such as déjà vu, or brief emotional symptoms, such as fear, if they impinge on the limbic system. Discharges on the lateral surface of the temporal lobe may cause auditory hallucinations, vertigo, or language disturbances (if on the left side). Well-defined limb or facial sensations or movements are not part of temporal lobe epilepsy.

792. The answer is A-Y, B-Y, C-N, D-N, E-N. *(Wilson, ed 12. chaps 349, 366.)* Conventional electromyography (EMG) and nerve conduction studies as well as muscle biopsy procedures are not useful in an evaluation of myasthenia gravis, because it is not a disease of muscle or nerve. (Electron microscopy of muscle can show unfolding of the postsynaptic muscle membrane, but this procedure is not commonly done.) Curare testing to precipitate myasthenic weakness is dangerous, undependable, and mainly of historical interest. Single-fiber EMG measures the timing of firing of two fibers in the same motor unit. The timing between pairs is inconsistent in myasthenia, giving rise to "jitter" in the oscilloscope tracing; this finding is virtually diagnostic of myasthenia. Repetitive stimulation of motor nerves to observe a decremental response also is a useful procedure in testing for myasthenia gravis.

793. The answer is A-Y, B-Y, C-N, D-Y, E-N. *(Wilson, ed 12. chap 19.)* Low back pain without ruptured disk or other nerve damage is common. It requires bed rest, administration of muscle relaxants, and time for recovery. It is often precipitated by lifting while the spine is flexed or laterally rotated. X-rays may show the nonspecific signs of paravertebral muscle spasm, i.e., straightening of the normal lumbar lordosis or scoliosis. Because of pain and spasm the patient cannot flex the spine normally. Signs of nervous system damage distinguish the patient with a more serious disorder. Bowel and bladder difficulty accompany damage to sacral roots or the spinal cord. Perineal sensation and rectal tone should be tested along with individual muscle strength, stretch reflexes, Babinski reflexes, and dermatomal sensation. Abnormal results on any of these tests suggest that there is nerve injury in addition to muscular strain.

794. The answer is A-N, B-Y, C-Y, D-Y, E-Y. *(Wilson, ed 12. chaps 25, 349, 362.)* Hypotonia or atonia is characteristic of denervated muscle. Muscle atrophy that occurs after destruction of a motor nerve is much more severe than simple disuse muscle atrophy; denervated muscle usually loses 70 to 80 percent of its original bulk within 90 days. Denervation of muscle produces Erb's reaction of degeneration, in which response to short-duration (faradic) stimulation is lost but response to long-duration (galvanic) stimulation is preserved. The isolated activity of individual muscle fibers (fibrillation) is a characteristic of denervated muscle. Fasciculations, on the other hand, occur when a motor neuron in the anterior horn of the spinal cord becomes diseased; because they depend on reinnervation of muscle by normal nerve fibers, fasciculations generally are not produced when a nerve is totally destroyed.

795. The answer is A-Y, B-N, C-N, D-N, E-Y. *(Wilson, ed 12. chap 25.)* The distinction between upper motor neuron and lower motor neuron lesions is critical in clinical medicine. Lesions proximal to the anterior horn cells (in general, the cerebral motor cortex or the corticospinal tract) produce the characteristic upper motor neuron syndrome of spasticity, increased reflexes, and an extensor plantar response (Babinski's sign). On the other hand, atrophy of muscles in a paretic limb suggests lower motor neuron disease. Such disorders, which may affect individual muscles, will be accompanied by fascicular twitches, which are manifestations of the hyperactivity of the diseased motor unit(s).

796. The answer is A-N, B-Y, C-Y, D-Y, E-N. *(Wilson, ed 12. chap 25.)* Rest tremor, frequently associated with Parkinson's disease, occurs at a rate of four to five beats per second. The rest tremor of Parkinson's disease is associated with flexed posture, slowness of movement, rigidity, postural instability, and suppression by willful activity. Many tremors that worsen during movement are exaggerations of the normal physiologic tremor. The essential-familial tremor is a faster action tremor (about 8 Hz) responsive to moderate doses of alcohol or beta-adrenergic blockade.

797. The answer is A-N, B-Y, C-N, D-Y, E-N. *(Wilson, ed 12. chap 30.)* It is important to search for treatable causes of dementia among the long list of conditions that account for this progressive and debilitating loss of cognitive function. Alzheimer's disease is by far the most common cause of dementia in this country. The diagnosis of this entity is based on the hallmark of progressive deterioration in mental and social functioning. Cases of vascular dementia—exemplified by multi-infarct dementia, which is usually the result of bilateral carotid disease—can be approached by anticoagulation and other strategies to lessen the risk of further small strokes. Patients with hypertension may develop another form of (theoretically treatable) vascular dementia known as Binswanger's disease (subcortical arteriosclerotic encephalopathy), which involves atherosclerosis-induced loss of subcortical white matter and ventricular enlargement. A host of chronic infections, some of which are treatable (e.g., syphilis, tuberculosis, and Whipple's disease), should be excluded during the workup of a patient with dementia. However, the courses of the dementias associated with human immunodeficiency virus or with slow-virus infection (Creutzfeldt-Jakob disease) have not yet been conclusively shown to be modified by treatment. Mass lesions, such as those caused by tumors, hematoma, or hydrocephalus, are partially remediable and should be excluded by anatomic imaging of the brain. Other potentially treatable causes of dementia that can be excluded by appropriate studies include the following: vasculitis, hypothyroidism, B_{12} deficiency, thiamine deficiency, nicotinic acid deficiency, adrenal insufficiency, Cushing's syndrome, chronic hypoglycemia, hypoparathyroidism, hyperparathyroidism, Wilson's disease, dialysis, and toxicities of drugs, alcohol, heavy metals, and organic metals.

798. The answer is A-N, B-Y, C-N, D-N, E-Y. *(Wilson, ed 12. chap 349.)* The electroencephalogram (EEG) is a useful tool in analyzing a host of conditions that affect the central nervous system, but it is specifically abnormal in relatively few nonepileptic conditions. Rapidly growing space-occupying lesions, cerebral contusions, or large infarcts may each produce focal slow waves. Bilateral slow waves may also be nonspecifically evident in a host of metabolic encephalopathies, including hypoxia, acidosis, hypoglycemia, hyponatremia, uremia, and hepatic coma. It should be noted that hepatic coma can sometimes also be associated with diagnostic bilateral triphasic waves. Moreover, barbiturate or benzodiazepine overdose can be associated with excess fast activity. Subacute sclerosing panencephalitis and Creutzfeldt-Jakob disease, two rapidly progressive diseases affecting the cerebral cortex, have fairly characteristic changes consisting of complex bursts of sharp and slow activity. If a patient is suspected of having herpes simplex encephalitis, a focal, temporal abnormality would be highly suggestive of this diagnosis. On the other hand, the EEG is frequently normal in many diseases that can have dramatic clinical presentations, including multiple sclerosis, delirium tremens, Wernicke-Korsakoff disease, bipolar affective disorders, schizophrenia, and withdrawal seizures.

799. The answer is A-Y, B-Y, C-Y, D-Y, E-N. *(Wilson, ed 12. chap 357.)* Dialysis "dementia" usually begins as a disorder of articulation, but general mental decline may be evident early as well. Electroencephalography may reveal bursts of slow waves or spikes; cerebrospinal fluid analysis and CT scan typically are normal. The illness is usually progressive to death, although some patients survive for several years. Except for clonazepam treatment of myoclonus and seizures, no effective therapy is known. It is currently believed that aluminum intoxication may be the cause.

800. The answer is A-N, B-Y, C-Y, D-Y, E-Y. *(Wilson, ed 12. chap 363.)* Acute mononeuropathy involving the oculomotor or peroneal nerves should prompt an investigation for diabetes. A neuropathy that is progressive, distal, and primarily sensory is most characteristic of diabetes but may also occur with an occult neoplasm. The autonomic neuropathy of diabetes usually coexists with the sensory type, but the latter may be mild. Relapsing neuropathy is more typical of idiopathic polyneuritis.

801. The answer is A-Y, B-Y, C-Y, D-N, E-N. *(Wilson, ed 12. chaps 359, 361.)* Several disorders produce chronic, progressive spinal cord disease with sensory and motor involvement. Syndromes of spinocerebellar degeneration may involve the motor and sensory spinal cord systems in addition to causing ataxia. Multiple sclerosis usually causes a relapsing illness but can cause a progressive, usually cervical myelopathy in elderly women. Cervical spondylosis, or bony compression of the cervical cord by osteophytic bars, is another common cause of myelopathy in the elderly. Lumbar disk compression of the cauda equina, which is made up of peripheral nerves, does not cause spinal cord signs. Amyotrophic lateral sclerosis is a disease of spinal cord motor neurons and corticospinal tracts, but has no sensory signs.

802. The answer is A-N, B-Y, C-N, D-N, E-Y. *(Wilson, ed 12. chaps 357, 360.)* Bilateral lateral-rectus palsies that develop acutely in alcoholic persons should suggest Wernicke's encephalopathy, which requires prompt treatment with thiamine. Bilateral sixth-nerve malfunction may be a falsely localizing sign from increased intracranial pressure, as in subdural hematoma, but does not occur as an isolated disturbance from intrinsic brainstem diseases (e.g., hemorrhage). Orbital fractures usually entrap the fourth nerve, less commonly the sixth; only rarely would the palsy be bilateral. Although neurosyphilis can cause cranial nerve palsies from adhesive meningitis, palsy of oculomotor-related nerves is a rarity.

803. The answer is A-N, B-Y, C-Y, D-Y, E-Y. *(Wilson, ed 12. chap 361.)* The finding of a clear sensory level above which pinprick is felt but below which sensation is absent is the *sine qua non* of spinal cord disease. The segmented level at which sensory loss begins also gives the corresponding cord level of the lesion. Other typical signs of spinal cord disease, such as hypertonicity and hyperreflexia, may be absent in acute lesions; bladder function, however, is invariably affected if the lesion is severe. Myelopathy due to deficiency of vitamin B_{12} only rarely gives a vague sensory level on the trunk.

804. The answer is A-N, B-Y, C-Y, D-N, E-Y. *(Wilson, ed 12. chap 351.)* Unilateral occlusion of a vertebral artery typically results in Wallenberg's lateral medullary syndrome. With an infarct on the left, this is likely to include damage to the left ninth and tenth cranial nerves, the left inferior cerebellar peduncle, and the spinothalamic fibers subserving pain and temperature on the right side. Vertigo and nystagmus are common since the lower vestibular complex may be affected. Horner's syndrome is also common with a smaller pupil and ptosis *ipsilateral* to the lesion. Only rarely is the medullary pyramid involved (Babinski-Nageotte syndrome) resulting in a *contralateral* hemiparesis sparing the face; hypoglossal weakness may then be present ipsilateral to the lesion. Lesions of the median longitudinal fasciculus producing internuclear ophthalmoplegia occur in the pons and midbrain in the territory of branches of the basilar artery.

805. The answer is A-Y, B-Y, C-N, D-N, E-Y. *(Wilson, ed 12. chap 360.)* Cranial nerves III, IV, and VI all pass through the cavernous sinus, so that complete ophthalmoplegia, including ptosis, may result from a disease process there. Since the supraorbital and maxillary divisions of the fifth nerve, but not the mandibular branch, pass through the cavernous sinus, the brow and cheek may be numb, but not the chin. The optic nerve will be involved only if the process extends superiorly.

806. The answer is A-Y, B-N, C-Y, D-Y, E-Y. *(Wilson, ed 12. chap 350. Callahan, N Engl J Med 318:942, 1988.)* Although many patients with epilepsy require anticonvulsants for life, about half will remain seizure-free long enough to warrant a trial off medications, many of which bear imposing side effects. Favorable prognostic factors for remaining seizure-free include few seizures before control is attained, control on single first-choice drug therapy, history of simple partial seizures or primary generalized seizures, and a normal EEG before drug withdrawal. Even if a patient has had a long seizure-free interval (> 2 years) and has a good chance of remaining seizure-free off anticonvulsants, the drug should be tapered over 3 to 6 months. Moreover, the patient and the physician should be aware of the consequences of relapse and be willing to accept the risk.

807. The answer is A-N, B-N, C-N, D-Y, E-N. *(Wilson, ed 12. chap 357. Charness, N Engl J Med 321:442, 1989.)* Wernicke's encephalopathy is a consequence of thiamine (vitamin B_1) deficiency. Though most commonly observed in chronic alcoholics in this country, well-documented cases have occurred in prisoners-of-war in whom alcohol played no role. Certain areas in the thalamus, hypothalamus, midbrain, floor of the fourth ventricle, and cerebellar vermis are prone to destruction as a consequence of thiamine deficiency. While most patients present with some form of abnormal mental functioning, the classic triad of ophthalmoplegia, confusion, and ataxia is rarely encountered. Based on autopsy series, many patients frequently go undiagnosed. When the diagnosis is suspected, thiamine should be administered before glucose, since the latter substance can precipitate worsening of the disease. Within hours thiamine will relieve the ocular palsies, although improvement in ataxia and in apathy and confusion takes longer. Many of those who recover from the acute encephalopathy will be left with a profound defect in memory and learning known as *Korsakoff's psychosis*.

808. The answer is A-N, B-N, C-Y, D-N, E-Y. *(Wilson, ed 12. chap 359.)* Parkinson's disease, characterized clinically by rest tremor, stooped posture, and akinesia, is associated with loss of dopaminergic neurons in the substantia nigra of the brainstem. There are several effective therapies for providing symptomatic relief. Anticholinergics, such as benztropine, block muscarinic receptors that inhibit the release of dopamine. Propranolol and metoprolol are beta-adrenergic blockers that can ameliorate the tremor, but have little effect on other pathogenetic features. Amantadine is effective in the early stages of Parkinson's disease because it promotes release of dopamine from nerve endings. The mainstay of treatment is levodopa-carbidopa (Sinemet). Levodopa, a source of replacement dopamine, is given along with carbidopa, which inhibits dopa decarboxylase, an enzyme that metabolizes levodopa in the periphery. The dopamine agonist bromocriptine acts directly upon dopamine receptors. Recently, deprenyl has been shown to slow the course of Parkinson's disease.

809. The answer is A-N, B-N, C-Y, D-Y, E-N. *(Wilson, ed 12. chap 369.)* Lithium has revolutionized the treatment of bipolar affective disorders. It is effective both during acute mania and in the prevention of recurrent attacks. Although side effects—particularly gastrointestinal upset, mild tremor, and thirst—are common, the drug is safe if used carefully. Lithium dosage should be titrated to serum levels: control of mania should be achieved at a level between 0.8 and 1.4 mmol/L and maintenance levels should be between 0.6 and 1.0 mmol/L. Lithium intoxication is manifested by depression of mental status; treatment is mainly supportive. Other important long-term side effects include hypothyroidism (by inhibiting secretion of thyroid hormone) and renal complications. Effects on the renal tubules produce nephrogenic diabetes insipidus with polyuria, polydipsia, and impaired urinary concentrating ability in about 25 percent of patients on the drug.

810. The answer is A-N, B-Y, C-Y, D-N, E-N. *(Wilson, ed 12. chap 367.)* Hypokalemic periodic paralysis is an autosomal dominant condition in two-thirds of cases; sporadic cases account for one-third of the incidence. It preferentially affects males. The pathogenesis of this disorder is unknown, but it is believed to involve excessive flux of potassium from blood into muscle during attacks. Furthermore, since attacks can occur when the potassium level is normal, factors other than hypokalemia alone must be important. Attacks generally involve proximal limb muscles. Between attacks the results of physical examination are normal except for persistent eyelid myotonia. Acute attacks can be managed successfully with oral or intravenous potassium and in most patients can be essentially abolished with the chronic administration of acetazolamide. Administration of potassium salts does not diminish the frequency of attacks.

811–814. The answers are: 811-D, 812-C, 813-C, 814-A. *(Wilson, ed 12. chap 19.)* In the assessment of uncomplicated disk protrusion, it is important to keep in mind that many lesions cause sciatica and that a protruding disk generally impinges on the nerve root that exits just below it (e.g., an ''L5-S1 disk'' most often compresses the S1 root). Walking on the toes requires a powerful gastrocnemius muscle, which is innervated by L5 and S1. When weakness in this maneuver is coupled with a depressed ankle reflex, an S1 compression is likely (protrusion of the L5-S1 disk). Compression of the L5 root by an L4-L5 disk does not affect knee or ankle reflexes but causes anterior tibial weakness (foot drop), extensor hallucis longus weakness, and weakness of foot inversion. The knee reflex is affected by an L3 or L4 radicular lesion (L2-L3 or L3-L4 disks, respectively), but hip flexors are affected by L2 and L3 only. These are the major lower extremity disk syndromes. In complex cases, several nerve roots are involved by protrusion of a single disk.

815–819. The answers are: 815-B, 816-A, 817-C, 818-E, 819-E. *(Wilson, ed 12. chaps 32, 33.)* Persons with large lesions of one or both of the frontal lobes or lesions of the central white matter and the anterior region of the corpus callosum may exhibit several clinical syndromes. Some affected persons develop what is known as the apathetic-akinetic-abulic state, which is characterized by decreased initiative and spontaneity combined with diminished speech and motor activity. Other syndromes include motor abnormalities, impaired intelligence, and personality changes.

Wernicke's aphasia occurs as a result of a lesion in the dominant temporal lobe. Affected persons are unable to read, write, or comprehend the speech of others. Quadrantic homonymous anopsia also may be associated with Wernicke's aphasia.

A lesion of the dominant parietal lobe can cause Gerstmann's syndrome. This syndrome is considered representative of an agnosia in that both the formulation and use of symbolic concepts are defective. As a result, affected persons are unable to write and calculate and to differentiate right from left.

Inability to recognize faces (prosopagnosia) results from a lesion in the visual association areas of the occipital lobe. This disorder can arise from either unilateral or, more frequently, bilateral involvement of the occipitotemporal regions. Visual acuity is intact in affected persons. A destructive lesion in one occipital lobe that destroys all terminal fibers in the geniculocalcarine pathway required for visual sensation would result in dense homonymous hemianopia.

820–824. The answers are: 820-A, 821-C, 822-B, 823-D, 824-E. *(Wilson, ed 12. chap 28.)* Sensory levels on physical examination can be used to pinpoint the spinal cord level affected in a variety of diseases. Each dermatomal level is associated with a major anatomic landmark. Sensory cervical spinal roots are associated with the following landmarks: posterior scalp (C2), neck (C3), clavicle (C4), shoulder (C5), thumb and forefinger (C6), middle finger (C7), and ring finger (C8). Key thoracic dermatomal landmarks include the axilla (T2 and T3), nipple (T4), and umbilicus (T10). Lumbar sensory levels include anterior thigh (L3), knee (L4), and lateral calf and great toe (L5), while sacral levels, which are harder to demarcate, include the posterior calf (S1) and posterior thigh (S2).

825–830. The answers are: 825-B, 826-B, 827-C, 828-B, 829-B, 830-D. *(Wilson, ed 12. chap 350.)* Rash and idiosyncratic bone marrow suppression are at times seen with phenobarbital, phenytoin, and carbamazepine; leukopenia and thrombocytopenia are most common with carbamazepine. Hepatotoxicity is a rare but feared effect of carbamazepine and an acute effect of valproic acid. In addition to the side effects listed in the question, phenytoin causes the appearance of a slightly prognathic jaw and coarsened facies. Phenytoin's neurologic side effects include ataxia. In fact, ataxia is a potential side effect of virtually all the anticonvulsants, including each of those listed in the question.

831–835. The answers are: 831-E, 832-A, 833-B, 834-D, 835-C. *(Wilson, ed 12. chap 23.)* Eye movement abnormalities occur as a result of a number of nervous system abnormalities. The pontine gaze center controls ipsilateral horizontal gaze. The medial longitudinal fasciculus (MLF) connects the gaze centers and the oculomotor nuclei. A lesion of the MLF results in an internuclear ophthalmoplegia—failure of adduction of the eye on the side of the lesion accompanied by contralateral nystagmus. Lesions of the frontal lobe gaze center cause a gaze preference to the side of the lesion, but the eyes can usually be made to cross the midline. The rostral interstitial nucleus of the MLF controls vertical gaze. Labyrinthine disorders cause vertigo and nystagmus, though nystagmus is also caused by a number of brainstem and cerebellar lesions.

Bibliography

Adelman M, Haponick EF, Bleecker ER, et al: Cryptogenic hemoptysis: Clinical features, bronchoscopic findings, and natural history in 67 patients. *Ann Intern Med* 102:829–834, 1985.

Adler SG, Cohen AH, Border WA: Hypersensitivity phenomena and the kidney: Role of drugs and environmental agents. *Am J Kidney Dis* 5:75–96, 1985.

Anderson RJ, Linas SL, Berns AS, et al: Nonoliguric acute renal failure. *N Engl J Med* 296:1134–1138, 1977.

Arbuthnott J, Bergdoll MS, Best GJ, et al (eds): International symposium on toxic shock syndrome. *Rev Infect Dis* 11 (suppl 1):S1–S333, 1989.

Arieff AI, Carroll HJ: Nonketotic hyperosmolar coma with hyperglycemia: Clinical features, pathophysiology, renal function, acid base balance, plasma-cerebrospinal fluid equilibria and the effects of therapy in 37 cases. *Medicine* 51:73–94, 1972.

Baloh RH, Honrubia V, Jacobson K: Benign positional vertigo: Clinical and oculographic features in 240 cases. *Neurology* 37:371–378, 1987.

Balow JE, Austin HA, Tsokos GC, et al: Lupus nephritis. *Ann Intern Med* 106:79–94, 1987.

Barnes PF, DeCock KM, Reynolds TN, et al: A comparison of amoebic and pyogenic abscess of the liver. *Medicine* 66:472–483, 1987.

Bishop JM: The molecular genetics of cancer. *Science* 235:305–311, 1987.

Bone RC, Fisher CJ Jr, Clemmer TP, et al: A controlled clinical trial of high-dose methylprednisolone in the treatment of severe sepsis and septic shock. *N Engl J Med* 317:653–658, 1987.

Bothwell TH, Charlton RW: A general approach to the problems of iron deficiency and iron overload in the population at large. *Semin Hematol* 19:54–69, 1982.

Bravo EL, Gifford RW: Pheochromocytoma: Diagnosis, localization and management. *N Engl J Med* 311:1298–1303, 1984.

Bray GA: Current status of intestinal bypass surgery in the treatment of obesity. *Diabetes* 26:1072–1079, 1977.

Broadus AE, Mangin M, Ikeda K, et al: Humoral hypercalcemia of cancer: Identification of a novel parathyroid hormone-like peptide. *N Engl J Med* 319:556–563, 1988.

Brownlee M, Vlassara H, Cerami A: Nonenzymatic glycosylation and the pathogenesis of diabetic complications. *Ann Intern Med* 101:527–537, 1984.

Byrne JJ, Moake JL: Thrombotic thrombocytopenic purpura and the hemolytic uremic syndrome: Evolving concepts of pathogenesis and therapy. *Baillieres Clin Haematol* 15:413–442, 1986.

Callahan N, Garrett A, Goggin T: Withdrawal of anticonvulsant drugs in patients free of seizures for two years: A prospective study. *N Engl J Med* 318:942–946, 1988.

Carmichael KA, Fallon MD, Dalinka M, et al: Osteomalacia and osteitis fibrosa in a man ingesting aluminum hydroxide antacid. *Am J Med* 76:1137–1143, 1984.

Carroll P, Matz R: Uncontrolled diabetes mellitus in adults: Experience in treating diabetic ketoacidosis and hyperosmolar treatment regimen. *Diabetes Care* 6:579–585, 1983.

Cello JP, Grendell JH, Crass RA, et al: Endoscopic sclerotherapy versus portacaval shunt in patients with severe cirrhosis and acute variceal hemorrhage. *N Engl J Med* 316:11–15, 1987.

Chaisson RE, Schecter GF, Thever CP, et al: Tuberculosis in patients with the acquired immunodeficiency syndrome. Clinical features, response to therapy and survival. *Am Rev Respir Dis* 136:570–574, 1987.

Charness ME, Simon RP, Greenberg DA, et al: Ethanol and the nervous system. *N Engl J Med* 321:442–454, 1989.

Chojkier M, Groszmann RJ, Atterbury CE, et al: A controlled comparison of continuous intra-arterial and intravenous infusions of vasopressin in hemorrhage from esophageal varices. *Gastroenterology* 77:540–546, 1979.

Chu KC, Smart CR, Tarone RE: Analysis of breast cancer mortality and stage distribution by age for the Health Insurance Plan clinical trial. *J Natl Cancer Inst* 80:1125–1132, 1988.

Cohn JN, Levine TB, Olvari MT, et al: Plasma norepinephrine as a guide to prognosis in patients with chronic congestive heart failure. *N Engl J Med* 311:819–823, 1984.

The CONSENSUS trial study group: Effects of enalapril on mortality in severe congestive heart failure: Results of the Cooperative North Scandinavian Enalapril Survival Study (CONSENSUS). *N Engl J Med* 316:1429–1435, 1987.

Coustan DR: Pregnancy in diabetic women. *N Engl J Med* 319:1663–1665, 1988.

Crawford ED, Eisenberger MA, McLeod DG, et al: A controlled trial of leuprolide with and without flutamide in prostatic carcinoma. *N Engl J Med* 321:419–424, 1989.

Crossley IR, Williams R: Spontaneous bacterial peritonitis. *Gut* 26:325–331, 1985.

Cryer PE, Binder C, Bolli GB: Hypoglycemia in IDDM. *Diabetes* 38:1193–1199, 1989.

Crystal RG, Bitterman PB, Rennard SF, et al: Interstitial lung diseases of unknown cause: Disorders characterized by chronic inflammation of the lower respiratory tract. *N Engl J Med* 310:154–166, 235–244, 1985.

Crystal RG, Brantley ML, Hubbard RC, et al: The alpha 1-antitrypsin gene and its mutations. Clinical consequences and strategies for therapy. *Chest* 95:196–208, 1989.

Curran JW, Jaffe HW, Hardy AM, et al: Epidemiology of HIV infection and AIDS in the United States. *Science* 239:610–616, 1988.

de Groat WC, Booth AM: Physiology of the urinary bladder and urethra. *Ann Intern Med* 92:312–315, 1980.

DeVita VT Jr. Hellmen S, Rosenberg SA: *Cancer: Principles and Practice of Oncology,* 3d ed. Philadelphia, Lippincott, 1989.

Dinarello CA, Cannon JG, Wolff SM: New concepts on the pathogenesis of fever. *Rev Infect Dis* 10:168–189, 1988.

Dooley CP, Cohen H: The clinical significance of *Campylobacter pylori. Ann Intern Med* 108:70–79, 1988.

Drew WL: Diagnosis of cytomegalovirus infection. *Rev Infect Dis* 10(S3):S468–S476, 1988.

Dyken PR: Subacute sclerosing panencephalitis. Current status. *Neurol Clin* 3:179–196, 1985.

Early Breast Cancer Trialists' Collaborative Group: Effects of adjuvant tamoxifen and of cytotoxic therapy on mortality in early breast cancer: An overview of 61 randomized trials among 28,896 women. *N Engl J Med* 319:1681–1692, 1988.

Eschback JW, Egrie JC, Downing MR, et al: Correction of the anemia of end-stage renal disease with recombinant human erythropoietin: Results of a combined Phase I and II clinical trial. *N Engl J Med* 316:73–78, 1987.

The Expert Panel: Report of the National Cholesterol Education Program Expert Panel on Detection, Evaluation and Treatment of High Blood Cholesterol in Adults. *Arch Intern Med* 148:36–69, 1988.

Fauci AS, Haynes BF, Katz P, et al: Wegener's granulomatosis: Prospective clinical and therapeutic experience with patients for 21 years. *Ann Intern Med* 98:76–85, 1983.

Feldman JM: Carcinoid tumors and syndrome. *Semin Oncol* 14:237–246, 1987.

Felig P, Baxter JD, Broadus AE, et al (eds): *Endocrinology and Metabolism,* 2d ed. New York, McGraw-Hill, 1987.

Ferner RE, Neil HA: Sulphonylureas and hypoglycaemia. *BMJ* 296:949–950, 1988.

Fischel MA, Richman DD, Grieco MH, et al: The efficacy of azidothymidine (AZT) in the treatment of patients with AIDS and AIDS-related complex: A double-blind, placebo-controlled trial. *N Engl J Med* 317:185–191, 1987.

Fisher CM: Lacunar strokes and infarcts: A review. *Neurology* 32:871–876, 1982.

Fitzpatrick TB, Eisen AZ, Wolff K, et al (eds): *Dermatology in General Medicine,* 3d ed. New York, McGraw-Hill, 1987.

Flier JS, Scully RE: Case records of the Massachusetts General Hospital (case 25-1982: Amenorrhea, virilization, and hyperpigmentation in a 15-year-old girl). *N Engl J Med* 306:1537–1544, 1982.

Foster DW, McGarry JD: The metabolic derangements and treatment of diabetic ketoacidosis. *N Engl J Med* 309:159–169, 1983.

Fox RI, Howell FV, Bone RC, et al: Primary Sjögren syndrome: Clinical and immunopathologic features. *Semin Arthritis Rheum* 14:77–105, 1984.

Fung CY, Garnick MB: Clinical Stage I carcinoma of the testis: A review. *J Clin Oncol* 6:734–750, 1988.

Gabuzda DH, Hirsch MS: Neurologic manifestations of infection with human immunodeficiency virus. Clinical features and pathogenesis. *Ann Intern Med* 107:383–391, 1987.

Girardin E, Grau GE, Dayer JM, et al: Tumor necrosis factor and interleukin-1 in the serum of children with severe infectious purpura. *N Engl J Med* 319:397–400, 1988.

Goldenberg DL, Reed JI: Bacterial arthritis. *N Engl J Med* 312:764–771, 1985.

Golomb HM: Treatment of hairy cell leukemia. *Blood* 69:979–983, 1987.

Greenberger PA, Patterson R: Allergic bronchopulmonary aspergillosis. Model of bronchopulmonary disease with defined serologic, radiologic, pathological and clinical findings from asthma to fatal destructive lung diseases. *Chest* 91(S6):165S–171S, 1987.

Haber DA, Mayer RJ: Primary gastrointestinal lymphoma. *Semin Oncol* 15:154–169, 1988.

Hainer BL: Cat-scratch disease. *J Fam Pract* 25:497–503, 1987.

Harrison LC, Campbell IL, Allison J, et al: MHC molecules and beta-cell destruction. Immune and nonimmune disorders. *Diabetes* 38:815–818, 1989.

Havel RJ: Lowering cholesterol, 1988. Rationale, mechanisms, and means. *J Clin Invest* 81:1653–1660, 1988.

Henderson ES, Lister TA (eds): *Leukemia,* 5th ed. Philadelphia, Saunders, 1990.

Hochberg FH, Miller DC: Primary central nervous system lymphoma. *J Neurosurg* 68:835–853, 1988.

Hollenberg NK: The treatment of renovascular hypertension: Surgery, angioplasty and medical therapy with converting enzyme inhibitors. *Am J Kidney Dis* 10(S1):52–60, 1987.

Hook EH, Holmes KK: Gonococcal infections. *Ann Intern Med* 102:229–243, 1985.

Jacobs RL, Freedman PM, Boswell RN: Nonallergic rhinitis with eosinophilia (NARES syndrome). Clinical and immunologic presentation. *J Allergy Clin Immunol* 67:253–262, 1981.

Jandl JH: *Blood—A Textbook of Hematology.* Boston, Little, Brown, 1987.

Jarcho JA, McKenna W, Pare JAP, et al: Mapping a gene for familial hypertrophic cardiomyopathy to chromosome 14q1. *N Engl J Med* 321:1372–1378, 1989.

Jordon RM, Kendall JW, Kerber CW: The primary empty sella syndrome: Analysis of the clinical characteristics, radiographic features, pituitary function and cerebrospinal fluid adenohypophyseal hormone concentrations. *Am J Med* 62:569–580, 1977.

Judd HL, Meldrum DR, Deftos LJ, et al: Estrogen replacement: Indications and complications. *Ann Intern Med* 98:195–205, 1983.

Kahn CR, White MF: The insulin receptor and the molecular mechanism of insulin action. *J Clin Invest* 82:1151–1156, 1988.

Keinath RD, Merrell DE, Vlietstra R, et al: Antibiotic treatment and relapse in Whipple's disease. Long-term follow-up of 88 patients. *Gastroenterology* 88:1867–1873, 1985.

Kelly WN, Harris ED Jr, Ruddy S, Sledge CB: *Textbook of Rheumatology.* Philadelphia, Saunders, 1989.

Kitabchi AE: Low-dose insulin therapy in diabetic ketoacidosis: Fact or fiction? *Diabetes Metab Rev* 5:337–363, 1989.

Kitchens CS, Van Mierop LHS: Envenomation by the Eastern coral snake (*Micrurus fulvius*): A study of 39 victims. *JAMA* 258:1615–1618, 1987.

Koeffler A, Friedler RM, Massry SG: Acute renal failure due to non-traumatic rhabdomyolysis. *Ann Intern Med* 85:23–28, 1976.

Koenig M, Hoffman EP, Bertelson CJ, et al: Complete cloning of the Duchenne muscular dystrophy (DMD) cDNA and preliminary genomic organization of the DMD gene in normal and affected individuals. *Cell* 50:509–517, 1987.

Korman N: Pemphigus. *J Am Acad Dermatol* 18:1219–1238, 1988.

Krockta WP, Barnes WC: Sexually transmitted diseases. Genital ulceration with regional adenopathy. *Infect Dis Clin North Am* 1:217–233, 1987.

Kurtz AB, Nabarro JN: Circulating insulin-binding antibodies. *Diabetologia* 19:329–334, 1980.

Kyle RA: Monoclonal gammopathy of undetermined significance: Natural history in 241 cases. *Am J Med* 64:814–826, 1978.

Lawly TJ, Bielory L, Gascon P, et al: A prospective clinical and immunologic analysis of patients with serum sickness. *N Engl J Med* 311:1407–1413, 1984.

Lebel MH, Freij BJ, Syrogiannopoulus GA, et al: Dexamethasone therapy for bacterial meningitis: Results of two double-blind, placebo control trials. *N Engl J Med* 319:964–971, 1988.

Lee GR: The anemia of chronic disease. *Semin Hematol* 20:61–80, 1983.

Malech HL, Gallin JI: Neutrophils in human diseases. *N Engl J Med* 317:687–694, 1987.

Martin JB, Gusella JF: Huntington's disease: Pathogenesis and management. *N Engl J Med* 315:1267–1276, 1986.

Meyers JD: Management of cytomegalovirus infections. *Am J Med* 85(2A):102–106, 1988.

Michet CJ, McKenna CH, Luthra HS, et al: Relapsing polychondritis: Survival and predictive role of early disease manifestations. *Ann Intern Med* 104:74–78, 1986.

Moylan JA, Evanson MA: Diagnosis and treatment of fat embolism. *Ann Rev Med* 28:85–90, 1977.

Muller JE, Rude RE, Braunwald EB, et al: Myocardial infarct extension: Occurrence, outcome, and risk factors in the multicenter investigation of limitation of infarct size. *Ann Intern Med* 108:1–6, 1988.

Narins RG, Jones ER, Stom MC, et al: Diagnostic strategies in disorders of fluid, electrolyte, and acid-base homeostasis. *Am J Med* 72:496–520, 1982.

Neu H: Ciprofloxacin: A major advance in quinolone chemotherapy. *Am J Med* 82(4A):1, 1987.

O'Grady JG, Williams R: Present position of liver transplantation and its impact on hepatological practice. *Gut* 29:560–570, 1988.

Olefsky JM, Kolterman OG, Scarlett JA: Insulin action and resistance in obesity and noninsulin-dependent type II diabetes mellitus. *Am J Physiol* 243:E15–E30, 1982.

Peppercorn MA: Sulfasalazine: Pharmacology, clinical use, toxicity and related new drug development. *Ann Intern Med* 101:377–386, 1984.

Pinals RS: Sulfasalazine in the rheumatic diseases. *Semin Arthritis Rheum* 17:246–259, 1988.

Pizzo PA, Commers J, Cotton D, et al: Approaching the controversies in antibacterial management of cancer patients. *Am J Med* 76:436–449, 1984.

Raffin TA: ARDS: Mechanisms and management. *Hosp Pract* 22 (Nov 15):65–80, 1987.

Ranshoff DF, Gracie WA: Assessment of prophylactic cholecystectomy and medical therapy for diabetics with silent gallstones. *Gastroenterology* 92:1588, 1987.

Reeders ST, Bruening MH, Davies KE, et al: A highly polymorphic DNA marker linked to adult polycystic kidney disease in chromosome 16. *Nature* 317:542–544, 1985.

Revler JB, Broudy VC, Cooney TG: Adult scurvy. *JAMA* 253:805–807, 1985.

Rich S: Primary pulmonary hypertension. *Prog Cardiovasc Dis* 31:205–238, 1988.

Rigel DS, Rivers JK, Koff AW, et al: Dysplastic nevi: Markers for increased risk from melanoma. *Cancer* 63:386–389, 1989.

Riordan JR, Rommens JM, Keren B, et al: Identification of the cystic fibrosis gene: Cloning and characterization of complementary DNA. *Science* 245:1066–1073, 1989.

Rojeski MT, Gharib H: Nodular thyroid disease: Evaluation and management. *N Engl J Med* 313:428–436, 1985.

Rosen FS, Cooper MD, Wedgewood RJP: The primary immunodeficiencies. *N Engl J Med* 311:235–242, 300–310, 1986.

Rosse WF, Parker CJ: Paroxysmal nocturnal hemoglobinuria. *Clin Haematol* 14:105–125, 1985.

Royer HD, Reinherz EL: Lymphocytes: Ontogeny, function and relevance to clinical disorders. *N Engl J Med* 317:1171, 1987.

Ryan EA, Reiss E: Oncogenous osteomalacia: Review of the world literature of 42 cases and report of two new cases. *Am J Med* 77:501–512, 1984.

Safian RD, Berman AP, Diver DJ, et al: Balloon aortic valvuloplasty in 170 consecutive patients. *N Engl J Med* 319:125–130, 1988.

Saudek CD, Felig P: The metabolic effects of starvation. *Am J Med* 60:117–126, 1976.

Schaefer EJ, Levy RI: Pathogenesis and management of lipoprotein disorders. *N Engl J Med* 312:1300–1310, 1985.

Schilsky RL: Renal and metabolic toxicities of cancer chemotherapy. *Semin Oncol* 9:75–83, 1982.

Schreiber AD: Paroxysmal nocturnal hemoglobinuria revisited. *N Engl J Med* 309:723–725, 1983.

Scriver CR, Baudet AL, Sly WS, et al (eds): *The Metabolic Basis of Inherited Disease,* 6th ed. New York, McGraw-Hill, 1989.

Seifter EJ, Ihde DC: Therapy of small cell lung cancer: A perspective on two decades of clinical research. *Semin Oncol* 15:278–299, 1988.

Sherrard DJ: Renal osteodystrophy. *Semin Nephrol* 12:56–67, 1988.

Shiau YF, Feldman GM, Resnick MA, et al: Stool electrolyte and osmolality measurements in the evaluation of diarrheal disorders. *Ann Intern Med* 102:773–775, 1985.

Slamon DJ, Godolphin W, Jones CA, et al: Studies of the HER-2/neu proto-oncogene in human breast and ovarian cancer. *Science* 244:707–712, 1989.

Snyder PJ: Gonadotroph cell adenomas of the pituitary. *Endocr Rev* 6:552–563, 1985.

Steere AC: Lyme disease. *N Engl J Med* 321:586–596, 1989.

Stunkard AJ, Sorensen TIA, Hanis C, et al: An adoption study of human obesity. *N Engl J Med* 314:193–198, 1986.

Summers RW, Switz DM, Sessions JT Jr, et al: National Cooperative Crohn's Disease Study: Results of drug treatment. *Gastroenterology* 77:847–869, 1979.

Tandan R, Bradley WG: Amyotrophic lateral sclerosis: Part I. Clinical features, pathology, and ethical issues in management. *Ann Neurol* 18:271–280, 1985.

Thawley SE: Surgical treatment of obstructive sleep apnea. *Med Clin North Am* 69:1337–1358, 1985.

The TIMI Study Group: Comparison of invasive and conservative strategies after treatment with intravenous tissue plasminogen activator in acute myocardial infarction: Results of the thrombolysis in myocardial infarction (TIMI) phase II trial. *N Engl J Med* 320:618–627, 1989.

Toronto Lung Transplant Group: Experience with single lung transplantation for pulmonary fibrosis. *JAMA* 259:2258–2262, 1988.

Trotman IF, Misiewicz JJ: Sigmoid motility in diverticular disease and the irritable bowel syndrome. *Gut* 29:218–222, 1988.

Ursing B, Alm T, Bergelin I, et al: A comparative study of metronidazole and sulfasalazine for active Crohn's disease: The cooperative Crohn's disease study in Sweden II. *Gastroenterology* 83:550–562, 1982.

Vanhoutte PM, Shimokawa H: Endothelium-derived relaxing factor and coronary vasospasm. *Circulation* 80:1–9, 1989.

Vogelstein B, Fearon ER, Hamilton SR, et al: Genetic alterations during colorectal-tumor development. *N Engl J Med* 319:525–532, 1988.

Wilson JD, Braunwald E, Isselbacher KJ, et al (eds): *Harrison's Principles of Internal Medicine,* 12th ed. New York, McGraw-Hill, 1990.

Wilson JD, Foster DW (eds): *Williams' Textbook of Endocrinology,* 7th ed. Philadelphia, Saunders, 1985.

Young GA, Vincent PC: Drug-induced agranulocytosis. *Clin Haematol* 9:483–504, 1980.

APPENDIX   LABORATORY VALUES OF CLINICAL IMPORTANCE

INTRODUCTORY COMMENTS

In preparing the Appendix, the editors have taken into account the fact that the system of international units (SI, système international d'unités) is now used in most countries and in virtually all medical and scientific journals including those in the United States.[1] However, many or most clinical laboratories in the United States continue to report values in traditional units. Therefore, in this book we utilize both systems for the Appendix and for the text itself. Values in SI units appear first, and *traditional units appear in parentheses* after the SI units. This dual approach is also used for the large part in the text. In those instances in which the numbers remain the same but only the terminology is changed (mmol/L for meq/L or IU/L for mIU/mL) only the SI units are given. In all other instances the SI unit is followed by the traditional unit in parentheses. The SI base units, SI derived units, other units of measure referred to in the Appendix, and SI prefixes are listed in Tables A-1 to A-3 at the end of the Appendix. Conversions from one system to another can be made as follows:

$$mmol/L = \frac{mg/dL \times 10}{atomic\ weight}$$

$$mg/dL = \frac{mmol/L \times atomic\ weight}{10}$$

BODY FLUIDS AND OTHER MASS DATA

Body fluid, total volume: 50 percent (in obese) to 70 percent (lean) of body weight
   Intracellular: 0.3–0.4 of body weight
   Extracellular: 0.2–0.3 of body weight
Blood:
   Total volume:
      Males: 69 mL per kg body weight
      Females: 65 mL per kg body weight
   Plasma volume:
      Males: 39 mL per kg body weight
      Females: 40 mL per kg body weight
   Red blood cell volume:
      Males: 30 mL per kg body weight (1.15–1.21 L/m² body surface area)
      Females: 25 mL per kg body weight (0.95–1.00 L/m² body surface area)

[1] Young DS: Implementation of SI Units for Clinical Laboratory Data. Ann Intern Med 106:114, 1987

[2] Since cerebrospinal fluid concentrations are equilibrium values, measurements of the same parameters in blood plasma obtained at the same time is recommended. However, there is a time lag in attainment of equilibrium, and cerebrospinal levels of plasma constituents that can fluctuate rapidly (such as plasma glucose) may not achieve stable values until after a significant lag phase.

CEREBROSPINAL FLUID[2]

		Conversion factor (CF) (C × CF = SI)
Osmolality	292–297 mosmol/kg (292–297 mosmol/L)	—
Electrolytes:		
Sodium	137–145 mmol/L (137–145 meq/L)	—
Potassium	2.7–3.9 mmol/L (2.7–3.9 meq/L)	—
Calcium	1–1.5 mmol/L (2.1–3.0 meq/L)	0.5
Magnesium	1–1.2 mmol/L (2.0–2.5 meq/L)	0.5
Chloride	116–122 mmol/L (116–122 meq/L)	—
CO_2 content	20–24 mmol/L (20–24 meq/L)	—
P_{CO_2}	6–7 kPa (45–49 mmHg)	0.1333
pH	7.31–7.34	—
Glucose	2.2–3.9 mmol/L (40–70 mg/dL)	0.05551
Lactate	1–2 mmol/L (10–20 mg/dL)	0.1110
Total protein:	0.2–0.4 g/L (20–40 mg/dL)	0.01
Prealbumin	2–6 percent	—
Albumin	56–75 percent	—
Alpha$_1$ globulin	2–7 percent	—
Alpha$_2$ globulin	4–12 percent	—
Beta globulin	8–16 percent	—
Gamma globulin	3–12 percent	—
IgG	0.01–0.014 g/L (1–1.4 mg/dL)	0.01
IgA	0.001–0.003 g/L (0.1–0.3 mg/dL)	0.01
IgM	0.0001–0.00012 g/L (0.01–0.012 mg/dL)	0.01
Ammonia	15–47 μmol/L (25–80 μg/dL)	0.5872
Creatinine	44–168 μmol/L (0.5–1.9 mg/dL)	88.40
Myelin basic protein	<4 μg/L	—
CSF pressure	50–180 mmH₂O	—
CSF volume (adult)	100–160 mL	—
Leukocytes:		
Total	<4 per mL	—
Differential:		
Lymphocytes	60–70 percent	—
Monocytes	30–50 percent	—
Neutrophils	1–3 percent	—

CHEMICAL CONSTITUENTS OF BLOOD

See also "Function Tests," especially "Metabolic and Endocrine."

	Conversion factor (CF) (C × CF = SI)
Acetoacetate, plasma: <100 μmol/L (<1 mg/dL)	97.95
Albumin, serum: 35–55 g/L (3.5–5.5 g/dL)	10
Aldolase: 0–100 nkat/L (0–6 U/L)	16.67
Alpha₁ antitrypsin, serum: 0.8–2.1 g/L (85–213 mg/dL)	0.01
Alpha fetoprotein (adult), serum: <30 μg/L (<30 ng/mL)	—
Aminotransferases, serum:	
Aspartate (AST, SGOT): 0–0.58 μkat/L (0–35 U/L)	0.01667
Alanine (ALT, SGPT): 0–0.58 μkat/L (0–35 U/L)	0.01667
Ammonia, whole blood, venous: 47–65 μmol/L (80–110 μg/dL)	0.5872
Amylase, serum: 0.8–3.2 μkat/L (60–180 U/L)	0.01667
Arterial blood gases:	
[HCO₃⁻]: 21–28 mmol/L (21–28 meq/L)	—
P_{CO₂}: 4.7–5.9 kPa (35–45 mmHg)	0.1333
pH: 7.38–7.44	—
P_{O₂}: 11–13 kPa (80–100 mmHg)	0.1333
Ascorbic acid (vitamin C), serum: 23–57 μmol/L (0.4–1.0 mg/dL)	56.78
Barbiturates, serum: normal, nondetectable	
Phenobarbital, "potentially fatal" level: approximately 390 μmol/L (9 mg/dL)	43.06
Most short-acting barbiturates, "potentially fatal" levels: approximately 150 μmol/L (35 mg/L)	4.419
Base, total, serum: 145–155 mmol/L (145–155 meq/L)	—
β-Hydroxybutyrate, plasma: <300 μmol/L (<3 mg/dL)	96.05
Bilirubin, total, serum (Malloy-Evelyn): 5.1–17 μmol/L (0.3–1.0 mg/dL)	17.10
Direct, serum: 1.7–5.1 μmol/L (0.1–0.3 mg/dL)	17.10
Indirect, serum: 3.4–12 μmol/L (0.2–0.7 mg/dL)	17.10
Bromides, serum: nondetectable	
Toxic levels: >17 mmol/L (>17 meq/L)	—
Bromsulphalein, BSP (5 mg per kg body weight, intravenously): 5 percent or less retention after 45 min	—
Calciferols (vitamin D), plasma:	
1,25-dihydroxyvitamin D [1,25(OH)₂D]: 5–14 nmol/L (20–60 pg/mL)	0.2400
25-hydroxyvitamin D [25(OH)D]: 20–100 nmol/L (8–42 ng/mL)	2.496
Calcium, ionized: 1.1–1.4 mmol/L (2.3–2.8 meq/L; 4.5–5.6 mg/dL)	0.2495
Calcium, plasma: 2.2–2.6 mmol/L (9–10.5 mg/dL)	0.2495
Carbon dioxide content, plasma (sea level): 21–30 mmol/L (21–30 meq/L)	—
Carbon dioxide tension (P_{CO₂}), arterial blood (sea level): 4.7–6.0 kPa (35–45 mmHg)	0.1333
Carbon monoxide content, blood: symptoms with over 20 percent saturation of hemoglobin	
Carotenoids, serum: 0.9–5.6 μmol/L (50–300 μg/dL)	0.01863
Ceruloplasmin, serum: 270–370 mg/L (27–37 mg/dL)	10
Chlorides, serum (as Cl⁻): 98–106 mmol/L (98–106 meq/L)	—
Cholesterol: see Table A-4	
Complement, serum:	
C3: 0.55–1.20 g/L (55–120 mg/dL)	0.01
C4: 0.20–0.50 g/L (20–50 mg/dL)	0.01

	Conversion factor (CF) (C × CF = SI)
Copper, serum: 11–22 μmol/L (70–140 μg/dL)	0.1574
Creatine phosphokinase, serum (total):	
Females: 0.17–1.17 μkat/L (10–70 U/L)	0.01667
Males: 0.42–1.50 μkat/L (25–90 U/L)	0.01667
Creatinine, serum: <133 μmol/L (<1.5 mg/dL)	88.40
Digoxin serum:	
Therapeutic level: 0.6–2.8 nmol/L (0.5–2.2 ng/mL)	1.281
Toxic level: >3.1 nmol/L (>2.4 ng/mL)	1.281
Ethanol, blood:	
Mild to moderate intoxication: 17–43 mmol/L (80–200 mg/dL)	0.2171
Marked intoxication: 54–87 mmol/L (250–400 mg/dL)	0.2171
Severe intoxication: >87 mmol/L (>400 mg/dL)	0.2171
Fatty acids, free (nonesterified), plasma: <180 mg/L (<18 mg/dL)	10
Ferritin, serum: 15–200 μg/L (15–200 ng/mL)	—
Fibrinogen, plasma: see "Platelets and Coagulation"	—
Fibrinogen split products: see "Platelets and Coagulation"	—
Folic acid, red cell: 340–1020 nmol/L cells (150–450 ng/mL cells)	2.266
Gastrin, serum: 40–200 ng/L (40–200 pg/mL)	—
Globulins, serum: 20–30 g/L (2.0–3.0 g/dL)	10
Glucose (fasting), plasma:	
Normal: 4.2–6.4 mmol/L (75–115 mg/dL)	0.05551
Diabetes mellitus: >7.8 mmol/L [>140 mg/dL (on more than one occasion)]	0.05551
Glucose, 2 h postprandial, plasma:	
Normal: <7.8 mmol/L (<140 mg/dL)	0.05551
Impaired glucose tolerance: 7.8–11.1 mmol/L (140–200 mg/dL)	0.05551
Diabetes mellitus: >11.1 mmol/L on more than one occasion (>200 mg/dL)	0.05551
Hemoglobin, blood (sea level):	
Male: 140–180 g/L (14–18 g/dL)	10
Female: 120–160 g/L (12–16 g/dL)	10
Hemoglobin A₁c: up to 6 percent of total hemoglobin	—
Immunoglobulins, serum:	
IgA: 0.9–3.2 g/L (90–325 mg/dL)	0.01
IgD: 0–0.08 g/L (0–8 mg/dL)	0.01
IgE: <0.00025 g/L (<0.025 mg/dL)	0.01
IgG: 8.0–15.0 g/L (800–1500 mg/dL)	0.01
IgM: 0.45–1.5 g/L (45–150 mg/dL)	0.01
Iron, serum: 14–32 μmol/L (80–180 μg/dL)	0.1791
Iron-binding capacity, serum: 45–82 μmol/L (250–460 μg/dL)	0.1791
Saturation: 0.2–0.45 (20–45 percent)	
Lactate dehydrogenase, serum:	
200–450 units/mL (Wrobleski)	—
60–100 units/mL (Wacker)	—
0.4–1.7 μkat/L (25–100 units/L)	0.01667
Lactic dehydrogenase isoenzymes, serum (agarose):	
Fraction 1 (of total): 0.14–0.25 (14–26 percent)	0.01
Fraction 2: 0.29–0.39 (29–39 percent)	0.01
Fraction 3: 0.20–0.25 (20–26 percent)	0.01
Fraction 4: 0.08–0.16 (8–16 percent)	0.01
Fraction 5: 0.06–0.16 (6–16 percent)	0.01
Lactate, venous plasma: 0.6–1.7 mmol/L (5–15 mg/dL)	0.1110
Lead, serum: <1.0 μmol/L (<20 μg/dL)	0.04826
Lipids: see Table A-4	—
Lipids, triglyceride, serum: see "Triglycerides"	

	Conversion factor (CF) (C × CF = SI)
Lipoprotein: see Table A-4	—
Lithium, serum:	
Therapeutic level: 0.6–1.2 mmol/L (0.6–1.2 meq/L)	—
Toxic level: >2 mmol/L (>2 meq/L)	—
Magnesium, serum: 0.8–1.2 mmol/L (2–3 mg/dL)	0.4114
Osmolality, plasma: 285–295 mosmol per kg serum water	—
Oxygen content:	
Arterial blood (sea level): 17–21 volume percent	—
Venous blood, arm (sea level): 10 to 16 volume percent	—
Oxygen percent saturation (sea level):	
Arterial blood: 0.97 mol/mol (97 percent)	0.01
Venous blood, arm: 0.60–0.85 mol/mol (60–85 percent)	0.01
Oxygen tension (P_{O_2}) blood: 11–13 kPa (80–100 mmHg)	0.1333
pH, blood: 7.38–7.44	—
Phenytoin, plasma:	
Therapeutic level: 40–80 μmol/L (10–20 mg/L)	3.964
Toxic level: >120 μmol/L (>30 mg/L)	3.964
Phosphorus, inorganic, serum: 1.0–1.4 mmol/L (3–4.5 mg/dL)	0.3229
Potassium, serum: 3.5–5.0 mmol/L (3.5–5.0 meq/L)	—
Proteins, total, serum: 55–80 g/L (5.5–8.0 g/dL)	10
Protein fractions, serum:	
Albumin: 35–55 g/L [3.5–5.5 g/dL (50–60 percent)]	10
Globulin: 20–35 g/L [2.0–3.5 g/dL (40–50 percent)]	10
Alpha$_1$: 2–4 g/L [0.2–0.4 g/dL (4.2–7.2 percent)]	10
Alpha$_2$: 5–9 g/L [0.5–0.9 g/dL (6.8–12 percent)]	10
Beta: 6–11 g/L [0.6–1.1 g/dL (9.3–15 percent)]	10
Gamma: 7–17 g/L [0.7–1.7 g/dL (13–23 percent)]	10
Pyruvate, venous, plasma: 60–170 μmol/L (0.5–1.5 mg/dL)	113.6
Quinidine, serum:	
Therapeutic range: 4.6–9.2 μmol/L (1.5–3 mg/L)	3.082
Toxic range: 15.4–18.5 μmol/L (5–6 mg/L)	3.082
Salicylate, plasma: 0 mmol/L	—
Therapeutic range: 1.4–1.8 mmol/L (20–25 mg/dL)	0.07240
Toxic range: >2.2 mmol/L (>30 mg/dL)	0.07240
Sodium, serum: 136–145 mmol/L (136–145 meq/L)	—
Steroids: see "Metabolic and Endocrine" under "Function Tests"	—
Triglycerides: <1.8 mmol/L (<160 mg/dL)	0.01129
Urea nitrogen, serum: 3.6–7.1 mmol/L (10–20 mg/dL)	0.3570
Uric acid, serum:	
Men: 150–480 μmol/L (2.5–8.0 mg/dL)	59.48
Women: 90–360 μmol/L (1.5–6.0 mg/dL)	59.48
Vitamin A, serum: 0.7–3.5 μmol/L (20–100 μg/dL)	0.03491
Vitamin B$_{12}$, serum: 148–443 pmol/L (200–600 pg/mL)	0.7378
Zinc, serum: 11.5–18.5 μmol/L (75–120 μg/dL)	0.1530

FUNCTION TESTS

Circulation

Arteriovenous oxygen difference: 30–50 mL/L
Cardiac output (Fick): 2.5–3.6 L/m² body surface area per min

	Conversion factor (CF) (C × CF = SI)
Contractility indexes:	
Maximum left ventricular dp/dt: 1650 ± 300 mmHg/s	
Maximum $(dp/dt)/p$: 44 ± 8.4 s^{-1}	
(dp/dt)/DP at DP = 40 mmHg: 37.6 ± 12.2 s^{-1} (DP = diastolic press.)	
Mean normalized systolic ejection rate (angiography): 3.32 ± 0.84 end-diastolic volumes per second	
Mean velocity of circumferential fiber shortening (angiography) 1.66 ± 0.42 circumferences per second	
Ejection fraction, stroke volume/end-diastolic volume (SV/EDV):	
Normal range: 0.55–0.78; average: 0.67	
End-diastolic volume: 75 ± 15 mL/m²	
End-systolic volume: 25 ± 8 mL/m²	
Left ventricular work:	
Stroke work index: 30–110 (g·m)/m²	
Left ventricular minute work index: 1.8–6.6 [(kg · m)/m²]/min	
Oxygen consumption index: 110–150 mL	
Pressures, intracardiac and intraarterial: see Table A-5	
Pulmonary vascular resistance: 2–12 (kPa·s)/L [20–120 (dyn·s)/cm⁵]	
Systemic vascular resistance: 77–150 (kPa·s)/L [770–1500 (dyn·s)/cm⁵]	
Systolic time intervals: see Table A-6	

Gastrointestinal See also "Stool."

Absorption tests:
  D-Xylose absorption test: After an overnight fast, 25 g xylose is given in aqueous solution by mouth. Urine collected for the following 5 h should contain 33–53 mmol (5–8 g) (or >20 percent of ingested dose). Serum xylose should be 1.7–2.7 mmol/L 1 h after the oral dose (25–40 mg per 100 mL).
  Vitamin A absorption test: A fasting blood specimen is obtained and 200,000 units of vitamin A in oil is given by mouth. Serum vitamin A levels should rise to twice fasting level in 3–5 h.

Bentiromide test (pancreatic function): 500 mg bentiromide (chymex) orally; p-aminobenzoic acid (PABA) measured in plasma and/or urine
  Plasma: >3.6(±1.1) mg/L at 90 min
  Urine: >50 percent recovered as PABA in 6 h

Gastric juice:

	Conversion factor (CF) (C × CF = SI)
Volume:	
24 h: 2–3 L	
Nocturnal: 600–700 mL	
Basal, fasting: 30–70 mL/h	
Reaction:	
pH: 1.6–1.8	
Titratable acidity of fasting juice: 4–9 μmol/s (15–35 meq/h)	0.261
Acid output:	
Basal:	
Females (mean ± 1 SD): 0.6 ± 0.5 μmol/s (2.0 ± 1.8 meq/h)	0.2778
Males (mean ± 1 SD): 0.8 ± 0.6 μmol/s (3.0 ± 2.0 meq/h)	0.2778
Maximal (after subcutaneous histamine acid phosphate 0.004 mg/kg body weight and preceded by 50 mg promethazine or after betazole 1.7 mg/kg body weight or pentagastrin 6 μg/kg body weight):	
Females (mean ± 1 SD): 4.4 ± 1.4 μmol/s (16 ± 5 meq/h)	0.2778
Males (mean ± 1 SD): 6.4 ± 1.4 μmol/s (23 ± 5 meq/h)	0.2778
Basal acid output/maximal acid output ratio: 0.6 or less	

	Conversion factor (CF) (C × CF = SI)

Gastrin, serum: 40–200 ng/L (40–200 pg/mL) — —

Secretin test (pancreatic exocrine function): 1 unit per kg body weight, intravenously

  Volume (pancreatic juice): >2.0 mL/kg in 80 min — —

  Bicarbonate concentration: >80 mmol/L (>80 meq/L) — —

  Bicarbonate output: >10 mmol in 30 min (>10 meq in 30 min) — —

Metabolic and endocrine

Adrenocorticotropin (ACTH) plasma, 8 A.M.: <18 pmol/L (<80 pg/mL) — 0.2202

Adrenal cortex function tests: see Chap. 317 — —

Adrenal medulla function tests: see Chap. 318 — —

Adrenal steroids, plasma:

  Aldosterone, 8 A.M.: <220 pmol/L (patient supine, 100 meq Na and 60–100 meq K intake) (<8 ng/dL) — 27.74

  Cortisol:

    8 A.M.: 140–690 nmol/L (5–25 μg/dL) — 27.59

    4 P.M.: 80–330 nmol/L (3–12 μg/dL) — 27.59

  Dehydroepiandrosterone (DHEA): 7–31 nmol/L (2–9 μg/L) — 3.467

  Dehydroepiandrosterone sulfate (DHEA sulfate): 1.3–6.7 μmol/L (500–2500 μg/L) — 0.002714

  11-Deoxycortisol (compound S): <30 nmol/L (<1 μg/dL) — 28.86

  17-Hydroxyprogesterone:

    Women: follicular phase, 0.6–3 nmol/L (0.20–1 μg/L); luteal phase, 1.5–10.6 nmol/L (0.5–3.5 μg/L) — 3.026

    Men: 0.2–9 nmol/L (0.06–3 μg/L) — 3.026

Adrenal steroids, urinary excretion:

  Aldosterone: 14–53 nmol/d (5–19 μg/d) — 2.774

  Cortisol, free: 55–275 nmol/d (20–100 μg/d) — 2.759

  17-Hydroxycorticosteroids: 5.5–28 μmol/d (2–10 mg/d) — 2.759

  17-Ketosteroids:

    Men: 24–88 μmol/d (7–25 mg/d) — 3.467

    Women: 14–52 μmol/d (4–15 mg/d) — 3.467

Angiotensin II, plasma, 8 A.M.: 10–30 nmol/L (10–30 pg/mL) — —

Arginine vasopressin (AVP), plasma:

  Random fluid intake: 2.3–7.4 pmol/L (2.5–8 ng/L) — 0.92

Calcitonin, plasma: <50 ng/L (<50 pg/mL) — —

Catecholamines, urinary excretion:

  Free catecholamines: <590 nmol/d (<100 μg/d) — 5.911

  Epinephrine: <275 nmol/d (<50 μg/d) — 5.458

  Metanephrines: <7 μmol/d (<1.3 mg/d) — 5.458

  Vanillylmandelic acid (VMA): <40 μmol/d (<8 mg/d) — 5.046

Glucagon, plasma: 50–100 ng/L (50–100 pg/mL) — —

Gonadal function tests: see Chaps. 321 and 322 — —

Gonadal steroids, plasma:

  Androstenedione:

    Women: 3.5–7.0 nmol/L (1–2 ng/ml) — 3.492

    Men: 3.0–5.0 mmol/L (0.8–1.3 ng/ml) — 3.492

  Estradiol:

    Women: 70–220 pmol/L (20–60 pg/mL), higher at ovulation — 3.671

    Men: <180 pmol/L (<50 pg/mL) — 3.671

  Progesterone:

    Men, prepubertal girls, preovulatory women, and postmenopausal women: <6 nmol/L (2 ng/mL) — 3.180

    Women, luteal, peak: >16 nmol/L (>5 ng/mL) — 3.180

Testosterone:

  Women: <3.5 nmol/L (<1 ng/mL) — 3.467

  Men: 10–35 nmol/L (3–10 ng/mL) — 3.467

  Prepubertal boys and girls: 0.17–0.7 nmol/L (0.05–0.2 ng/mL) — 3.467

Gonadotropins, plasma:

  Women, mature, premenopausal, except at ovulation:

    FSH: 5–20 IU/L (5–20 mIU/mL) — —

    LH: 5–25 IU/L (5–25 mIU/mL) — —

  Ovulatory surge:

    FSH: 12–30 IU/L (12–30 mIU/mL) — —

    LH: 25–100 IU/L (25–100 mIU/mL) — —

  Postmenopausal women:

    FSH: >12–30 IU/L (>12–30 mIU/mL) — —

    LH: >50 IU/L (>50 mIU/mL) — —

  Men, mature:

    FSH: 5–20 IU/L (5–20 mIU/mL) — —

    LH: 5–20 IU/L (5–20 mIU/mL) — —

  Children of both sexes, prepubertal:

    FSH: <5 IU/L (<5 mIU/mL) — —

Growth hormone, after 100 g glucose by mouth: <5 μg/L (<5 ng/mL) — —

Human chorionic gonadotropin, β subunit (β-hCG), plasma:

  Men and nonpregnant women: <3 IU/L (<3 mIU/mL) — —

Insulin, serum or plasma, fasting: 43–186 pmol/L (6–26 μU/mL) — 7.175

Insulin-like growth factor 1 (somatomedin C, IGF-1/SM-C): see Chap. 314 — —

Oxytocin:

  Random: 1–4 pmol/L (1.25–5 ng/L) — 0.80

  Ovulatory peak in women: 4–8 pmol/L (5–10 ng/L) — 0.80

Pancreatic islet function tests: see Chap. 319 — —

Parathyroid function tests: see Chap. 340 — —

Pituitary function tests: see Chaps. 313 to 315 — —

Pregnancy tests: see Chap. 322 — —

Prolactin, serum: 2–15 μg/L (2–15 ng/mL) — —

Renin-angiotensin function tests: see Chap. 317 — —

Semen analysis: see Chap. 321 — —

Thyroid function tests:

  Dynamic tests of thyroid function: see Chap. 316 — —

  Radioactive iodine uptake, 24 h: 5–30 percent (range varies in different areas due to variations in iodine intake) — —

  Resin T_3 uptake: 0.25–0.35 (25–35 percent) (varies among laboratories; for calculation of indexes of resin T_3 uptake, see Chap. 316) — 0.01

  Reverse triiodothyronine (rT_3), plasma: 0.15–0.61 nmol/L (10–40 ng/dL) — 0.01536

  Thyroid-stimulating hormone (TSH): 0.4–5 mU/L (0.4–5 μU/mL) — —

  Thyroxine (T_4), serum radioimmunoassay: 64–154 nmol/L (5–12 μg/dL) — 12.86

  Triiodothyronine (T_3), plasma: 1.1–2.9 nmol/L (70–190) ng/dL) — 0.01536

Pulmonary See Tables A-9 and A-10.

Renal

Clearances (corrected to 1.72 m² body surface area):

  Measures of glomerular filtration rate:

    Inulin clearance (C1):

      Males (mean ± 1 SD): 2.1 ± 0.4 mL/s (124 ± 25.8 mL/min) — 0.01667

	Conversion factor (CF) (C × CF = SI)

Females (mean ± 1 SD): 2.0 ± 0.2 mL/s (119 ± 12.8 mL/min) — 0.01667

Endogenous creatinine clearance: 1.5–2.2 mL/s (91–130 mL/min) — 0.01667

Urea: 1.0–1.7 mL/s (60–100 mL/min) — 0.01667

Measures of effective renal plasma flow and tubular function:

p-Aminohippuric acid clearance (Cl_{PAH}):

Males (mean ± 1 SD): 10.9 ± 2.7 mL/s (654 ± 163 mL/min) — 0.01667

Females (mean ± 1 SD): 9.9 ± 1.7 mL/s (594 ± 102 mL/min) — 0.01667

Concentration and dilution test:

Specific gravity of urine:

After 12-h fluid restriction: 1.025 or more — —

After 12-h deliberate water intake: 1.003 or less — —

Protein excretion, urine: <0.15 g/d (<150 mg/d) — 0.001

Males: 0–0.06 g/d (0–60 mg/d) — 0.001

Females: 0–0.09 g/d (0–90 mg/d) — 0.001

Specific gravity, maximal range: 1.002–1.028 — —

Tubular reabsorption, phosphorus: 79–94 percent of filtered load — —

HEMATOLOGIC EXAMINATIONS

See also "Chemical Constituents of Blood."

Bone marrow See Table A-12.

Erythrocytes and hemoglobin See also Table A-12.

Carboxyhemoblogin:

Nonsmoker: 0–0.023 (0–2.3 percent) — 0.01

Smoker: 0.021–0.042 (2.1–4.2 percent) — 0.01

Erythrocyte "life span":

Normal survival: 120 days — —

Chromium-labeled, half-life ($t_{\frac{1}{2}}$): 28 days — —

Glucose-6-phosphate dehydrogenase: 12.1 ± 2 IU/gHb (WHO) — —

Ham's test (acid serum): negative — —

Haptoglobin, serum 0.5–2.2 g/L (50–220 mg/dL) — 0.01

Hemoglobin, plasma: 0.01–0.05 g/L (1–5 mg/dL) — 0.01

Hemoglobin A_2 (HbA_2): 0.015–0.035 (1.5–3.5 percent) — 0.01

Hemoglobin, fetal (HbF): <0.02 (<2 percent) — 0.01

Hemoglobin H prep: negative — —

Methemoglobin: <0.017 (<1.7 percent) — 0.01

Osmotic fragility:

Slight hemolysis: 0.45–0.39 percent — —

Complete hemolysis: 0.33–0.30 percent — —

Plasma iron turnover: 20–42 mg/d or 0.45 mg/kg body weight per day — —

Protoporphyrin, free erythrocyte (FEP): 0.28–0.64 μmol/L of red blood cells (16–36 μg/dL of red blood cells) — 0.0177

Red cell distribution width (Coulter): 13 ± 1.5 percent

Sedimentation rate:

Westergren, <50 years of age:

Males: 0–15 mm/h

Females: 0–20 mm/h

Westergren, >50 years of age:

Males: 0–20 mm/h

Females: 0–30 mm/h

Sucrose hemolysis: negative

Leukocytes See Table A-13.

Platelets and coagulation

Alpha$_2$ antiplasmin: 70–130 percent

Antithrombin III: 80–120 percent

Bleeding time:

Duke method: <4 min

Simplate: <7 min

Clot retraction, qualitative: apparent in 60 min, complete <24 h, usually <6 h

Euglobulin lysis time: >2 h

Factor II: 60–100 percent

Factor V: 60–100 percent

Factor VII: 60–100 percent

Factor IX: 60–100 percent

Factor X: 60–100 percent

Factor XI: 60–100 percent

Factor XII: 60–100 percent

Factor XIII: clot stable in urea

Fibrinogen: 2.0–4.0 g/L (200–400 mg/dL) — 0.01

Fibrin split products: <10 mg/L (<10 μg/mL) — —

Plasminogen: 2.4–4.4 CTA U/mL

Protein C (antigenic assay): 58–148 percent

Protein S (antigenic assay): 58–148 percent

Partial thromboplastin time (activated PTT): comparable to control

Prothrombin time (quick one-stage): control ± 1 s

Protamine paracoagulation (3P) test: negative

Platelets: 130,000–400,000 per microliter

Thrombin time: control ± 3 s

von Willebrand's antigen: 60–150 percent

Miscellaneous

Leukocyte alkaline phosphatase (LAP): 0.2–1.6 μkat/L (13–100 U/L) — 0.01667

Lysozyme (muramidase), serum: 5–25 mg/L (5–25 μg/mL) — —

Lysozyme, urine: <2 mg/L (<2 μg/mL) — —

Schilling test: excretion in urine of orally administered radioactive vitamin B_{12}: 7–40 percent — —

Viscosity, plasma: 1.7–2.1 — —

Viscosity, serum: 1.4–1.8 — —

STOOL

Bulk:

Wet weight: <197.5 (115 ± 41) g/d — —

Dry weight: <66.4 (34 ± 15) g/d — —

Alpha$_1$ antitrypsin: 0.98 (±0.17) mg/g dry weight stool — —

Coproporphyrin: 600–1500 nmol/d (400–1000 μg/d) — 1.527

Fat (on diet containing at least 50 g fat): <6.0 (4.0 ± 1.5) g/d when measured on a 3-day (or longer) collection

Percent of dry weight: <0.30 (<30.4 percent) — 0.01

Coefficient of fat absorption: >0.95 (>95 percent) — 0.01

Fatty acid:

Free: 0.01–0.10 (1–10 percent of dry matter) — 0.01

Combined as soap: 0.005–0.12 (0.5–12 percent of dry matter) — 0.01

Nitrogen: <1.7 (1.4 ± 0.2) g/d — —

Protein content: minimal — —

Urobilinogen: 68–470 μmol/d (40–280 mg/d) — 1.693

Water: 0.65 (approximately 65 percent) — 0.01

URINE

See also "Metabolic and Endocrine" under "Function Tests."

	Conversion factor (CF) (C × CF = SI)
Acidity, titratable: 20–40 mmol/d (20–40 meq/d)	—
Ammonia: 30–50 mmol/d (30–50 meq/d)	—
Amylase: 35–260 Somogyi units/h	—
Amylase/creatinine clearance ratio [(Cl$_{am}$/Cl$_{cr}$) × 100]: 1–5	—
Bentiromide (pancreatic function): 50 percent excreted in 6 h as p-amino benzoic acid (PABA) after 500 mg oral bentiromide	—
Calcium (10 meq/d or 200-mg/d calcium diet): <3.8 mmol/d (<7.5 meq/d)	0.5
Catecholamines: <600 nmol/d (<100 μg/d)	5.911
Copper: 0–0.4 μmol/d (0–25 μg/d)	0.01574
Coproporphyrins (types I and III): 150–460 nmol/d (100–300 μg/d)	1.527
Creatine, as creatinine:	
Adult males: <380 pmol/d (<50 mg/d)	7.625
Adult females: <760 pmol/d (<100 mg/d)	7.625
Creatinine: 8.8–14 mmol/d (1.0–1.6 g/d)	8.840
Glucose, true (oxidase method): 0.3–1.7 mmol/d (50–300 mg/d)	0.5551
5-Hydroxyindoleacetic acid (5-HIAA): 10–47 μmol/d (2–9 mg/d)	5.230
Lead: <0.4 μmol/d (<80 μg/d)	0.004826
Protein: <0.15 g/d (<150 mg/d)	0.1
Porphobilinogen: none	—
Potassium: 25–100 mmol/d [25–100 meq/d (varies with intake)]	—
Sodium: 100–260 mmol/d [100–260 meq/d (varies with intake)]	—
Urobilinogen: 1.7–5.9 μmol/d (1–3.5 mg/d)	1.693
Vanillylmandelic acid (VMA): <40 μmol/d (<8 mg/d)	5.046
D-Xylose excretion: 5 to 8 g within 5 h after oral dose of 25 g	—

TABLE A-1 SI and other units

Quantity	Name of unit	Symbol for unit	Derivation of units
SI BASE UNITS			
Length	meter	m	
Mass	kilogram	kg	
Time	second	s	
Thermodynamic temperature	Kelvin	K	
Amount of substance	mole	mol	
SI DERIVED UNITS			
Area	square meter	m^2	
Force	newton	N	(m·kg)/g^2
Pressure	pascal	Pa	N·m^2
Work, energy	joule	J	N·m
Celsius temperature	degree Celsius	°C	K
OTHER UNITS RETAINED FOR USE			
Time	minute	min	
	hour	h	
	day	d	
Volume	liter	L	

TABLE A-2 Radiation derived units

Quantity	Old unit	SI unit	Name for SI unit (and abbreviation)	Conversion
Activity	curie (Ci)	Disintegrations per second (dρs)	becquerel (Bq)	1 Ci = 3.7 × 10^{10} Bq 1 mCi = 37 mBq 1 μCi = 0.037 MBq or 37 GBq 1 Bq = 2.703 × 10^{-11} Ci
Absorbed dose	rad	joule per kilogram (J/kg)	gray (Gy)	1 Gy = 100 rad 1 rad = 0.01 Gy 1 mrad = 10^{-3} cGy
Exposure	roentgen (R)	coulomb per kilogram (C/kg)	—	1 C/kg = 3876 R 1 R = 2.58 × 10^{-4} C/kg 1 mR = 258 pC/kg
Dose equivalent	rem	joule per kilogram (J/kg)	sievert (Sv)	1 Sv = 100 rem 1 rem = 0.01 Sv 1 mrem = 10 μSv

TABLE A-3 SI prefixes and their symbols

Factor	Prefix	Symbol for prefix
10^9	giga	G
10^6	mega	M
10^3	kilo	k
10^2	hecto	h
10^1	deka	da
10^{-1}	deci	d
10^{-2}	centi	c
10^{-3}	milli	m
10^{-6}	micro	μ
10^{-9}	nano	n
10^{-12}	pico	p
10^{-15}	femto	f
10^{-18}	alto	a

TABLE A-4 Classification of total cholesterol and LDL-cholesterol values

	Total plasma cholesterol	LDL-cholesterol	Conversion factor (C to SI)
Desirable	<5.20 mmol/L (<200 mg/dL)	<3.36 mmol/L (<130 mg/dL)	0.02586
Borderline high	5.20–6.18 mmol/L (200–239 mg/dL)	3.36–4.11 mmol/L (130–159 mg/dL)	0.02586
High	≥6.21 mmol/L (≥240 mg/dL)	≥4.14 mmol/L (≥160 mg/dL)	0.02586

SOURCE: The Expert Panel. Report of the National Cholesterol Education Program Expert Panel on Detection, Evaluation, and Treatment of High Blood Cholesterol in Adults. Arch Intern Med 148:36, 1988

TABLE A-5 Hemodynamic values

Pressures (mmHg):	
Systemic arterial:	
Peak systolic/end-diastolic	100–140/60–90
Mean	70–105
Left ventricle:	
Peak systolic/end-diastolic	100–140/3–12
Left atrium (or pulmonary capillary wedge):	
Mean	2–12
a wave	3–10
v wave	3–15
Pulmonary artery:	
Peak systolic/end-diastolic	15–30/4–14
Mean	9–17
Right ventricle:	
Peak systolic/end-diastolic	15–30/2–7
Right atrium:	
Mean	2–6
a wave	2–8
v wave	2–7
Resistances [(dyn·s)/cm⁵]:	
Systemic vascular resistance	700–1600
Total pulmonary resistance	100–300
Pulmonary vascular resistance	30–130
Flows:	
Cardiac index (liters per minute per square meter)	2.4–3.8
Stroke index (milliliters per beat per square meter)	30–65
Oxygen consumption (liters per minute per square meter)	110–150
Arteriovenous oxygen difference (milliliters per liter)	30–50

TABLE A-6 Systolic time intervals in normal individuals (in milliseconds)

Regression equation		SD of index
QS₂ (M)	= −2.1 HR + 546	14
QS₂ (F)	= −2.0 HR + 549	14
PEP (M)	= −0.4 HR + 131	13
PEP (F)	= −0.4 HR + 133	11
LVET (M)	= −1.7 HR + 413	10
LVET (F)	= −1.6 HR + 418	10

NOTE: QS₂ = total electromechanical systole, PEP = preejection phase, LVET = left ventricular ejection time, HR = heart rate, M = male, F = female, SD = standard deviation of the systolic time interval index. Systolic ejection period = 220–320 ms per beat; diastolic filling period = 380–500 ms per beat.
SOURCE: AM Weissler, CL Garrard, Mod Concepts Cardiovasc Dis 40:1, 1971.

TABLE A-7 Normal values of echocardiographic measurements in adults*

	Range, cm	Mean, cm	Number of subjects
Age (years)	13 to 54	26	134
Body surface area (m²)	1.45 to 2.22	1.8	130
RVD—flat	0.7 to 2.3	1.5	84
RVD—left lateral	0.9 to 2.6	1.7	83
LVID—flat	3.7 to 5.6	4.7	82
LVID—left lateral	3.5 to 5.7	4.7	81
Posterior LV wall thickness	0.6 to 1.1	0.9	137
Posterior LV wall amplitude	0.9 to 1.4	1.2	48
IVS wall thickness	0.6 to 1.1	0.9	137
Mid IVS amplitude	0.3 to 0.8	0.5	10
Apical IVS amplitude	0.5 to 1.2	0.7	38
Left atrial dimension	1.9 to 4.0	2.9	133
Aortic root dimension	2.0 to 3.7	2.7	121
Aortic cusps' separation	1.5 to 2.6	1.9	93
Percentage of fractional shortening†	34 to 44%	36%	20
Mean rate of circumferential shortening (Vcf)‡, or mean normalized shortening velocity	1.02 to 1.94 circ/s	1.3 circ/s	38

* RVD = right ventricular dimension; LVID = left ventricular internal dimension; d = end diastole; s = end systole; LV = left ventricle; IVS = interventricular septum.

† $\dfrac{\text{LVIDd} - \text{LVIDs}}{\text{LVIDd}}$

‡ $\dfrac{\text{LVIDd} - \text{LVIDs}}{\text{LVIDd} \times \text{ejection time}}$

SOURCE: From H Feigenbaum, Echocardiography, in *Heart Disease—A Textbook of Cardiovascular Medicine*, E Braunwald (ed), Philadelphia, Saunders, 1980.

TABLE A-8 Amplitude of Q, R, S, and T waves in scalar electrocardiogram of 100 normal adults*

	I	II	III	aV_R	aV_L	aV_F	V₁	V₅	V₆
Patients with Q wave	38%	41%	50%	—	38%	40%	0%	60%	75%
Q amplitude:									
Mean	0.4	0.6	0.9	—	0.4	0.7	0	0.3	0.3
Range	0 to 0.10	0 to 1.6	0 to 2.3	—	0 to 1.1	0 to 1.7	0	0 to 1.8	0 to 1.8
R amplitude:									
Mean	5.6	8.9	4.5	1.3	3.4	6.0	1.9	12.6	10.2
Range	1.0 to 10.0	2.0 to 16.9	1.0 to 12.1	0 to 2.9	0 to 8.2	0 to 13.8	1.0 to 6.0	7.0 to 21.0	5.0 to 18.0
S amplitude:									
Mean	2.0	2.1	2.4	7.0	2.6	—	8.0	2.5	1.3
Range	0 to 5.0	0 to 3.7	0 to 6.4	2.2 to 11.8	0 to 5.8	—	3.0 to 13.0	0 to 5.0	0 to 2.0
T amplitude:									
Mean	1.9	2.3	1.0	—	0.3	1.7	1.0	3.3	1.0
Range	1.0 to 3.0	1.0 to 4.0	−2.0 to 2.0	—	−1.0 to 2.0	0 to 4.0	−2.0 to 2.0	2.0 to 7.0	1.0 to 4.0

* Values of Q, R, S, and T amplitudes are in millimeters (1 mm = 0.1 mv).
SOURCE: From J D Cooksey et al, *Clinical Vectorcardiography and Electrocardiography*, 2d ed, Chicago, Year Book Medical Publishers, 1977. Used by permission.

TABLE A-9 Summary of values useful in pulmonary physiology

	Symbol	Typical values	
		Men	Women
PULMONARY MECHANICS			
Spirometry—volume-time curves:			
Forced vital capacity	FVC	$\geq$4.0 liters	$\geq$3.0 liters
Forced expiratory volume in 1 s	FEV_1	>3.0 liters	>2.0 liters
FEV_1/FVC	$FEV_1\%$	>60%	>70%
Maximal midexpiratory flow	MMF (FEF 25–27)	>2.0 liters per second	>1.6 liters per second
Maximal expiratory flow rate	MEFR (FEF 200–1200)	>3.5 liters per second	>3.0 liters per second
Spirometry—flow-volume curves:			
Maximal expiratory flow at 50% of expired vital capacity	$\dot{V}_{max}$ 50 (FEF 50%)	>2.5 liters per second	>2.0 liters per second
Maximal expiratory flow at 75% of expired vital capacity	$\dot{V}_{max}$ 75 (FEF 75%)	>1.5 liters per second	>1.0 liters per second
Resistance to airflow:			
Pulmonary resistance	RL (R_L)	<3.0 cmH_2O/s per liter	
Airway resistance	Raw	<2.5 cmH_2O/s per liter	
Specific conductance	SGaw	>0.13 cmH_2O/s	
Pulmonary compliance:			
Static recoil pressure at total lung capacity	Pst TLC	25 $\pm$ 5 cmH_2O	
Compliance of lungs (static)	CL	0.2 L/cmH_2O	
Compliance of lungs and thorax	C(L + T)	0.1 L/cmH_2O	
Dynamic compliance of 20 breaths per minute	C dyn 20	0.25 $\pm$ 0.05 liters per cmH_2O	
Maximal static respiratory pressures:			
Maximal inspiratory pressure	MIP	>90 cmH_2O	>50 cmH_2O
Maximal expiratory pressure	MEP	>150 cmH_2O	>120 cmH_2O
LUNG VOLUMES			
Total lung capacity	TLC	6–7 liters	5–6 liters
Functional residual capacity	FRC	2–3 liters	2–3 liters
Residual volume	RV	1–2 liters	1–2 liters
Inspiratory capacity	IC	2–4 liters	2–4 liters
Expiratory reserve volume	ERV	1–2 liters	1–2 liters
Vital capacity	VC	4–5 liters	3–4 liters
GAS EXCHANGE (SEA LEVEL)			
Arterial O_2 tension	Pa_{O_2}	95 $\pm$ 5 mmHg	
Arterial CO_2 tension	Pa_{CO_2}	40 $\pm$ 2 mmHg	
Arterial O_2 saturation	Sa_{O_2}	97 $\pm$ 2%	
Arterial blood pH	pH	7.40 $\pm$ 0.02	
Arterial bicarbonate	HCO_3^-	24 $\pm$ 2 mmol/L	
Base excess	BE	0 $\pm$ 2 mmol/L	
Diffusing capacity for carbon monoxide (single breath)	DL_{CO}	25 mL CO/min/mmHg	
Dead space volume	V_D	50 $\pm$ 25 mL	
Physiologic dead space: dead space-tidal volume ratio (rest) (exercise)	V_D/V_T	$\leq$35% V_T $\leq$20% V_T	
Alveolar-arterial difference for O_2	A-a D_{O_2}	$\leq$20 mmHg	

TABLE A-10 **Prediction equations for spirometric tests, lung volumes, and gas exchange in adults**

Variable	Sex	Age (A)	Height (H)	Weight (W)	Constant (C)	Standard deviation (SD)
PULMONARY MECHANICS						
Spirometry—volume-time curves* (H in inches):						
FVC	M	−0.025	+0.148	—	−4.241	0.74
	F	−0.024	+0.115	—	−2.852	0.52
FEV$_1$	M	−0.032	+0.092	—	−1.260	0.55
	F	−0.025	+0.089	—	−1.932	0.47
MEFR	M	−0.047	+0.109	—	+2.010	1.66
(FEF 200–1200)	F	−0.036	+0.145	—	−2.532	1.19
MMF	M	−0.045	+0.047	—	+2.513	1.12
(FEF 25–75)	F	−0.030	+0.060	—	+0.551	0.80
Spirometry—flow-volume curves† (H in centimeters):						
V̇$_{max}$ 50	M	−0.015	+0.069	—	−5.400	1.422
(FEF 50%)	F	−0.013	+0.035	—	−0.444	1.22
V̇$_{max}$ 75	M	−0.012	+0.044	—	−4.143	1.026
(FEF 75%)	F	−0.014	—	—	+3.042	0.936
Lung volumes‡ (H in meters; W in kilograms):						
TLC	M	—	+6.92	−0.017	−4.30	0.67
	F	−0.015	+6.71	—	−5.77	0.48
FRC	M	+0.015	+5.30	−0.037	−3.89	0.56
	F	—	+5.13	−0.028	−4.50	0.41
RV	M	+0.022	+1.98	−0.015	−1.54	0.38
	F	+0.007	+2.68	—	−3.42	0.32
VC	M	−0.020	+4.81	—	−2.81	0.50
	F	−0.022	+4.04	—	−2.35	0.40
Gas exchange§ (H in meters; W in kilograms):						
DL$_{CO}$	M	−0.20	+32.5	—	−17.6	5.1
	F	−0.16	+21.2	—	− 2.66	3.6

NOTE: Answer = (A × age) + (H × height) + (W × weight) + C ± 2 SD. Example: The normal value and lower limit for the FEV$_1$ are sought in a man, age 40 years, height 183 cm, and weight 91 kg. The following equation gives the normal value:
FEV$_1$ = (−0.032 × 40) + (0.092 × 72) + (−1.260) = 4.08 liters
The lower limit of normal:
4.08 − (2 × SD) = 4.08 − (2 × 0.55) = 2.98 liters
Only 2.5% of a normal population will fall below this value (2 SD below the mean).
For other abbreviations, see Table A-9.
* Morris et al, Am Rev Respir Dis 103:57, 1971.
† Knudson et al, Am Rev Respir Dis 113:587, 1976.
‡ Grimby G, Söderholm B, Acta Med Scand 173:199, 1963.
§ Coates JE, *Lung Function and Application in Medicine*, Philadelphia, Davis, 1965.

TABLE A-11 **Differential nucleated cell counts of bone marrow**

	Normal, mean%*	Range, %†
Myeloid:	56.7	
Neutrophilic series:	53.6	
Myeloblast	0.9	0.2–1.5
Promyelocyte	3.3	2.1–4.1
Myelocyte	12.7	8.2–15.7
Metamyelocyte	15.9	9.6–24.6
Band	12.4	9.5–15.3
Segmented		
Eosinophilic series	3.1	1.2–5.3
Basophilic series	<0.1	0–0.2
Erythroid:	25.6	
Pronormoblasts	0.6	0.2–1.3
Basophilic normoblasts	1.4	0.5–2.4
Polychromatophilic normoblasts	21.6	17.9–29.2
Orthochromatic normoblasts	2.0	0.4–4.6
Megakaryocytes	<0.1	
Lymphoreticular	17.8	
Lymphocytes	16.2	11.1–23.2
Plasma cells	2.3	0.4–3.9
Reticulum cells	0.3	0–0.9

* From MM Wintrobe et al, *Clinical Hematology*, 8th ed, Philadelphia, Lea & Febiger, 1981.
† Range observed in 12 healthy men.

TABLE A-12 Erythrocytes and hemoglobin: Normal values at various ages

Age	Red blood cell count,* 10^{12}/L	Hemoglobin,* g/L (g/dL)	Vol. packed RBCs,* mL/dL	MCV, fL	MCH, pg	MCHC, g/L (g/dL)	MCD, µm
Days 1–13	5.1 ± 1.0	195 ± 50 (19.5 ± 5)	54.0 ± 10.0	106–98	38–33	340–360 (36–34)	8.6
Days 14–60	4.7 ± 0.9	140 ± 33 (14 ± 3.3)	42.0 ± 7.0	90	30	330 (33)	8.1
3 months to 10 years	4.5 ± 0.7	122 ± 23 (12.2 ± 2.3)	36.0 ± 5.0	80	27	340 (34)	7.7
11–15 years	4.8	131 (13.14)	39.0	82	28	340 (34)	
Adults:							
Females	4.8 ± 0.6	140 ± 20 (14 ± 2)	42.0 ± 5.0	90 ± 7	29 ± 2	340 ± 20 (34 ± 2)	7.5 ± 0.3
Males	5.4 ± 0.9	160 ± 20 (16 ± 2)	47.0 ± 5.0	90 ± 7	29 ± 2	340 ± 20 (34 ± 2)	7.5 ± 0.3

* The range of values represents almost the extremes of observed variations (93 percent or more) at sea level. The blood values of healthy persons should fall well within these mean ± SD figures.

NOTE: MCV = mean corpuscular volume, MCH = mean corpuscular hemoglobin, MCHC = mean corpuscular hemoglobin concentration, MCD = mean corpuscular diameter.

SOURCE: MM Wintrobe et al, *Clinical Hematology,* 8th ed, Philadelphia, Lea & Febiger, 1981.

TABLE A-13 Normal leukocyte count, differential count, and hemoglobin concentration at various ages

Age	Leukocytes, total	Neutrophils Total	Band	Segmented	Eosinophils	Basophils	Lymphocytes	Monocytes
12 mo	11.4(6.0–17.5)	3.5(1.5–8.5)	0.35	3.2	0.3(0.05–0.7)	0.05(0–0.20)	7.0(4.0–10.5)	0.55(0.05–1.1)
		31	3.1	28	0.4	0.4	61	4.8
4 yr	9.1(5.5–15.5)	3.8(1.5–8.5)	0.27(0–1.0)	3.5(1.5–7.5)	0.25(0.02–0.65)	0.05(0–0.20)	4.5(2.0–8.0)	0.45(0–0.8)
		42	3.0	39	2.8	0.6	50	5.0
6 yr	8.5(5.0–14.5)	4.3(1.5–8.0)	0.25(0–1.0)	4.0(1.5–7.0)	0.23(0–0.65)	0.05(0–0.20)	3.5(1.5–7.0)	0.40(0–0.8)
		51	3.0	48	2.7	0.6	42	4.7
10 yr	8.1(4.5–13.5)	4.4(1.8–8.0)	0.24(0–1.0)	4.2(1.8–7.0)	0.20(0–0.60)	0.04(0–0.20)	3.1(1.5–6.5)	0.35(0–0.8)
		54	3.0	51	2.4	0.5	38	4.3
21 yr	7.4(4.5–11.0)	4.4(1.8–7.7)	0.22(0–0.7)	4.2(1.8–7.0)	0.20(0–0.45)	0.04(0–0.20)	2.5(1.0–4.8)	0.30(0–0.8)
		59	3.0	56	2.7	0.5	34	4.0

NOTE: Values are expressed as "cells × 10^9/L." The numbers underlined are percentages.

SOURCE: WJ Williams et al (eds), *Hematology,* 3d ed, New York, McGraw-Hill, 1983. By permission.

Color Plates

Color Plates

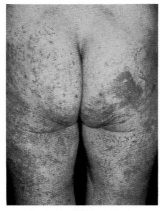

A (QUESTION 368)

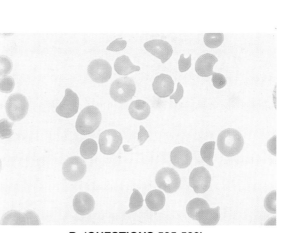

B (QUESTIONS 525-529)

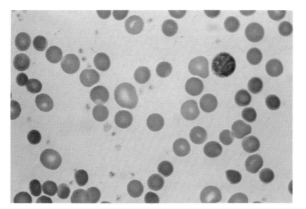

C (QUESTIONS 525-529)

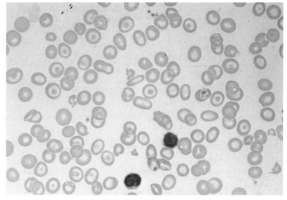

D (QUESTIONS 525-529)

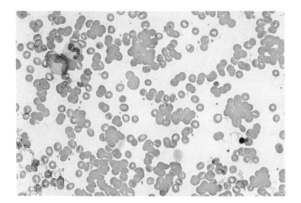

E (QUESTIONS 525-529)

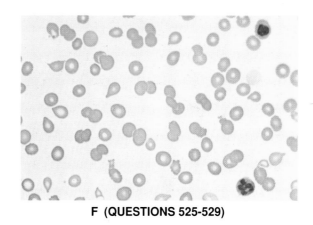

F (QUESTIONS 525-529)

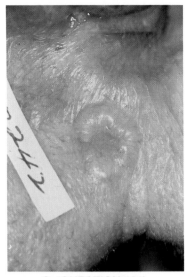

G (QUESTION 531)

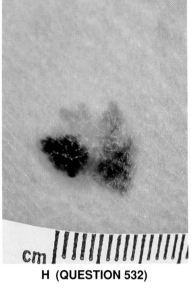

H (QUESTION 532)

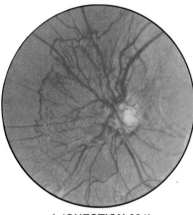

I (QUESTION 621)

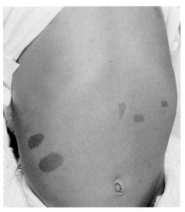

J (QUESTION 703)

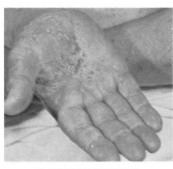

K (QUESTION 704)

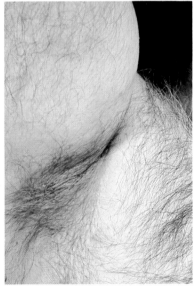

L (QUESTION 705)

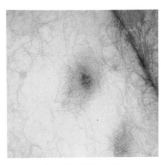

M (QUESTION 706)

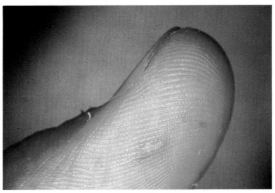

N (QUESTION 707)

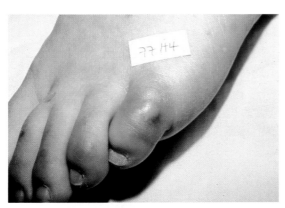

O (QUESTION 708)

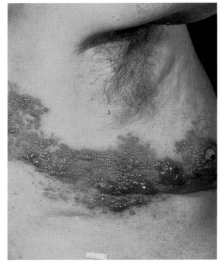

P (QUESTIONS 709-710)

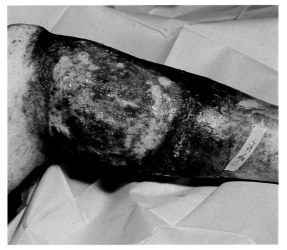

Q (QUESTION 711)

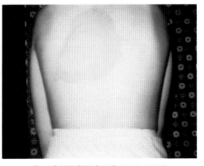

R (QUESTIONS 712-713)

(From Steere AC et al: Ann Intern Med 86:685, 1977; with permission)

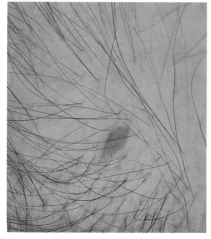

S (QUESTION 714)

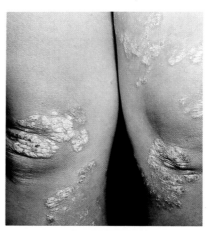

T (QUESTION 715)

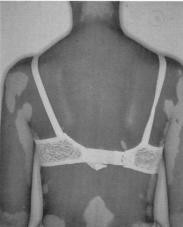

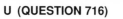

U (QUESTION 716)

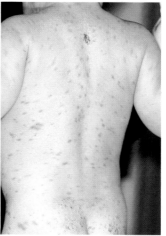

V (QUESTION 718)

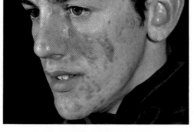

W (QUESTION 719)

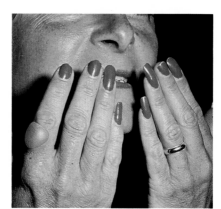

X (QUESTIONS 720-721)